Voices of Trauma:
Treating Psychological
Trauma Across Cultures

Voices of Trauma

Treating Psychological Trauma Across Cultures

Edited by

Boris Drožđek
Psychotrauma Centrum Zuid Nederland/Reinier van Arkel groep
's-Hertogenbosch, the Netherlands

John P. Wilson
Cleveland State University
Ohio, USA

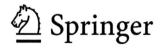 Springer

Corresponding Editor:

Boris Drožđek, MD, MA, Psychiatrist
Reinier van Arkel groep
Psychotrauma Centrum Zuid Nederland
Bethaniestraat 10
Postbus 70058,
5211 LJ
The Netherlands
E-mail: B.Drozdek@Rvagroep.nl

ISBN-13: 978-0-387-69794-9   e-ISBN-13: 978-0-387-69797-0

Library of Congress Control Number: 2007926433

Printed on acid-free paper.

9 8 7 6 5 4 3 2 1

springer.com

Foreword

By Laurence J. Kirmayer

There is increasing recognition that culture profoundly shapes the experience of suffering and healing. Indeed, current guidelines for trauma intervention in international work recommend cultural adaptation, but the details of how to accomplish this remain unclear. In this volume, Boris Droždek and John P. Wilson have brought together an exceptional group of creative clinicians whose work illuminates the issues at stake in taking culture seriously.

Intercultural work confronts us with many kinds of difference: the unique lifeworld of another person, the unusual experiences of psychiatric disorder, the distinctive history of the stranger from a distant place. Although people from diverse backgrounds may live in the same society, they also participate in distinct cultural communities, both local and transnational. How clinicians approach these differences reflects their clinical skills and orientation, but it also depends on larger social values and institutions that allow us to meet others in a place of safety and mutual respect.

Listening empathetically builds bridges across the divides of experience and identity. Empathy brings us close to those who suffer and allows us to understand something of their predicament. But empathy has its limits, beyond which imagination falters, notably in the face of the extremities of torture and other forms of violence. Much writing in the field of trauma, including previous work by the editors of this volume, has explored the challenge of maintaining empathy in the context of histories of violence and ongoing threats to safety and a coherent world. In the clinical encounter, steadfast respect and a commitment to facing the other's predicament allow us to work together to make sense of the ruptures, fear and uncertainty that trauma brings.

When people come from different backgrounds there may be specific difficulties in understanding and empathizing with their experience. We need cultural knowledge to stock our imaginations with the stories and images that emerge from others' ways of life. Ethnography teaches us that culture is not some surplus meaning tacked on to a common core of human experience, but something essential to our nature. Certainly, there are existential universals that transcend the vagaries of time and place, but these are always framed in terms of cultural particulars that are deeply rooted in habits, embodied ways of knowing, and our most sacred and serious commitments.

Cultural assumptions are also present in mental health theories and practices. The metaphors used to think about a clinical situation have a cultural history and convey specific values. They serve to illuminate some facets of experience but inevitably cast other aspects into shadow. The metaphor of trauma, for example, focuses attention on the impact of discrete events, making an analogy between physical injury and the psychological effects of violence or sudden loss. An emphasis on trauma, however, diverts attention from the everyday struggles and concerns that may dominate the lives of people living in harsh and uncertain circumstances or those who face the challenge of reconstructing their lives after migration. While much of the literature on the treatment of trauma considers people living in wealthy countries, the largest numbers of people exposed to severe trauma continue to live in low-income countries with ongoing violence, social conflict, and instability. In such situations of protracted conflict, the mental health effects of violence and social strife are not primarily due to discrete traumatic events, but to more pervasive losses of meaning, order, relationships, community and the sense of a just social world.

Diagnostic constructs also work as metaphors, both in terms of their explicit use as conceptual models and their implicit connotations as labels that affect social relations between people. The construct of PTSD, which has dominated discussions of the treatment of trauma in recent years, emphasizes the enduring effects of fear conditioning on subsequent adjustment and response to later stressors. But PTSD is a limited construct that captures only part of the impact of violence, ignoring issues of loss, injustice, meaning and identity that may be of greater concern to traumatized individuals and to their families and children or later generations.

The choice of conceptual vocabulary in the clinic is always part of larger narratives of suffering and healing with implications both for individual outcomes and for the ways that patients are seen in the larger society. So it is with terms like *refugee* or *asylum seeker*. These categories, created by international conventions, capture only one facet of the experience of the person in transition. More broadly, describing someone as a victim, survivor, or perpetrator positions them socially and politically, and assigns moral meaning to their suffering that shapes the ways they tell their own story.

A clinical focus on the symptoms of distress presented by the refugee, survivor, or victim may divert attention from the social contexts that define their identities and possibilities. As time wears on, the salient concerns for survivors become less focused on the meaning of the past than on the realities of the present, and possibilities for the future. For refugees, this shift in temporal perspective underscores the crucial importance of their place in the host society where they have found refuge. The quality of hospitality and the opportunities to rebuild a life in a new place are central to the healing process for immigrants and refugees. A crucial part of the refugee's story depends on the local politics of their place of asylum and resettlement. Of course, in the contemporary world, the relevant contexts extend far beyond this local world: new technologies for communication and transportation allow transnational networks to play an increasingly important role in identity and community for those who migrate, linking distant communities and events in planetary networks, as the local and the global are reciprocally inscribed.

The ways we understand trauma and identity shape the goals and methods of clinical intervention. Although it would be more than enough for clinicians to be of help to suffering individuals, intercultural clinical work has implications beyond the well-being of individuals. Working through the grief of loss and fear of trauma can help individuals avoid the psychic scars that lead to a thirst for revenge, the tendency to see the world in polarized terms of black and white, and the righteous anger that undermines clear thinking and compassion for others.

The attentiveness and respect toward others essential to intercultural work are an essential counter to the fear-built walls and moats that separate us from each other. The history of colonialism, slavery, exploitation and social exclusion form an inescapable backdrop to the clinical encounter with traumatized individuals. The growing inequality between rich and poor nations—as well as the increasing disparities within some of the wealthiest of nations—contribute to a mounting sense of injustice. The microcosm of the clinical encounter then becomes not only a place for bearing witness and healing wounds but also a crucible in which new possibilities for civil society can be forged.

Rebuilding a social world requires both a renewed commitment to justice and specific acts of contrition, atonement and restitution—but forgiveness follows different protocols in different cultures and traditions. What helps at the level of individual psychology, may not have equal efficacy at the levels of family interaction or community reconstruction. We need more work that explores the broader social and cultural implications of clinical intervention. The case studies in this volume are an important step in elaborating the range of responses that can help individuals, families, and ultimately, whole communities work through their suffering to a place of strength, solidarity, and creative vitality.

Laurence J. Kirmayer, MD

James McGill Professor & Director

Division of Social & Transcultural Psychiatry

McGill University

Editor-in-Chief, *Transcultural Psychiatry*

Director, Culture & Mental Health Research Unit

Institute of Community & Family Psychiatry

Sir Mortimer B. Davis—Jewish General
Hospital, Montreal, Quebec, Canada

Preface

VOICES OF TRAUMA ACROSS CULTURES: TREATMENT OF POSTTRAUMATIC STATES IN GLOBAL PERSPECTIVE

By Boris Droždek

Whatever You Do, Don't Forget the "Helicopter View"

This publication aims at presenting a theoretical framework and guidelines for intercultural treatment of complex posttraumatic states and PTSD, together with a set of illustrative case presentations of treatment encounters in different settings throughout the world. It aims at combining knowledge from psychiatry, anthropology, and social psychology in an in-depth analysis of complex treatment tasks emerging in a culturally sensitive treatment of complex trauma reactions and PTSD. It takes into account both intrapersonal and interpersonal, as well as societal factors that shape the individual's experience of trauma, determine its reactions to traumatic events and coping strategies, and influence healing process. This publication is also meant to be a "source book" supporting mental health workers in assessment, diagnosis and treatment of traumatized clients with different cultural backgrounds, as it describes how an authentic and productive intercultural encounter in trauma therapy gradually takes place. Description of this encounter, and the raise of shared concepts of disease, illness and healing, by gradually "peeling off the onion layers" of cultural backgrounds in both client and therapist, is the most important focus of the case presentations in this publication. As we all know, while peeling the onion one gets tears in the eyes. Therefore, issues of transference and countertransference in trauma treatment are discussed as well, together with the topic of culturally sensitive intervision and supervision of trauma workers.

Why Read This Book?

Mental health problems of victims of natural and man-made disasters have become a major public health issue worldwide. Many of these victims have being traumatized in their own country in a context of war or political violence and submitted to forced migration afterwards. They sought shelter in other countries of the world, and were confronted with different cultures, and sets of sometimes very different norms and values, languages and religions. When seeking help they are often facing a difference between their own explanatory models of illness and health with those of their helpers. They are also confronted with models of healing that sometimes differ from those they are accustomed to and expect to have beneficiary effects for their well being.

In multicultural societies, victims of traumatic events face dilemmas when seeking help, as do their helpers, mental health workers, taught to provide healing based on traditions and worldviews that are culturally dependent, and not always enough culturally sensitive.

Rescue workers and NGO personnel operating in disaster areas around the world can face the same problems. They often work in cultures different from their own, and should establish a healing setting combining the knowledge they have with the needs and expectations of their clients.

Modern psychiatry shows serious gaps and problems when practiced in situations where helpers and victims have different cultural backgrounds, and different assumptions about disease, illness, and healing. Scientifically grounded, evidence-based treatments do not always work in these cases, frustrating the therapists. On the other hand, trauma victims feel misunderstood when seeking help for their fears, shame or guilt, expecting social justice, signs of forgiveness and rehabilitation, and receiving drugs or protocolized treatments in return.

In intercultural encounters, it is critical to understand the importance of cultural and societal issues, while defining and framing the clients' problems and structuring adequate treatment strategies.

This publication is a joint effort of professionals from different parts of the world to accentuate the importance of contextual thinking in psychiatry in general and in intercultural treatment of complex posttraumatic states in particular.

Chapter by Chapter, Voice by Voice

In chapter 1, Boris Droždek reviews the literature on the genesis of contextual/ systemic thinking in science in general, and in psychiatry in particular. He discusses the interplay of culture and posttraumatic states. He presents the critique of the concept of PTSD based on knowledge from anthropology and cultural psychiatry. He focuses on the implementation of contextual thinking in intercultural treatment of posttraumatic states and its importance in defining and framing of the victim's problems, assessment of trauma damage, creation of the healing environment and treatment interventions.

In chapter 2, Michael Harris Bond presents the contribution of social psychology in understanding the phenomenon of evil and destruction in humans. He discusses the definitions, scope and costs of collective violence. He elaborates how one gets encultured to violence and describes the universal processes leading to and potentiating collective violence. He analyzes how cultures mobilize and orchestrate the evolutionary predisposition for violence in humans, as well as the role of culture in proposing solutions for reducing of savagery.

In chapter 3, Robert Jay Lifton provides us with an in-depth psychohistorical analysis of the Japanese fanatical religious cult leader involved in the attack on the passengers of the Tokyo subway in 1995. His analysis focuses on the individual psychology of the cult leader and the group psychological processes within the cult as well as on historical and sociological backgrounds that created the context wherein the cult arose and operated violently. Lifton's chapter shows us clearly how important it is to understand the context that created violence and explore possible interventions to prevent such events.

Chapters 4 to 15 contain case presentations of encounters between victims and healers. These chapters give voice to both parties. They explore the ways of helping those who were subjected to "psychological, social and economic amputation" as a consequence of profound immersion in man-made violence and death. These case histories were shared within the safe seclusion and privacy of therapeutic settings. They tell us about the world we live in and the dark sides of humankind, but also about resiliency and survival strategies of those who managed to stay alive upon meeting death and annihilation.

In these chapters the reader will meet a former child soldier from Cambodia, an Afghan refugee in Australia, an Armenian young man from Azerbaijan who does not want to forget his past, a Chechen family migrating through several countries, a woman from Kosovo and her baby and a female survivor of sexual violence from South Sudan. One can learn about the life of a former political activist from Mauritania, the struggles of a Congolese adolescent unable to find internal peace in Canada, about an Egyptian family migrating together with ghosts and a Chinese woman in Hong Kong in search for balance between her individual and collective sense of the self. Last, but not least, we can read how a plane crash affected the Dominican community in New York and the therapists involved in helping them, and how traditional American Indian healing rituals impacted a Caucasian American trauma therapist.

The authors focus on several topics relevant to intercultural treatment of trauma. Jaswant Guzder (chapter 5) and Catherine So-kum Tang (chapter 6) discuss the combination of western and non-western methods in trauma treatment and the importance of the awareness of limitations of psychology and psychiatry. Cécile Rousseau and Déogratias Bagilishya (chapter 12) present the process of intertwining of cultural and political signifiers, in both trauma and the reconstruction process. They combine different treatment approaches and show the importance of extending interventions beyond the therapy setting to co-working with different agencies in the society. The contextual approach is also highlighted in the works of Robin Bowles and Nooria Mehrabi (chapter 14) and Nino Makhashvili and Lela Tsiskarishvili (chapter 11). They show us how healing is possible even when therapists do not have a complete insight into trauma stories of their clients. They highlight the importance of trust and empathy to facilitate self-disclosure. These chapters illustrate how victims with a collectivist sense of the self can regain strength by re-establishing of their social roles and without processing of traumatic experiences on the intrapsychic level. Boris Drožđek (chapter 7) presents a culturally sensitive way of applying psychodynamic psychotherapy of trauma within a bio-psycho-social treatment model. He also reflects on the issue of PTSD diagnosis as a continuum, with anxiety and psychotic features on the extremes, and underlying changes in victims' personality. Gesine Sturm, Thierry Baubet and Marie Rose Moro (chapter 10) focus on mobilization of social and symbolic resources in intercultural trauma treatment. As transcultural therapies confront therapists with an extremely complex field of interrelations between different cultural and political contexts, therapists should consider these variables and try to understand the unique way their clients try to deal with them. Accepting the impact of "outer reality" on their subjectivity, as well as taking into account the subjective experience and the unique way the individuals perceives their individual traumatic experience, are of crucial value in the healing process. Marian Tankink and Annemiek Richters (chapter 9) provide a discussion of gender specific considerations in treatment. They also focus on silence as a coping strategy and cultural censorship in victims of sexual violence and the role of gossiping in refugee communities. Elizabeth Batista Pinto Wiese (chapter 13) presents how intercultural trauma therapy functions on the principle of the "building blocks," targeting different levels of client's functioning and shifting between them during course of treatment. She describes a mother/infant treatment process, wherein psychotherapy is combined with the Sandplay therapy. Eduard Hauff (chapter 8) presents a brief psychotherapy of a victim of childhood war trauma. He shows how to deal with client's fragmented trauma stories and co-morbid conditions. John Wilson (chapter 4) provides us with yet another, unorthodox perspective of intercultural trauma treatment, describing his own experience of being submitted to traditional healing rituals. He discusses the universal and culture-specific components of healing rituals, and reminds us not to forget to learn from our clients. David Lindy, Rebecca Morales and Jacob Lindy (chapter 15) examine reactions of a community on disaster trauma. They introduce and discuss topics like the myth of sameness, the bicultural self and the trauma membrane. They also focus on the countertransference reactions in mental health workers involved in helping families of the disaster victims. In chapter 16, Ton Haans, Johan Lansen and Han ten Brummelhuis extend the ideas presented in chapter 15. Their chapter provides a detailed discussion of critical issues for the supervision process. Their unique contribution examines the differences and characteristics of providing intercultural clinical supervision to trauma helpers both in the western and non-western societies.

In the closing, chapter 17, John Wilson and Boris Drožđek discuss the issues of convergence and divergence between healing principles across cultures and describe how the themes of trauma are metabolized in the great mythologies. They examine fundamental questions on relationships among trauma, culture and posttraumatic states, and propose some directions for future research.

The goal of this volume is to collect and structure knowledge in the field of intercultural trauma treatment that has proliferated worldwide. It provides the reader with the opportunity to hear the voices of trauma victims struggling to reshape their lives, and get a closer look at a large spectrum of healing practices. Contributors to this volume are the messengers. They are taught to hear and understand the pain of their clients. They are willing to share this knowledge to broaden the basis of collective understanding on a global basis.

Acknowledgments

Many people have helped us on the way during this interesting journey with their love, support and comments.

First, we want to extend our gratitude and thanks to Tony Marsella, the editor of this series for Springer Publishers, who believed in the project from its very beginnings.

Second, our thanks to Laurence Kirmayer for his insightful preface, the knowledge and inspiration that he has shared with us throughout the years.

Third, we are very thankful to all the voices of trauma across cultures, the victims of political violence and war worldwide, which were willing to share their intimate life stories and make this book a reality.

Also, we want to thank Ms. Kathleen Letizio, assistant to Dr. Wilson, for her commitment and dedication.

Finally, we extend deep gratitude to our families who had, yet again, supported, loved and understood us at times that our attention was stolen from them by this collaboration.

Boris Drożdek

John P. Wilson

Table of Contents

ISSUES FOR FUTURE RESEARCH
AND CLINICAL INTERVENTIONS

About the Editors

Boris Drožđek, M.D., M.A., is psychiatrist at Psychotrauma Centrum Zuid Nederland/Reinier van Arkel groep, 's-Hertogenbosch, the Netherlands, an international centre for treatment of victims of political and war violence. He is leading the residency training in social psychiatry, collaborating with different NGO's in post-war areas, teaching and giving trainings in psychotraumatology and transcultural psychiatry on a regular basis in the Netherlands and abroad. He is international director of the International Summer School of Psychotrauma in Dubrovnik, Croatia. He is author of several scientific publications and chapters to books and, together with John P. Wilson, editor of the *Broken Spirits: The Treatment of Traumatized Asylum Seekers, Refugees, War and Torture Victims* (New York: Brunner-Routledge, 2004).

John P. Wilson, Ph.D., is currently Professor of Psychology at Cleveland State University in Cleveland, Ohio, U.S.A. He is a founding member and Past President of the International Society for Traumatic Stress Studies (ISTSS) and a Fellow of the American Institute of Stress. He is a Diplomate and Fellow of the American Academy of Experts in Traumatic Stress, a Fulbright Scholar and the International Director of the International Summer School of Psychotrauma in Dubrovnik, Croatia. Dr. Wilson is the author of ten books and over 30 monographs and chapters on traumatic stress syndromes. Research and clinical work developed by Dr. Wilson have led to consultations with different national and international agencies like the U.S. Army and Navy, Department of Veterans Affairs, The White House and The World Health Organization, where he developed mental health programs during the war in Bosnia in 1994/1995., and more recently in Croatia to aid victims of war trauma.

Contributors

Déogratias Bagilishya is a psychologist working at the Montreal Children's Hospital, Montreal, Canada and in private practice. He specializes in transcultural psychiatry and treatment of refugees and migrants who have undergone persecution and violence. He also works as a cultural mediator in cases of intercultural conflict.

Thierry Baubet is a senior psychiatrist at the University of Paris and Director of the trauma team in the Department of Child and Adolescent Psychiatry at Avicenne Hospital (AP-HP). He also work with Doctors Without Borders.

Michael Harris Bond has been practicing social psychology for the last three decades at the Chinese University of Hong Kong where he is Professor of Psychology. He is fascinated by culture, having been initially socialized into a Torontonian English Canadian one, followed by an American graduate education in California, and an extended cross-cultural immersion as a Research Associate from 1971–74 at Kwansei Gakuin University in Japan. His writing on the interface of culture and social psychology may be found in a book he co-authored with Peter Smith and Cigdem Kagitcibasi, *Understanding social behavior across cultures: Living and working with others in a changing world* (Sage, London, 2006)

Robin Bowles (BSW (Hons) MSW) began working with refugee survivors of torture and trauma approximately 18 years ago at STARTTS, Sydney, Australia, soon after the service began in 1988. She works as a psychotherapist and a senior clinical supervisor, and also has a small private practice in Sydney. Her research and practice interests include the interface of psychoanalysis, culture, politics, trauma and working with interpreters in psychotherapy. She is currently a trainee in the Adult Psychotherapy Training Program with the NSW Institute of Psychoanalytic Psychotherapy.

Han ten Brummelhuis is an anthropologist affiliated with the Universiteit van Amsterdam, the Netherlands. His research interests are focused on Southeast Asia. In the last ten years part of his teaching was concentrated on the connections between anthropology and psychiatry.

Jaswant Guzder is an associate professor in the Department of Psychiatry, McGill University. She is active in the Divisions of Social and Transcultural Psychiatry and Child Psychiatry. She is Head of Child Psychiatry, Director of Childhood Disorders Day Hospital and former director of the Cultural Consultation Service at the Jewish General Hospital in Montreal, with teaching and research commitments at McGill and Concordia University. She is a third generation South Asian migrant, an artist and a mother.

Ton Haans is psychologist and psychotherapist. He is trainer and supervisor for the Dutch Society of Group Dynamics and Group Psychotherapy. He is accredited supervisor of the German Supervision Association. At the moment he has a private consultation and supervision practice for workers in the field of intercultural trauma and group treatments.

Edvard Hauff M.D., Ph.D., is a psychiatrist, Professor of Transcultural Psychiatry and Head of the Institute, Institute of Psychiatry, University of Oslo, Norway. He is also Director of Psychiatric Education, Ulleval Hospital. One of his main professional interests is the development of mental health services in low-income countries, and since 1993 he has been involved in training psychiatrists and establishing mental health services in Cambodia, where he is also Honorary Professor at the University of Health Sciences. He has for many years conducted research, worked clinically and served as an international consultant in the field of forced migration and mental health.

Johan Lansen M.D., is a psychiatrist, trained psychoanalyst and group psychotherapist. He is the emeritus director of the Sinai Center in the Netherlands for treatment of victims of the Nazi Holocaust and their children. He has many years of experience in clinical supervision. He has been treating victims of man-made disaster for many years and is a trainer and supervisor to centers treating refugees in Europe. Together with Ton Haans he is involved in training courses for experienced therapists to become supervisors in this field. He is involved in research on the emotional impact of trauma therapy on therapists and has developed with Ton Haans a particular model of structured supervision in this field.

Robert Jay Lifton is a psychiatrist at Harvard Medical School and the author of many volumes on psychology and history. His most recent books are *Superpower Syndrome: America's Apocalyptic Confrontation with the World* (winner of the National Book Award), *Crimes of War: Iraq* and *Destroying the World to Save it: Aum Shinriky, Apocalyptic Violence, and the New Global Terrorism.*

David C. Lindy, M.D., is Clinical Director/Chief Psychiatrist of the Visiting Nurse Service of New York's division of Community Mental Health Services. He participated in the mental health response to major disasters in New York City, including the attacks on the World Trade Center (1993, 2001) and the crash of American Airlines flight 587. Dr. Lindy is also Associate Clinical Professor of Psychiatry, College of Physicians & Surgeons, Columbia University, in New York City, and is on the faculty of the Columbia University Center for Psychoanalytic Training & Research.

Jacob D. Lindy, M.D., is a psychiatrist and psychoanalyst, co-director of the Cincinnati Psychoanalytic Institute, training and supervising analyst and past president of the International Society for Traumatic Stress Studies and the Liaison to Eastern Europe. He is author of many scientific publications on posttraumatic states, and was involved in consultations and providing services for survivors of different disasters in the past 30 years.

Nino Makhashvili, M.D., is a psychiatrist and psychotherapist working in Tbilisi, Georgia. She is a founder and a past medical director of the Georgian Center for Psychosocial and Medical Rehabilitation of Torture Victims. At present she is a director of Global Initiative on Psychiatry –Tbilisi. She has been working in the field of psychotraumatology with refugees and IDPs, prisoners and victims of domestic violence and serving as a supervisor and consultant to trauma therapists. She is author and co-author of 4 books and various articles.

Nooria Mehraby (M.D Kabul, M.M Pathology(Kabul)M.M counsel UWS) herself a refugee, is a senior clinician with STARTTS, Sydney, who has more then 18 years work experience with refugees both overseas and in Australia. She is the author of many publications (including two textbook chapters). Her particular interest is on developing cross –cultural therapeutic interventions with refugees. She is also the editor of Interface Column in the national journal of Psychotherapy in Australia. This column explores differences in psychotherapy across cultures, gender, age, religion and different groups of clients.

Rebecca Morales, LCSW-R, received her BSW from the College of New Rochelle, her MSW from Fordham University School of Social Service, and training in psychoanalysis from Riverdale Seminars in Modern Psychoanalysis. She is the Bronx Borough Director of the Visiting Nurse Service of New York's Community Mental Health Services, and is very interested in promoting Hispanic mental health.

Marie Rose Moro is Professor of psychiatry at the University of Paris, France and Chief of the Department of Child and Adolescent Psychiatry at Avicenne Hospital. She equally directs the Center of transcultural Studies in Bobigny, France, and she is the editor of the transcultural review L'Autre, www.clinic–transcultural.org

Annemiek Richters, M.D., Ph.D., a physician and medical anthropologist, is professor of Culture, Health and Illness at Leiden University Medical Center (Department of Public health and Primary care, Discipline Group Medical Anthropology) in the Netherlands. Her research and teaching focuses on issues in the area of health and human rights; gender violence, trauma and healing, social-cultural aspects of HIV/AIDS, and reproductive health care for migrant women in the Netherlands.

Cécile Rousseau, M.D., M.sc., is Associate Professor in the Department of Psychiatry at McGill University, and Director of the Transcultural Child Psychiatry Team of the Division of Social and Transcultural Psychiatry centers on the assessment and treatment of survivors of torture, political violence and persecution.

Gesine Sturm is a clinical psychologist and anthropologist who was trained in Germany and in France. At present she works in the trauma team at the Avicenne Hospital and she is the coordinator of the Diplome Universitaire in transcultural psychiatry at the University of Paris Nord.

Catherine So-kum Tang is currently Professor at the Department of Psychology, the Chinese University of Hong Kong (CUHK). She is also the Director of the following postgraduate trauma-related programs at the CUHK: MA in Trauma Psychology, Postgraduate Diploma in Family Violence, and Postgraduate Diploma in Life Adversities; which are first of such programs in the Asia-Pacific Region.

Marian Tankink, M.A., a former community psychiatric nurse, is a medical anthropologist at Leiden University Medical Center (Department of Public health and Primary care, Discipline Group Medical Anthropology), the Netherlands. She is working on her PhD thesis on research among refugee women from Afghanistan, Bosnia, and South-Sudan who experienced sexual violence as part of the conflict in their countries of origin or during their flight. Her main research focus is differences and similarities in meaning production and health-seeking strategies among these women.

Lela Tsiskarishvili is a clinical psychologist working in Tbilisi, Georgia. She has worked as a child psychotherapist at the Georgian Center for Psychosocial and Medical Rehabilitation of Torture Victims (GCRT). At present she is the Executive Director of GCRT.

Elizabeth Wiese-Batista Pinto, PhD, was working as a psychotherapist at the Catholic University of Sao Paulo and at the Institute of Psychology of the University of Sao Paulo, Brasil. She also worked as a Visiting Professor at the University of Rouen, France and she specialized in Transcultural Psychiatry at the University of Paris XIII. Her research and publications focus on the assessment of children from 1 to 12 months old, children emotional development, play therapy, mother/child psychotherapy and transcultural psychotherapy. Currently, she works as a psychotherapist at the Psychotrauma Centrum Zuid Nederland/The International Centre for Victims of War, Trauma and Political Violence and at the Infant Psychiatry unit of the Reinier van Arkel Groep in 's-Hertogenbosch, the Netherlands.

1
The Rebirth of Contextual Thinking in Psychotraumatology

Boris Drožđek

Introduction

In this time of information proliferation (revolution), globalization, multiculturalism and interconnectedness, it seems important to re-evaluate the impact of politics, economics, and other societal issues on the human psyche. Focussing predominantly on the intrapsychic or the neurobiological dimensions of human experiences in psychiatry enables a more manageable conceptualization of mental illness and health, although at cost of fully understanding of their complexity. The interaction between the outside world and the individual should be analysed in order to understand human psychology more accurately.

Western psychiatry, being a product of societies with long-lasting democracies, and rooted in its tradition and culture of individualism, seems to have overlooked the fact that in other corners of the world daily life of individuals is more heavily influenced and impacted by history and politics. Being brought up in a family tackled by Cultural Revolution in China or the cleansing actions of the Stalin regime in the former Soviet Union or becoming entangled in political activism and terror in many other countries with totalitarian regimes in the world, determines ways individuals perceive life, think of it and define their roles and expectations. Besides this, in collectivist societies, the existence of an individual is much more depending and relying on larger systems than in individualistic ones, and individual actions can seldom be properly understood when not related to a broader context.

While in developmental psychiatry, social psychiatry, and systemic therapy, the importance of contextual thinking has being acknowledged, and has formed a firm fundament for theory and practice, other schools and streams within psychiatry have developed in a different way throughout the past. A huge amount of knowledge about different aspects of mental health problems (neurobiological, intrapsychic, clinical, etc.) has being produced, and many different, well-paved roads towards better understanding of human psychology have being constructed. However, "the big picture" somehow seems to fade. Therefore, it is necessary to unite these different roads in a larger avenue that will lead us to a more complete perception of the complexity of human psyche, and to more efficient treatments of those whose spirits are seriously wounded or broken.

The Parts or the Whole: The Context of the Evolution of Contextual Thinking

The systemic/contextual thinking suggests that the only way to understand the major problems of our time is to approach them in a holistic way. The problems are interconnected and interdependent, and cannot be understood in isolation. The whole is more than the mere sum of its parts, and the connections between the parts add a new and distinct quality and dimension to the whole. While the focus of the mechanistic, reductionist approach is on the parts, the contextual approach emphasizes the whole.

The contextual thinking is not a product of the modern era. The change from mechanistic to the holistic paradigm has proceeded in different forms and at different speeds in the various fields of science throughout the history.

In ancient Greek times, the Pythagoreans distinguished a pattern from matter, and viewed it as something that limits matter and gives it shape. In order to create understanding of the phenomena and the world they inquired into pattern rather than into substance or matter.

Aristotle made a distinction between matter and form, and he linked the two through a process of development. Matter does not exist separately from form, and vice versa. According to Aristotle, matter contains the essence of all things, but only by means of form this essence becomes real. Aristotle created a formal system of logic that has dominated Western thought and science for a long time.

In the sixteenth and seventeenth centuries, the radical change of this worldview emerged, because of the discoveries in mathematics, astronomy, and physics by Newton, Galileo and Copernicus. The dominant metaphor of that, so called, Cartesian era became the one of the "world as a machine". The notion of the universe as spiritual, organic, and living was changed.

The first strong opposition to the Cartesian mechanistic paradigm occurred only in the late eighteenth and nineteenth centuries, through the Romanticist Movement in art and philosophy. Aristotelian tradition made its comeback, and one conceived of form as a pattern of relationships within an organized whole. This conception is a basis of the contemporary systemic thinking.

In the second half of the nineteenth century due to remarkable advances in biology, like the perfection of microscope and the formulation of cell theory, the mechanism became a dominant paradigm again. These discoveries have opened the doors of understanding of the structures on the cell level, but biology remained ignorant of the activities that coordinate and integrate different operations into the functioning of the cell as a whole.

The critics of mechanism (schools of vitalism and organicism in biology) maintained that the reductionist concepts are applicable to organisms, but insufficient to fully understand the phenomenon of life. They pointed out that the missing ingredient is the understanding of organization or organizing relations. Only in the early twentieth century, the concept of organization gradually replaced the old notion of function. The importance of connectedness, relationships and context came into focus again. As Capra (1996, p. 29) wrote in his book about scientific understanding of life and living systems, "The great shock of twentieth-century science has been that systems cannot be understood by analysis. The properties of the parts are not intrinsic properties but can be understood only within the context of the larger whole. Thus the relationship between the parts and the whole has been reversed. Accordingly, systems thinking concentrates not on basic building blocks, but on basic principles of organization. Systems thinking is "contextual", which is the opposite of analytical thinking. Analysis means taking something apart in order to understand it; systems thinking means putting it into the context of a larger whole."

The application of systemic thinking in science makes our knowledge maybe less manageable, and more complex, but it helps us understanding life in a better and more adequate way. Also, this approach raises an important question. If everything is connected to everything else, how can we hope to understand anything? Hereby it is important to introduce the term approximate knowledge (Capra, 1996, p. 41). While the mechanistic paradigm is based on a belief in the certainty of scientific knowledge, the systemic one recognizes that all scientific theories are limited and approximate, and that science cannot provide definitive understanding.

The more recent research (Pert, 1999) indicates that in the humans the nervous, the immune, and the endocrine system are not separately operating, and are not serving different functions. It is also difficult to understand their interconnectedness when studying them separately in neuroscience, endocrinology and immunology. These three systems form together a single cognitive, psychosomatic network interconnected by the peptides as molecular messengers. Peptides interlink and integrate mental, biological, and emotional activities of the humans. These molecules are the biochemical manifestations of emotions and they alter behaviour and mood states. The limbic system is highly enriched with peptides, but they are also found in intestines. While the limbic system is traditionally associated with emotions, this finding implies that cognition expands throughout the organism, and that humans can feel their emotions in the "guts", too. According to systemic thinking, a dynamic balance within organism represents health, while an imbalance, overemphasizing one and neglecting other tendencies, is unhealthy.

In order to understand why systemic thinking still lacks firm anchoring in the Western science one should analyse the modern culture of the Western world. The Western industrial culture overemphasizes the self-assertive and neglects the integrative tendencies. This culture prefers rational over intuitive thinking, analysis over synthesis, reductionism over holistic approach and linear over nonlinear thinking. In terms of values, the Western culture favours expansion, competition, quantity and domination, and neglects conservation, cooperation, quality and partnership (Capra, 1996).

As showed, at times when reductionist approach does not generate enough understanding of phenomena around us, a pendulum swings back to the other side, and a need towards integrative knowledge and values emerges. I believe this time has come yet again.

Is there more than Just the Brain?: The Context of the Development of Cultural Psychiatry

In his overview of the sociocultural foundations of psychopathology and the development of cultural psychiatry, Marsella (1993) pointed out the important role of Jean Jacques Rousseau, the famous French philosopher, who was a part of the Romanticist Movement more than two and a half centuries ago. He claimed that humans are by nature good, and that only the institutions have made them bad. These words launched a new era of thought directed toward better understanding of the role of society in harming the human condition. While at those times the prevailing thoughts on insanity linked the sickness with religious and moral perspectives, Rousseau's followers introduced psychosocial models, and were calling for massive social reforms in the conceptualization and treatment of insanity. From these early efforts, the study of culture and psychopathology emerged as a new academic and professional field. On the top of this, Rousseau even attributed poor health to social corruption and inequity anticipating the public health and social medicine movements that were to follow almost a century later on.

Rousseau's ideas were further developed by Thomas Hobbes (1588–1679), who brought a new consciousness about the role of society as a powerful and ever-changing determinant of human behaviour and John Locke (1632–1704), who proposed that the human mind was a blank slate, a tabula rasa, upon which were imprinted the experiences of life.

By the early nineteenth century, a number of medical theorists and practitioners had extended and applied Rousseau's thoughts to psychiatric problems. In 1851, John Jarvis, an American psychiatrist, made an effort to link brain function and process to the events within the macrosocial, microsocial and psychosocial spheres of human activity. He wrote that "insanity is a part of the price we pay for civilization. Civilization brings with more opportunities for great and excessive mental action, more uncertain and hazardous employment, and consequently more disappointments, more means and provocations for sensual indulgences, more accidents and injuries, more groundless hopes, and more painful struggle to obtain that which is beyond reach or to effect that which is impossible" (Rosen, 1959, p. 21). Jarvis anticipated contemporary systems theorists.

Although mainly focused on the intrapsychic determinates of mental health problems, Freud and psychoanalysis gave some important contributions to understanding of relationship between culture and psychopathology. Freud (1930) changed his theories frequently throughout his lifetime, but his view that mankind was doomed to an eternal neurosis because of the inevitable struggle created by the imposition of societal restraints upon the biological nature has remained a hallmark across time. Malinowski's anthropological study (1924) of the universality of the oedipus complex launched scores of explorations into the psychoanalysis-anthropology relationship.

Parallel to the work of organismic biologists by the 1930s, German psychologists started developing the basis of the school of Gestalt psychology. The ideas of this school became later on the fundaments of systems theory in psychology. The Gestalt school focused on a clearly different pathway towards the understanding of the psyche than the psychoanalytic school.

Later on, the interpersonal school of psychiatry purposively sought to integrate anthropology, sociology, social psychology, psychoanalysis, and psychiatry while applying Freudian principles.

Parallel to these developments in the history of psychiatry, there still existed the assumption that psychiatric symptoms and diseases are universal all over the world, and that their expressions are not dependant of patients' cultural backgrounds. At the same time, throughout the years a set of culture-bound syndromes has being described and added to psychiatric textbooks as kinds of rare, exotic phenomena. These developments both mirror an implicit racism in developmental hierarchies, and a colonial attitude of the western science towards all other, non-western worldviews.

According to Marsella (1993), in the period since 1970, there has been a proliferation of theory and research that has launched the study of socio-cultural aspects of psychopathology into the mainstreams of scientific inquiry and clinical application. This was a consequence of a growth of interest in medical anthropology, psychological anthropology, and psychiatric anthropology, the development of cross-cultural psychology and ethnic minority psychology, and the emergence of transcultural psychiatry, social psychiatry, and community psychiatry. The anthropology started criticising western ethnocentric medical theory and practice. It offered valuable knowledge through comparative studies of non-western ethno-psychiatric practices. Major achievements were the acknowledgement of cultural relativity in standards of normality and abnormality, and the cultural determination of personality via variations in child rearing, social processes, conceptions of personhood, and basic values structures. The awareness emerged that the process of diagnosis introduces the risk of error because of variations in the ethnicity of the patient, the diagnostician, and the diagnostic system which is being used.

To a large extent, the developments of the post-1970 period (Marsella, 1993) "have been a result of a heightened sensitivity to the socio-cultural factors encouraged by (1) international collaborative studies (e.g., the World Health Organization Pilot Study of Schizophrenia), (2) increases in the number of ethnic minority mental health professionals interested in the socio-cultural foundations of psychopathology, (3) the growing disaffection of non-Western mental health professionals with the ethnocentrism and bias of Western psychiatry, (4) increased social awareness of the pathological sequelae of racism, sexism, imperialism, colonialism, and other "isms", (5) increased awareness of the pernicious consequences of war, urbanization, poverty, and other socio-cultural phenomena for mental health, and (6) a growing awareness of the multiple and interactive determinants of psychopathology (e.g., biology, psychology, sociology)".

More recently, because of globalization, with its mass migrations, rapid transportation, and new, fast telecommunications, mental health services for immigrants and refugees are developing. Studies of the issues of migration, flight and resettlement, raise awareness of the impact of culture on psychiatric problems. More understanding for influences of culture on psychopathology, conceptualization of illnesses, illness behaviour, and expectations from treatment in different cultural settings is generated. The theories of cultural relativism confront the universalistic attitude in psychiatry. In addition, western psychiatry becomes aware of the impact of its own cultural context on the forming of psychiatric thinking throughout its development. Only by being confronted with the "other", one gets awareness of its own identity. Nowadays, one should not think any more of cultural or transcultural psychiatry, but of intercultural encounters as a paradigm of psychiatric treatment in a modern multicultural world.

The Interplay of Culture and Psyche

Kroeber and Kluckhohn (1962) identified more than 150 different definitions of the term culture. Within the study of culture and psychopathology, the most important factor in the conceptualization and definition of culture was the recognition that normal and abnormal human behaviour were both a product and a determinant of culture.

The concept of culture is about the process of being and becoming a social creature, about the rules of a society, and about the ways in which these are enacted, experienced, and transmitted. Spirituality and religion in each cultural context are important for providing meaning to life as well as a means to deal with death, suffering, pain, injustice, tragedy, and stressful experiences (Pargament, 1997). Marsella (1988, p. 8) defines culture as a shared learned behaviour that is transmitted from one generation to another to promote individual and group adjustment and adaptation. Culture is presented externally as artefacts, roles, and institutions, and is represented internally as values, beliefs, attitudes, cognitive styles, epistemologies, and conscious patterns. Inevitably, any interpersonal transaction involves an encounter of cultures. Kirmayer (2005) thinks of culture as a biological construct. Culture is a name for the ways in which human beings organize themselves over time through social systems to adapt to natural and self-created environments, with the brain being an instrument of culture. At the same time, biology is a cultural construction, with understanding of and attitudes towards the body being shaped by cultural models and values.

While in the past one perceived culture as a closed, static, homogeneous and homeostatic system, nowadays we conceptualize it as a changing, permeable, dynamic system, allowing a broad range of varieties and transitional forms not only between cultures, but within one culture as well.

From the viewpoint of cultural history, cultures can be divided into the individualistic (guilt), and collectivistic (shame) cultures (Dodds, 1951). These two forms of societies shape the self and self schemas of individuals in different ways. For example, while in individualistic societies there is a tendency of explaining events in life in terms of people's enduring qualities, in collectivistic ones is locus of causality usually externalized, and explanations for behaviour are situational. In individualistic societies individual's self esteem is related to competitiveness, while in collectivistic ones it is related to cooperative behaviour. Even the super ego is in some collectivistic societies a collective one, meaning that individual is not feeling responsible only for his deeds, but for those of his ancestors, too. According to ethnoanalysts the same phenomena are observed with the ego and the id (Parin, Morgenthaler, & Parin-Mattéy, 1963).

Culture impacts the regulation and expression of emotions, sets limits of tolerance of specific and strong emotions, and provides lay theories and strategies about handling emotions. For example, some Asians can express their emotions in accordance with the balance of yin and yang. Besides that in their cultures, it is quite common that disturbances of mood, affect, and anxiety are not viewed as mental health problems, but as social or moral problems (Kirmayer, 1989).

Cultures shape individual expressions and perceptions of how to suffer under stress, and these modes are taught and learned sometimes openly, sometimes indirectly (Kleinman & Kleinman, 1997). Grief and shame provide good examples of the influence of culture on coping. While in individualistic societies problems are expressed more in a psychological way, and a concept of counselling is introduced, in collectivistic societies grieving takes place in an interaction between individual and the supernatural, including the ancestors and the living (de Jong, 2004).

In collectivistic (shame) societies a sin becomes a sin only at the moment of public revelation. As long as it remains hidden, it does not have to be considered a sin. In addition, cause of a sin must in the first place be found outside the person of a sinner, who is considered just partially responsible for his deeds. One can restore social balance after occurrence of a shameful incident by blood feud (vendetta) or reconciliation with ghosts through, for example, following instructions given by traditional healers.

In more extreme forms of individualistic (guilt) societies preoccupation with guilt leads to a collective Christian guilt neurosis (Stroeken, 1988), with Victorian moral and Calvinism as examples. According to protestant moral, one is born as a sinner, and penance does not help to get rid of a sin. But also, in Islam is guilt an important issue. One has to pray several times a day in order to prove his devotion to God, and plead him/herself free from sins. In guilt-cultures, values of individual reality, individual identity, and individual responsibility as ethical principle are propagated (Mansfeld, 1981).

Some western societies nowadays are good, and in some aspects, extreme examples of the tension within an individualistic culture (Drožđek, Turkovic, & Wilson, 2006). These societies are characterized by shifting of responsibilities from individual to a collective level. At the same time on a collective level responsibilities are not taken and are shifted away to the next higher level of global politics and economy. In the context where individualization and liberalization are the highest collective values, intrinsic individual values and moral norms get gradually substituted by the values and norms of market economy.

Culture also shapes the ways the self or personhood is constructed. In Chinese and Japanese culture the social construction of personhood is described as a number of concentric layers involving the unconscious, the interpersonal, the intimate and wider society (Hsu, 1971). The Lohorung in Nepal perceive the self as an interaction of an ancestral substance with a live-bringing concept (Hardman, 2000). In West Africa (Horton, 1993; Kwasi, 1980) and in the African-Surinamese-Caribbean tradition a human being consists of a biological part of body and blood, and a spiritual part.

Culture influences the help seeking behaviour and the access to counselling, that is, talking with a stranger as a way of solving problems. Culture not only defines pain and suffering but also what is seen as private and public pain (Helman, 1994), what should be shared with others and what must remain a secret.

Of course, beside the highly polarized and somehow exotic examples of societal organisations, there is a whole range of transitional societies, with their own specificities, and fused forms of schemas that are reflecting themselves on conceptualisation of emotional experiences, as well as on expectations of how the most adequate healing process should look like.

The Interplay of Culture and Posttraumatic Reactions (PTSD)

In all cultures, humans are locked into the way their culture formulates social reality, because feelings and thoughts are what culture ultimately bequeaths to individuals to feel and think (Rubenfeld, 2005). Trauma and culture are intertwined because traumatic experiences are part of the life cycle, universal in manifestation and occurrence, and typically demand a response from culture in terms of healing, treatment, and interventions.

The ways in which culture influences health in general, mental health, and PTSD in particular, are multidimensional. In the first place, accounts for traumatic incidents and posttraumatic damage can be different in every society. For example, traditional Buddhists, who believe in karma, often show more acceptance of terrible events than Westerners do. Islamic patients, who believe that their fate is in Allah's hands, may feel less of a need to actually strive for any relief.

Further, through socio- and psycho physiological processes culture influences symptoms, course and outcome of PTSD, determines clinical presentation of problems and help-seeking behaviour. In addition, culture shapes the ways individual, family, and larger systems cope with, and adapt to consequences of trauma. It also determines understanding and conceptualizing of suffering, as well as making of a hierarchy of values and needs that underlie decision-making, and influence expectations from support and treatment. Last but not least, culture shapes the therapist-patient relationship. Hereby is important to mention that both, cultural backgrounds of the patient and the one of the therapist, shape the encounter within treatment and are responsible for the opening of the portals towards healing.

Yet there are some universal phenomena in reactions to trauma, too. Joseph Campbell's (1949) study of mythology has identified universal themes of the heroic figure whose journey of self-transformation in the life cycle upon survival of traumatic experiences is above the story of the individual trauma survivor (Wilson, 2006). Further on, scientific evidence, especially neurobiological studies, have documented that affect dysregulation, right hemisphere alterations in brain functioning, and strong kindling phenomena are universal in PTSD (Schore, 2003; Friedman, 2001). The core symptoms of posttraumatic reactions are also much more similar than different in all cultures. Victims describe having problems re-experiencing traumatic events, having nightmares and intrusive thoughts. They are suffering from hyper arousal, including poor sleep, poor concentration, and irritability. Avoidance symptoms are also common, especially those involving reminders that trigger memories of the past and violence. Numbing and social withdrawal, however, can vary depending on individual or situational differences. In addition, depressive symptoms seem to be universal in all the cultural groups.

Critique of the PTSD Concept: Contributions from Cultural Psychiatry and Anthropology

The PTSD concept has been criticized for its failure to fully account for all the changes and co-morbid presentations that are common among victims of multiple and prolonged trauma (Steel, 2001). The PTSD concept, the way it is described in the DSM-IV (APA, 1994), is a reduced one. It does not take into account the whole spectrum of posttraumtic damage, including core beliefs changes (Janoff-Bulman, 1985), dissociative moments, ruptures in growth and development of victim's personality, and co-morbidity like depression or substance abuse. It also ignores the socio-political-cultural context in which trauma occurs. However, the context is central to how people respond to, comprehend, and recover from trauma (Wilson, 1989). The context of trauma is shaped, and in turn shapes, worldviews, cultural norms, and constructions of society and individual victims. Trauma is therefore not a disembodied construct, as suggested by DSM-IV (APA, 1994), but a cultural and historical reality that must be entered into by the clinician.

Eisenbruch (1991) coined the term "cultural bereavement," when describing the complexity of trauma in refugees. This relates to the loss of home, material possessions, social networks, and the sense of social and spiritual belonging and connection to a land, its symbols, and its people.

Anthropologist Young (1995) defines PTSD just as one phase in a dynamic process of individual adaptation on adversities in life, and not as a final, well-defined diagnostic entity. In his interactive model of individual reaction to trauma, Chemtob (1996) describes the reaction of an individual as an interaction of the universal aspects of reactions on trauma and violence with the culture-bound reactions, and the personal history of the trauma victim.

Yet another interesting discussion of cultural relevance of the PTSD concept deserves to be mentioned. Reviewing the trauma literature, Steel (2001) identified two diverging views; one that focussed on the importance of the PTSD concept, and argued that psychological traumatization and its aftermath are the most important factors impeding reconstruction efforts in post conflict situations, and an opposing view that identifies trauma and PTSD as concepts imposed by Western traumatologists on post-war non-western victims populations in what amounts to a new form of cultural colonialism (Summerfield, 1997). In the latter view, the focus on individual pathology is dangerous, because of its potential to hide the political and social reality of repression and political violence (Summerfield, 1997).

The impact of posttraumatic damage must not be individualized, medicalized and reified (Dijk van, 2006). The individualization takes place when one focuses exclusively on the impact of trauma on the individual intrapsychic level, overseeing the posttraumatic destruction of the society. The medicalization of social suffering has being discussed at large by Summerfield (1999). He states that all refugees need social justice, and just some need psychological treatment. Unfortunately, western governments offer more often medical aid, both to refugees seeking asylum and in the form of humanitarian aid to other countries, than social justice. Kleinman (1995) wrote that "trauma stories become the currency in health care interactions to obtain access to social commodities and to achieve a new status as political refugee." The reification is about the concept of PTSD as a universal and timeless phenomenon not bound with time and social constructs.

The importance of contextual thinking in understanding and treating complex posttraumatic states is evident when one does not think of PTSD a universal, but as a culture-bound phenomenon. Bracken (2001) wrote that PTSD is not a consequence of trauma, but a result of interaction between trauma and culture, in this case the individualized, Judeo-Christian, post-modern culture of the western world. In this world, cultural and societal institutions that shape meanings of their members are weakened, and the experience of an individual human being is central to the culture. The typical assumption in this culture is that traumatic life-events and violence cause PTSD, and that talking therapies are the most efficient methods of healing. Only recently, Moodley and West (2005) discussed the limitations of verbal therapies and presented a rationale for the integration of traditional, culturally sensitive healing practices into counselling and psychotherapy.

One can imagine a traumatized individual being a spider anchored in a complex and often invisible web. When looking at it, one sees the spider clearly, and does not have to see the web at all. However, the spider does not exist and cannot live without the web. The web must not be overlooked. The web is the metaphor for the victim's context, for all those intrapsychic, interpersonal, and socio-political domains that define him/her.

Summarizing, the PTSD concept should be broadened and has to address a broader spectrum of posttraumatic damage, and incorporate contextual issues, including the ethno-cultural and societal aspects.

Contextual Thinking in Intercultural Trauma Treatment

In treating psychological sequels of trauma, one should acknowledge the necessity of focussing both on the intrapsychic and biological dimensions of traumatic experience, and on the interpersonal, and the socio-political dimensions. In addition, it is sometimes necessary to bring into account transgenerationally transmitted experiences, myths, or stories from the past that shape worldviews, and a formation of basic assumptions of an individual. With other words, one has to take into consideration both, the "hardware" and the "software" of trauma victims, and to explore the impact of trauma on different levels of human existence.

Bronfenbrenner (1981, pp. 22–26) calls these levels "the ecological environment" and describes them as a nested arrangement of concentric structures, each contained within the next. These structures are referred to as the micro, meso, exo, and macrosystems. A microsystem is defined as " . . .a pattern of activities, roles, and interpersonal relations experienced by the developing person in a given setting with particular physical and material characteristics." . . ."A mesosystem comprises the interrelations among two or more settings in which the developing person actively participates (such as, for a child, the relations among home, school, and neighbourhood peer group; for an adult, among family, work, and social life). . . .An exosystem refers to one or more settings that do not involve the developing person as an active participant, but in which events occur that affect, or are affected by, what happens in the setting containing the developing person . . . . . .The macrosystem refers to consistencies, in the form and content of lower-order systems (micro-, meso-, and exo-) that exist, or could exist, at the level of the subculture or the culture as a whole, along with any belief systems or ideology underlying such consistencies."

Since trauma does not take place in a vacuum or only in a head or brain of the victim, but in a "real world", and in a society that surrounds him/her, treatment should not take place in a vacuum either, and must address the often very complex array of factors that affect both origins of trauma, and healing. Without paying attention to these factors psychiatric interventions are very aggressive and haughty, they can be experienced as distant by the users, and users, our traumatized clients with psychological and psychiatric problems, will not admit professionals into the "private world" of their psyche. One cannot reduce personality and individuality only to biology of the brain. Humans are anchored in sociocultural contexts that both give them ways to react and bind them, they are born and bred in relations, they are inevitably influenced and influencers (Rubenfeld, 2005).

How to Define and Frame the Victim's Problems?

In intercultural trauma treatment, mental health providers confront a large spectrum of problems their clients are presenting. These problems can be defined as psychological, but yet at the same time as medical, social, political, cultural, existential, or as multidimensional. A mental health provider must transcend the either/or attitude and search for a broad conceptual frame (Bala, 2004). Kaleidoscopic conceptual lenses, instead of a prism have to be used in order to allow the understanding of the complex problems and cultural diversities, and explore the interplay of internal and external influences that hinder or facilitate development. The mental heath professional needs an integrated and flexible perspective to identify and evaluate the risk factors and the protective factors in both the developmental and socio-environmental context (Cicchetti & Cohen, 1995; Bala, 2004).

Trauma profoundly affects both communities and individuals. Therefore, its consequences can be seen as individual problems, but also as problems on the family and societal levels. Interventions should also target all these different levels. Before intervening, it is of crucial importance to first assess the clients' explanatory models, their interpretations of the past and current events that have affected and still affect their lives, and their expectations from the healing process. Thereby it is important to explore the interaction between the internal and the external meaning systems, and understand how the dominant beliefs rooted in culture colour the experience (Dallos, 1997; Bala, 2004). In intercultural trauma therapy "the question is not how many people are in the room, but how many are in the therapist's head" (Haley, 1981). And beyond this, one has to be aware of the people that are in client's head, too, and of the experiences, stories, and myths that both therapist and clients bring with into the encounter of the healing.

Marsella (2005, p. 3) has noted that healing sub-cultures have at least five distinct elements: "(1) a set of assumptions about the nature and causes of problems specific to their world view and construction of reality; (2) a set of assumptions about the context, settings, and requirements for healing to occur; (3) a set of assumptions and procedures to elicit particular expectations, emotions, and behaviours: (4) a set of requirements for activity and participation levels and/or roles for patient, family, and therapist; and (5) specific requirements for therapist training and skills expertise criteria."

When planning interventions, the mental health professional together with the client has to rank the priority areas of change. In some cases, where the "mental engineering" of individual problems is the highest ranked one, the professional is offered a space to work on the integration of fragmented traumatic experiences. This task is the closest one to the "classically" defined professional role of the western (psycho) therapist. In other cases, where the "social engineering" and the reparation of the damaged social tissue deserve the most attention, practical aid must be offered in combination with symptom control, aiming at stabilization of the client as a necessary precondition for further healing. Reparation of the social tissue empowers social coherence, and mobilizes social support, enabling trauma victim to re-enter his/her social group. In the latter case, the professional has to expand and redefine boundaries of his professional role.

The interest of mental health professionals in the last decades has been predominantly focused on the pathological dimensions of exposure to trauma and losses. The tendency to approach posttraumatic states in terms of strength and potentials for growth is of more recent date, and will definitely help better understanding of trauma victims. While assessing and treating posttraumatic states, the mental health professional has to explore both the damage, and the remaining healthy capacities, and to be aware of both the sources of vulnerabilities, and the sources of protection and resilience in trauma victims. The contextual thinking and broadening of narrow conceptualizations of posttraumatic states is hereby again of great importance. The empowering of resilience is crucial in treating trauma where some of the factors that create problems in victim's life cannot be directly influenced. The protective processes have a synergetic, cumulative effect (Bala, 2004), and resilience can be forged even when problems cannot be solved immediately (Walsh, 1998).

The mapping of the victims' problems, psychological, social and economic damage, and the available sources of resilience, together with their interpretation within the contexts of the victims' past, present, and future outlooks, and the planning of interventions, makes the contextual view necessary and unavoidable. The contextual view helps to defuse the purported "objectivity" and "detachment" of the mental health professional, and allows him/her to encounter the trauma client as a "subject" in relation, while at the same time sustaining the important therapeutic roles as a commentator, consultant, and authentic, empathic helper (Fosshage, 2003; Schermer, 2005). The standpoint of engagement allows the humanity and self-experience of the professional in more resilient ways in the context of healing (Schermer, 2005). The intercultural treatment of complex posttraumatic states must be a balancing act, between personal and socio-political domains, between private and public, between pain and empowerment (Bala, 2004).

To conclude with, there can be no experience of psychological trauma without a cultural history, grounding or continuity of background. Further on, there is no individual sense of personal identity without a cultural reference point (Wilson, 2004). In a related way, globalization, driven by economic and political forces, is also creating the emergence of "global culture" which enables the prospect of fusing cross-cultural modalities and treatment and subjecting them to scientific measures of efficacy (Wilson, 2006).

Assessment of Trauma

In assessing trauma it is important to be attentive to possible culture-bound idiomatic and nonverbal expressions relevant to the presenting problem. It is also vital to ensure that the procedures used allow exploration of ethnocultural issues that can impact the presenting problem or significant areas of the client's life and identity. The assessment process should also allow space to explore the impact of critical settlement, cultural transition, and ethnocultural issues at various levels of the system (Aroche & Coello, 2004).

Several issues are of great importance when planning the assessment procedure. First of all one must bear in mind that Western psychodiagnostic categories, as defined in DSM-IV (APA, 1994) or ICD-10 (WHO, 1992), are often not appropriate in non-Western cultures. Therefore, other tools like the Cultural Formulation of Diagnosis (CFD)(Mezzich, Kleinman, Fabrega, & Parron, 1996) can be very useful. CFD helps clinician to understand the identity of patient, his/her explanation of illness, the influence of psychosocial environment on patient's problems and the level of patient's functioning in daily life. It also helps getting insight into dynamics of the patient-clinician relationship.

Another useful instrument that can be used is the Explanatory Model Interview (Kleinman, 1978) that provides questions for eliciting patient's explanatory models for disease, illness, and healing. Using culturally sensitive instruments prevents clinician being trapped into, what Kleinman (1977) calls, a category fallacy. That is, one first defines the Western category, then starts looking for that category in a non-Western culture, and subsequently finds what was defined earlier, leading to that what had to be proven. However, if one would carefully listen to people's narratives, the reported complaints might not match the Western category.

The other important issue is the one of the language, and verbal expression of emotions in different cultures. The vocabulary for different emotions is not the same all over the world, and is sometimes very different from the one used, for example, in English language, the language of diagnostic instruments and classifications. Therefore, one has to carefully make an inventory of the expressions of distress in other cultures (the "idioms of distress") before the conclusion that the way people perceive their problem is the same as described in the DSM/ICD categories, can be made.

The third important issue is the need for standardization of diagnostic instruments across cultures. Instruments have to be tested for their content, semantic, conceptual, and technical validity. How to properly adapt instruments has been described elsewhere (de Jong & van Ommeren, 2002; van Ommeren et al., 1999). In clinical settings there is often a need to use self-report questionnaires. Many have been used in cross-cultural settings. The Harvard Trauma Questionnaire (Mollica er al., 1992), the Hopkins Symptom Checklist (Mouantounoua & Brown, 1995), and the SIP (Hovens, Bramsen, & van der Ploeg, 2002) are instruments that has been used widely in refugee populations and whose facility has been widely demonstrated. Also measures such as the PCL and the IES-R (Asukai et al., 2002) have equally been utilized in many different cultural settings with disaster and refugee populations.

The fourth important issue is the use of interpreters during assessment. They should be trained in the refinement of the assessment process as this can sensitize them to the nuances of language necessary for understanding the world of emotional suffering and fear (McFarlane, 2004). More on the use of interpreters has being discussed elsewhere (Bot & Waddensjo, 2004).

How to Create a Safe Sanctuary/The Therapist Variable

In creation of a safe context for an intercultural encounter in trauma treatment, the issues of treatment environment, therapist's attitude, and cultural sensitivity are of utmost importance.

As Aroche and Coello (2004) point out, the environment where treatment takes place is important, both because it is likely to provide the very first impression about the therapist and the agency he or she represents, and because it provides important clues about the quality of the personal or agency commitment to the client. The authors plead in their intercultural work with refugees for an environment that appears flexible and fairly informal, that places the comfort and needs of the client in a high priority, and that portrays, through its décor and ambience, a readiness to be inspired by other cultural influences.

For many clients coming from cultures where disclosing personal problems to a professional stranger is not a common way of healing, the first contact with an agency or a therapist can be a fearful experience. For many of them is the first contact with the therapist the closest encounter that they have ever had with a "representative" from the culture of the host country. Therefore it is important, that the therapist in the first sessions provides client in a pro-active way with all needed information on agency's work, makes an initial assessment of problems and shares it with the client, and compares his/her and the client's explanatory models of problems. Also, therapist explains transparently the possibilities and risks of the treatment process, and tries, in case of traumatized clients, to alleviate the stigma of being a psychiatric patient. This is also the time to check the validity of the assumptions made at the time of referral about language and cultural issues impacting the choice of therapist, interpreter, and any other relevant variables (Aroche & Coello, 2004).

Droždek and Wilson (2004, p. 251) defined five important factors that are of critical significance in establishing a therapeutic alliance. "First, a mutually respectful relationship between therapist and client is needed. Second, the creation of trust and safety is essential and promoted by transparency, calmness, and predictability of action. The clinical program, with its different phases, goals, interventions, and expectations from clients should be presented to clients before treatment begins. Third, program guidelines have to be respected and "secret agendas" are not permitted. Fourth, therapists exhibit tolerance and have the capacity to "decode messages" from their clients. These messages are sometimes "hidden" due to different cultural backgrounds. Fifth, a culturally sensitive attitude must be adopted by therapists."

Cultural sensitivity is one of the important foundations of the intercultural trauma treatment. It is not about a specific treatment technique, but about the attitude of the therapist. This attitude can be summarized as the one wherein therapist combines his knowledge on healing with authentic curiosity about his/her own and the patient's cultural background. Therapist is aware of own identity, and at the same time sensible for explanatory models of illness, disease, and healing that patient brings with into treatment. Therapist leads and structures the treatment, but lets the patient be his guide whenever it comes to culture related issues that he/she can not place into the own worldview. All other aspects of therapist's cultural competence, like language skills or specific knowledge of patient's culture are welcome, but not of crucial importance.

Some practical tips help therapists to establish a better contact. Being familiar with culturally appropriate greetings and styles of interaction can be of great help. For example, signs of respect that client shows towards therapist can vary from culture to culture – from putting a hand on the chest after shaking hands in the Middle East or North Africa; kissing hands in Afghanistan; to kissing a shoulder in Iran. Never entering a session room before the therapist is also a sign of respect clients may show. These customs convey some understanding between client and therapist that goes beyond words.

The Context of Recovery and Healing

In the same way that trauma does not happen in a vacuum, neither does healing. Healing and recovery do not take place only within the walls of a session room or a clinic, and do not depend on psychotherapeutic interventions only. The outside, "real world" surrounding both a traumatized victim and therapist impacts this processes, too. The outside world does not, sometimes, value adequately a victim's personal trauma, and reacts adversely to it. It can be a world where a victim coming from another culture struggles to find a place in the new society. The attitude of the environment towards the new arrivals influences the course of cultural transition. A refugee, for example, has to find a new modus of survival in a world where he/she is no longer the target of persecution, and where, being a part of civil society, there are also new rights and obligations to be obtained and respected. Some survival strategies obtained in the original surrounding of the home country can be very maladaptive in the context of the host country. This phenomenon should come into focus of the treatment. It can be also a world of racism, colonialism, criminality, and a world of secondary victimisation of an already traumatized migrant or refugee. Yet at the same time it is a world of opportunities, expansion of horizons, inspiring mixtures of cultures, norms, values and traditions. Taking into account the influence of the outside world on intrapsychic life of a traumatized client is therefore of utmost importance. In addition, sometimes a therapist has to adopt a pro-active attitude towards influencing client's social surrounding in the course of treatment. A good example is advocacy in case of asylum seekers clients, where therapist cannot permit him/herself to focus exclusively on the intrapsychic wounds of the client. Client is suffering not only from a psychological breakdown, but from a social and economical breakdown, too, and a responsible treatment strategy includes interventions on all mentioned levels.

Treatment of trauma in refugees and migrants has to take care of processes of adaptation to migration (Akthar, 1999)(whether it is a forced one or not), and their impact on the psyche of trauma victim. It is important to keep in mind that complex arrays of tensions play themselves within and between different social systems a victim is a part of. Within the family, for example, different individuals are likely to become acculturated at different levels, depending on age, gender, and circumstance. This can lead to intergenerational conflicts. They evolve when parents tend to retain traditional values related to appropriate role behaviours and standards of conduct for their children, while children tend to adopt the norms and values of the new host culture more rapidly than parents because of their enrolment in school, greater language facility, and friendship with children who are members of the new culture (De Santis & Ugarriza, 1995). Adaptation to migration can result in complete immersion into host culture, or preservation of original cultural backgrounds in their previous form. Also, different levels of transitional forms of adaptation, with combinations of "old" and "new" cultural traits and values occur. The resulting tensions and anxieties can play an important role in the expression of symptoms associated with traumatic events experienced prior to resettlement.

Berry (1991) defined factors influencing the relationship between acculturation and stress: (1) modes of acculturation: integration, assimilation, separation, marginalization; (2) phases of acculturation: contact, conflict, crisis, adaptation; (3) nature of larger society: multicultural versus assimilationist, prejudicial, discriminatory; (4) characteristics of acculturating group: age, social status, social support; and (5) characteristics of the acculturating individual: appraisal, coping, attitudes, contact.

The other important issue in intercultural treatment of trauma is the attitude of therapist, as described earlier in this chapter, which seems to be even important for the success of treatment as the kind of treatment selected. In other words, what one does is just as important as how one does it.

The use of different treatment methods in intercultural trauma treatment has being documented elsewhere (Wilson & Droždek, 2004). Both verbal and non-verbal (experiential) techniques have proved their value in treatment of traumatized migrants and refugees. Feeling relieved after verbally expressing the distress due to traumatic experiences, seems to be a universal phenomenon not depending on cultural background. However, experiential therapies are of great value here because of communication problems (language) present and universal difficulties that victims face when trying to find words to describe feelings associated with the horror of traumatic experiences. The use of psychomotor therapy (de Winter & Droždek, 2004), music (Orth, Doorschodt, Verburgt, & Droždek, 2004) and art therapy (Wertheim-Cahen, van Dijk, Schouten, Roozen, & Droždek, 2004), as well as body psychotherapy (Kärcher, 2004) has being well described in literature.

Both group and individual treatments can be applied, and where possible group settings are favoured over individual ones (Droždek & Wilson, 2004). However, treatment interventions have to be modified in a culturally sensitive way. For example, some clients need therapists with a more authoritarian approach, due to both, the existence of posttraumatic damage and their cultural background. This can cause difficulties for a western educated clinician, taught to prefer an egalitarian therapeutic relationship to a hierarchical one.

Techniques to stimulate storming in group psychotherapy by asking members to comment on each other's "good" and "bad" characteristics as observed in the group (Yalom, 1995), can lead in a non-western group to large group conflicts, and may have a disastrous effect on group cohesion (Drožđek & Wilson, 2004).

Finally, in some groups is the dynamics strongly influenced by cultural norms of group members. In groups of clients coming from cultures where age is traditionally more valued than experience or education, respect for the elderly and their viewpoints is an important norm. In such a group, for example, it can take serious amount of time until another group member takes leadership when the oldest client is not able or willing to do this. More examples of dynamics within intercultural trauma treatment can be found elsewhere (Drožđek & Wilson, 2004).

In order to further develop and enrich intercultural trauma treatment it is important to be curious towards traditional, culture-bound healing methods, and to combine them, where necessary and possible, with methods rooted in western scientific tradition. Traditional healing methods can be a source of inspiration, and create more understanding of expectations clients from different cultures may have of trauma treatment. Although traditional healing is not being condensed in academic writings, healers have impressed researchers by the wide variety of psychotherapeutic interventions they use (de Jong, 2004; Okpaku, 1998; Peltzer, 1995). For example, in Mozambique and Sierra Leone healers perform cleansing rituals that allow ex-child soldiers to be reintegrated in society. In Uganda rituals were used to assist rebels who had been looting and plundering for years to reintegrate into civil post-war society (de Jong, 2000). In Uganda and Sudan healers perform rituals that allow female rape survivors to continue their lives without the social stigma of being blamed for the rape or without cancelling previous marriage arrangements (de Jong, 2004). In Christian and Islamic post-war societies religion provides individuals and communities with a platform for healing through prayers, pilgrimage or the use of amulets with Koran texts. Unfortunately, only a few studies exist that evaluate the treatment effects of healers, and more research has to be done in order to make their knowledge accessible to a wider audience.

Yet another important aspect of intercultural trauma treatment is a shift of focus from pathology to health. This includes awareness of clients' self-empowerment and self-management and autonomy of trauma victims in structuring daily activities and psychosocial activities that foster coping and resiliency (Pearson, Lopez, & Cunningham, 1998). This approach offers an exit from the medicalization of social and political problems, and should be used in healing of intrapsychic posttraumatic wounds.

Some powerful factors leading to exclusion of traumatized migrants and refugees from treatment has to be mentioned as well. Training of the mental health professionals in dealing with complexities that this population presents is not always adequate. Further on, transference and countertransference issues play an important role in trauma treatment, and clinicians present difficulties in working with clients presenting strong and different political convictions of their own, or they might have to work with representatives of ethnic groups who are collectively accused of being perpetrators (Ekblad & Jaranson, 2004). On the same continuum, therapists find extremely difficult to work with perpetrators of violence or with clients being both victims and perpetrators at different times of their lives. Another reason to exclude specific groups from services is that survivors could be stigmatized, like rape survivors or people with a physical and/or mental handicap being perceived as the product of magic-religious forces (Ekblad & Jaranson, 2004). Finally, western clinicians can be influenced by stereotyped opinions by stating that non-westerners do not want to discuss the past, and that they somatize rather than psychologize their distress, even though there is a substantial body of evidence supporting the view that somatizing is the rule rather than the exception around the globe (Üstun & Sartorius, 1995).

Conclusion

To conclude with, it is important to be aware of the fact that confronting culture-bounded issues in trauma treatment must not become a goal by itself, but rather a means to promote recovery and healing. The healing process must be a balancing act. The recovery occurs when a "new" balance between resiliency and damage emerges, a balance that enriches victim's quality of life. This can sometimes be realized by diminishing of survivor's suffering from nightmares and flashbacks, and at other times by influencing his/her living arrangements or solving marital and familial conflicts. In all cases, it is of crucial importance to be aware of the different levels of human existence that trauma impacts and destroys, to assess them and to focus interventions on. The ability to shift back and forth between these levels in the course of treatment is an important skill, too.

Although the application of contextual thinking on intercultural trauma treatment makes us aware of the complexity of the problem, we must bare in mind that, as Aroche and Coello (2004) state, in the end we are all humans, and the similarities are far greater than the differences. But the differences should not be neglected and overlooked.

Intercultural trauma treatment is a new field – one whose time has come. It reminds us yet again of the basic values of human encounters, beyond all sophisticated treatment techniques and devices, and it offers ways for expanding the borders of our profession as mental health workers.

Appendix

MODIFIED CULTURAL FORMULATION OF DIAGNOSIS

English version from DSM-IV (APA, 1994) with socio-psychological issues added

I   CLINICAL HISTORY
>   1 Patient identification
>   2 History of present illness
>   3 Psychiatric history and previous treatment
>   4 Social and developmental history
>   5 Family history
>   6 Course and outcome
>   7 Diagnostic formulation (axes I–V)

II   SOCIAL PSYCHOLOGICAL DIMENSION (how are individual's thoughts, feelings, and behaviour influenced by other people)

A   *Socio-political/historical comments on the context of the trauma*
B   *Societal dimension*

>   1 Native and host culture analysis (individual vs. collectivist vs. transitional, locus of causality (internal vs. external), conformity vs. independence, controllability of life, stability vs. instability of causality, adherence to tradition, social norms, prejudices, respect for authority, marriages (ex. arranged or not), differences in childrearing, self-disclosure culture or not, schemas for storytelling or not, non verbal communication patterns)
>   2 Collective self/social roles of the patient
>   3 Self categorisation of the social identity/self concept of the patient (part of self which derives from membership in a social group(s), together with the value and emotional significance attached to it), self schemas (independence vs. interdependence, explanations for behaviour, ego or "other" focussed emotions, sources of self esteem)

C   *Cultural identity of the patient (intra and interpersonal dimensions)*

>   1 Cultural reference group(s) (derived from B 3)
>   2 Language
>   3 Cultural factors in development
>   4 Involvement with culture of origin (ethnic identity)
>   5 Involvement with host culture (integration, marginalisation, assimilation, separation/dissociation)(in case of migration)

III   CULTURAL FORMULATION OF DIAGNOSIS
A   *Cultural explanations of the illness*

>   1 Predominant idioms of distress and local illness categories
>   2 Meaning and severity of symptoms in relation to cultural norms

3 Perceived causes and explanatory models

4 Help-seeking experience and plans

B   *Cultural factors related to psychosocial environment and levels of functioning*

1 Social stressors

2 Social supports

3 Levels of functioning and disability

C   *Cultural elements of the clinician-patient relationship, the dynamics of the intercultural encounter in treatment* (both therapist's and client's cultural identity and background)

D   *Overall cultural assessment*

E   *Final comments (what worked, and what did not, and why?)*

Arthur Kleinman's eight questions for eliciting the patient's explanatory model (EM) of his/her illness (Kleinman, 1978)

1. What do you think has caused your problem?
2. Why do you think it started when it did?
3. What do you think your sickness does to you? How does it work?
4. How severe is your sickness? Will it have a short or long course?
5. What kind of treatment should you receive?
6. What are the most important results you hope to receive from this treatment?
7. What are the chief problems your sickness has caused for you?
8. What do you fear most about your sickness?

References

Akthar, S. (1999). *Immigration and identity: turmoil, treatment and transformation.* Northvale, NJ: Jason Aronson.

American Psychiatric Association (APA). (1994). *Diagnostic and statistical manual of mental disorders* (4th ed.). Washington DC: APA.

Aroche, J., & Coello, M. J. (2004). Ethnocultural considerations in the treatment of refugees and asylum seekers. In J. P.Wilson & B. Droždek (Eds.), *Broken Spirits: The treatment of traumatized asylum seekers, refugees, war and torture victims* (pp. 53–80). New York: Brunner-Routledge.

Asukai, N., Kato, H., Kawamura, N., Kim, Y., Yamamoto, K., Kishimoto, J., et al. (2002). Reliability and validity of the Japanese-language version of the impact of event scale-revised (IES-R-J): four studies of different traumatic events. *Journal of Nervous and Mental Disorders, 190*, 175–182.

Bala, J. (2004). Beyond the personal pain: integrating social and political concerns in therapy with refugees. In: D. Ingleby (Ed.), *Forced migration and mental health: rethinking the care of refugees and displaced persons* (pp. 169–182). New York: Springer.

Berry, J. (1991). Managing the process of acculturation for problem prevention. In: J. Westermeyer, C. Williams, & A. Nguyen (Eds.), *Mental health services for refugees* (pp.189–204). Washington, DC: Government Printing Office.

Bot, H., & Waddensjo, C. (2004). The presence of a third party: a dialogical view on interpreter-assisted treatment. In J. P.Wilson & B. Drožđek (Eds.), *Broken Spirits: The treatment of traumatized asylum seekers, refugees, war and torture victims* (pp. 355– 378). New York: Brunner-Routledge.

Bracken, P. (2001). Post-modernity and posttraumatic stress disorder. *Social Science and Medicine, 53,* 733–743.

Bronfenbrenner, U. (1981). *The ecology of human development; experiments by nature and design* (4th ed.). Cambridge: Harvard University Press.

Campbell, J. (1949). *Hero with a thousand faces.* New York: Penguin Books.

Capra, F. (1996). *The web of life.* Anchor/Doubleday: New York.

Chemtob, C. (1996). Posttraumatic stress disorder, trauma and culture. In: F. Lieh Mak & C. Nadelson (Eds.), *International review of psychiatry* (pp. 257–292). Washington: APA.

Cicchetti, D., & Cohen, D. J. (1995). Perspectives on developmental psychopathology. In: D. Cicchetti & D. J. Cohen (Eds.), *Developmental psychopathology, theory and methods* (pp. 753–800). New York: Wiley.

Dallos, R. (1997). *Interacting stories. Narratives, family beliefs and therapy.* London: Karnac Books.

DeSantis, L., & Ugarriza, D. N. (1995). Potential for intergenerational conflict in Cuban and Haitian immigrant families. *Archives of Psychiatric Nursing, 6,* 354–364.

Dijk van, R. (2006). Cultuur, trauma en PTSS: kanttekeningen bij de cultuurgebondenheid van de posttraumatische stressstoorniss. *Cultuur Migratie en Gezondheid,* 4/5, 20–31.

Dodds, E. R. (1951). *The Greeks and the irrational.* Berkeley/Los Angeles: University of California Press.

Drožđek, B., & Wilson, J. P. (2004). Uncovering: trauma-focused treatment techniques with asylum seekers. In J. P.Wilson & B. Drožđek (Eds.), *Broken Spirits: The treatment of traumatized asylum seekers, refugees, war and torture victims* (pp. 243–276). New York: Brunner-Routledge.

Drožđek, B., Turkovic, S., & Wilson, J. P. (2006). Posttraumatic shame and guilt: culture and the posttraumatic self. In J. P.Wilson (Ed.), *The posttraumatic self: restoring meaning and wholeness to personality* (pp. 333–368). New York: Routledge.

Eisenbruch, M. (1991). From post-traumatic stress disorder to cultural bereavement: diagnosis of Southeast Asian refugees. *Social Science & Medicine, 33,* 673–680.

Ekblad, S., & Jaranson, J. M. (2004). Psychosocial rehabilitation. In J. P.Wilson & B. Drožđek (Eds.), *Broken Spirits: The treatment of traumatized asylum seekers, refugees, war and torture victims* (pp. 609–636). New York: Brunner-Routledge.

Fosshage, J. L. (2003). Contextualizing self psychology and relational psychoanalysis: Bi-directional influence and proposed synthesis. *Contemporary Psychoanalysis, 39,* 411–448.

Freud, S. (1930; 1962). *Civilization and its discontents.* (Strachey Edition). New York: W.W. Norton.

Friedman, M. J. (2001). Allostatic versus empirical perspectives on pharmacotherapy. In J. P. Wilson, M. J. Friedman, & J. D. Lindy (Eds.), *Treating psychological trauma and PTSD* (pp. 94–125). New York: Guilford Press.

Haley, J. (1981). *Reflections on therapy.* Washington: The Family Therapy Institute.

Hardman, C. E. (2000). Other worlds: notions of self and emotions among the Lohorung Rai. *Berg,* 320.

Helman, C. G. (1994). *Culture, health and illness.* Butterworth Heineman Ltd.

Horton, R. (1993). *Patterns of thought in Africa and the west.* Cambridge: Cambridge University Press.

Hovens, J., Bramsen, I., & van der Ploeg, H. (2002). Self-rating inventory for posttraumatic stress disorder: review of the psychometric properties of a new brief Dutch screening instrument. *Perceptual and Motor Skills, 94*, 996–1008.

Hsu, F. L. (1971). Psychosocial homeostasis and Jen: conceptual tools for advancing psychological anthropology. *American Anthropologist, 73*, 23–44.

Janoff-Bulman, R. (1985). The aftermath of victimisation: Rebuilding shattered assumptions. In C. R.Figley (Ed.), *Trauma and its wake (Vol. 1): the study and treatment of posttraumatic stress disorder* (pp. 15–35). New York: Brunner/Mazel.

de Jong, J. T. V. M. (2000). Traumatic Stress among Ex-combatants. In N. Pauwels (Ed.), *War force to work force: global perspectives on demobilization and reintegration*. Baden-Baden: Nomos Verlag.

de Jong, J. T. V. M., & van Ommeren, M. H. (2002). Toward A Culturally Informed Epidemiology: A Pragmatic Model For Qualitative and Quantitative Psychiatric Research In Cross-Cultural Contexts. *Transcultural Psychiatry, 39*, 4.

de Jong, J. T. V. M. (2004). Public mental health and culture: disasters as a challenge to western mental health care models, the self, and PTSD. In J. P.Wilson & B. Droždek (Eds.), *Broken Spirits: The treatment of traumatized asylum seekers, refugees, war and torture victims* (pp. 159–178). New York: Brunner-Routledge.

Kärcher, S. (2004). Body psychotherapy with survivors of torture. In J. P.Wilson & B. Droždek (Eds.), *Broken Spirits: The treatment of traumatized asylum seekers, refugees, war and torture victims* (pp. 403–418). New York: Brunner-Routledge.

Kirmayer, L. J. (1989). Cultural variations in the response to psychiatric disorders and emotional distress. *Social Science & Medicine, 29*, 327–339.

Kirmayer, L. J. (2005). personal communication.

Kleijn, W. C., Hovens, J. E., & Rodenburg, J. J. (2001). Posttraumatic stress symptoms in refugees: assessments with the Harvard Trauma Questionnaire and the Hopkins Symptom Checklist-25 in different languages. *Psychological Reports, 88*, 527–532.

Kleinman, A. (1977). Depression, somatization and the new cross-cultural psychiatry. *Social Science and Medicine, 11*, 3–10.

Kleinman, A. (1978). Concepts and a model for the comparison of medical systems as cultural systems. *Social Science & Medicine, 12*, 85–93.

Kleinman, A. (1995). *Writing at the margin*. Berkeley: University of California Press.

Kleinman, A., & Kleinman J. (1997). The appeal of experience, the dismay of images: cultural appropriations of suffering in our times. In A. Kleinman, V. Das, & M. Lock. (Eds.), *Social suffering* (pp. 1–23). Berkeley: University of California Press.

Kroeber, A., & Kluckhohn, C. (1962). *Culture: A critical review of concepts and definitions*. New York: Random House.

Kwasi, W. (1980). *Philosophy and an African culture*. Cambridge: Cambridge University Press.

Malinowski, B. (1924). Psychoanalysis and anthropology. *Psyche, 4*, 293–332.

Mansfeld, J. (1981). Protagoras on epistemological obstacles and persons. In G. B. Kerferd (Ed.), *The sophists and their legacy* (pp. 38–53). Wiesbaden: Franz Steiner Verlag.

Marsella, A. J. (1993). Sociocultural foundations of psychopathology: A pre-1970 historical overview. *Transcultural Psychiatric Research and Review, 30*, 97–142.

Marsella, A. J. (1988). Cross-cultural research on severe mental disorder: issues and findings. *Acta Psychiatrica Scandinavica Supplementum, 344*, 7–22.

Marsella, A. J. (2005). Rethinking the 'talking cures' in a global era. *Contemporary Psychology, 11*, 2–12.

McFarlane, A. C. (2004). Assessing PTSD and comorbidity: issues in differential diagnosis. In J. P.Wilson & B. Droždek (Eds.), *Broken Spirits: The treatment of traumatized asylum seekers, refugees, war and torture victims* (pp. 81–104). New York: Brunner-Routledge.

Mezzich, J. E., Kleinman, A., Fabrega, H., & Parron, D. (Eds.). (1996). *Culture and Psychiatric Diagnosis, a DSM-IV perspective*. Washington DC: American Psychiatric Press.

Mollica R. F, Caspi-Yavin Y, Bollini P, Truong T, Tor S, & Lavelle J. (1992). The Harvard Trauma Questionnaire. Validating a cross-cultural instrument for measuring torture, trauma, and posttraumatic stress disorder in Indochinese refugees. *Journal of Nervous and Mental Disorders, 180*, 111–116.

Moodley, R., & West, W. (2005). *Integrating traditional healing practice into counselling and psychotherapy*. Thousand Oaks, CA: Sage Productions.

Mouantounoua, V. L., & Brown, L. G. (1995). Hopkins Symptom Checklist-25, Hmong version: a screening instrument for psychological distress. *Journal of Personality Assessment, 64*, 376–383.

Okpaku, S. O. (Ed.). (1998). *Clinical methods in transcultural psychiatry*. Washington DC: APA.

Orth, J., Doorschodt, L., Verburgt, J., & Droždek, B. (2004). Sounds of trauma: an introduction to methodology in music therapy with traumatized refugees in clinical and outpatient settings. In J. P.Wilson & B. Droždek (Eds.), *Broken Spirits: The treatment of traumatized asylum seekers, refugees, war and torture victims* (pp. 443–480). New York: Brunner-Routledge.

Pargament, K. I. (1997). *The psychology of religion and coping: Theory, research, practice*. New York: Guilford Press.

Parin, P., Morgenthaler, F., & Parin-Mattéy, G. (1963). *Die Weissen denken zuviel*. Zürich: Atlantis.

Pearson, N., Lopez, J.P., & Cunningham, M. (Eds.). (1998). *Recipes for healing*. Manila: PST/CIDS/Copenhagen: IRCT.

Peltzer, K. ((Ed.). (1995). *Psychology and health in African cultures*. Frankfurt/Main, IKO.

Pert, C. B. (1999). *Molecules Of Emotion: The Science Behind Mind-Body Medicine*. New York: Scribner.

Rosen, G. (1959). Social stress and mental disease from the 18th century to the present. *The Milbank Memorial Fund Quarterly, 11*, 1–31.

Rubenfeld, S. (2005). Relational perspectives regarding countertransference in group and trauma. *International Journal of Group Psychotherapy, 55*, 115–136.

Schermer, V. L. (2005). Introduction. *International Journal of Group Psychotherapy, 55*, 1–30.

Schore, A. N. (2003). *Affect dysregulation and the repair of the self*. New York: Norton.

Steel, Z. (2001). Beyond PTSD: towards a more adequate understanding of the multiple effects of complex trauma. In C. Moser, D. Nyfeler, & M. Verwey. (Eds.), *Traumatiserungen von Flüchtlingen und Asyl Schenden: Einflus des politischen, sozialen und medizinischen Kontextes.* (pp. 66–84). Zürich: Seismo.

Stroeken, H. P. J. (1988). Cultuur zonder schuld en schaamte? In P. J. G. Mettrop, M. L. van Thiel, & E. M. Wiersema (Eds.), *Schuld en schaamte: Psychoanalytische opstellen* (pp. 31–44). Meppel/Amsterdam: Boom.

Summerfield, D. (1997). The impact of war and atrocity on civilian populations. In D. Black, M. Newman, J. Harris-Hendricks, & G. Mezey (Eds.), *Psychological trauma: a developmental approach* (pp. 148–155). London: Gaskell.

Summerfield, D. (1999, April). *Lecture*. Paper presented at the conference Het buitengewone van de hulp aan asielzoekers, Utrecht, The Netherlands.

Üstun, T. B., & Sartorius, N. (Eds.). (1995). *Mental illness in general health care*. Chichester: Wiley.

Van Ommeren, M., Sharma, B., Thapa, S., Makaju, R., Prasain, D., Bhattarai, R., et al.(1999). Preparing instruments for transcultural research: use of the translation monitoring form with Nepali-speaking Bhutanese refugees. *Transcultural Psychiatry, 36*, 285–301.

Walsh, F. (1998). Beliefs, spirituality and transcendence: Keys to Family Resilience In: McGoldric M. (Ed.), *Re-visioning family therapy. Race, Culture and Gender in Clinical Practice* (pp. 62–78). New York: The Guilford Press.

Wertheim-Cahen, T., van Dijk, M., Schouten, M., Roozen, I., & Drožđek, B. (2004). About a wheeping willow, a Phoenix rising from its ashes, and building a house. . . . Art therapy with refugees: three different perspectives. In J.P.Wilson & B. Drožđek (Eds.), *Broken Spirits: The treatment of traumatized asylum seekers, refugees, war and torture victims* (pp. 419–442). New York: Brunner-Routledge.

Wilson, J. P. (Ed.). (1989). *Trauma, Transformation and Healing*. New York: Brunner/Mazel.

Wilson, J. P., & Drožđek, B. (Eds.). (2004). *Broken Spirits: The treatment of traumatized asylum seekers, refugees, war and torture victims*. New York: Brunner-Routledge.

Wilson, J. P. (2004). *The abyss experience and the trauma complex*. New York: Brunner-Routledge.

Wilson, J. P. (2006). *The posttraumatic self: Restoring meaning and wholeness to personality*. New York: Brunner-Routledge.

Winter de, B., & Drožđek, B. (2004). Psychomotor therapy: healing by action. In J. P. Wilson & B. Drožđek (Eds.), *Broken Spirits: the treatment of traumatized asylum seekers, refugees, war and torture* victims (pp. 385–402). New York: Brunner-Routledge.

World Health Organization (WHO). (1992). *The ICD-10 classification of mental and behavioral disorders clinical descriptions and diagnostic guidelines*. Geneva: World Health Organization.

Yalom, I. D. (1995). *The Theory and Practice of Group Psychotherapy*. New York: Basic Books.

Young, A. (1995). *The harmony of illusions. Inventing posttraumatic stress disorder*. New Jersey: Princeton University Press.

2
Culture and Collective Violence: How Good People, Usually Men, do Bad Things

Michael Harris Bond

"Little by little, we were taught all these things. We grew into them."

Adolf Eichmann

We are taught to love; we are taught to hate. We build; we destroy. We give life; we kill. These human activities are the consequences of culture, our birth culture and the individual translation of that cultural heritage we all absorb and carry into our future, further socializing those who associate with us. Culture is profoundly implicated in all we do, and is responsible for legitimating the violence we perpetrate against one another. It answers Mao Tse Tung's opening question in his *Selected works* (Mao, 1960), "Who are our friends; who are our enemies?" By providing the answer to this basic social probe and legitimizing our responses, culture becomes the culprit, responsible for the collective violence we perpetrate together against others. Or, for the peace we wage . . .

In this essay, I will develop the theme of culture as educator, as motivator, as roadmap, as coordinator and as legitimizer of the evil we do in the name of good. Culture provides the plausibility structures (Berger & Luckman, 1966) for these essential supports to the collective violence we wreak upon one another, but culture is not the agent of the carnage; it is we as social agents acting in concert who provide the daily, proximal supports for the orchestration of collective violence. We reward and we punish those who act with us or against us or who by-stand, thereby motivating ourselves and others to act in accordance with those plausibility structures. Culture proposes; man (usually) disposes.

Many contemporary cultures encompass, however, a rich cornucopia of possibilities, providing ample opportunities for cooperative initiatives, non-violent responses to provocation, and joint consultation for peaceful alternatives. These alternative responses are taught within any cultural group for dealing with in-group members, with the teaching especially designed to promote the female role. These responses are also taught in some cultural sub-groups in terms of social philosophy and guidance, and occasionally become cultural and even national policy, implemented through agencies of socialization.

However, these non-violent alternatives are especially difficult to enact whenever a cultural group considers itself under threat of destruction. So, it is in times of peace that we must act to build institutions for the non-violent resolution of the inevitable problems arising from inter-dependency and our habitation of this single, imperiled planet. Ironically, this integrative process will be prompted when members of a culture are educated to appreciate the enormity of collective violence.

The Enormity of Collective Violence

Most of us recoil from the brutality and the carnage and the suffering occasioned by collective violence, although sanitized and fictionalized versions of violence in the media fascinate many viewers. Our revulsion often takes this or other forms of turning away from the sobering facts concerning the real havoc that we wreak upon one another. We are well conditioned to find the pain and distress of violence, along with their accompanying embodiments in coagulated blood, amputated limbs, emaciated frames, severed limbs, and death masks, abhorrent. This is an understandable, but dangerous reaction. If we cannot confront the specter of collective savagery, even at a remove, how can we be strongly enough motivated to "wage peace"? A reminder of our human downside is a salutary incentive to avoid the downward spiral that leads to the organized destruction of other people.

A Definition of Collective Violence

In Chapter 8 of its 2002 Report on violence and health, the World Health Organization (p. 215) supplied a definition of collective violence that will suffice for present purposes. It is:

"the instrumental use of violence by people who identify themselves as members of a group – whether this group is transitory or has a more permanent identity – against another group or set of individuals, in order to achieve political, economic or social objectives."

We are considering *collective* violence, so the group nature of the violence must be underscored. We are in the realm of social movement theory (Garner, 1997). Not only are people identifying themselves as individual members of a group acting against members of another group; they are *acting together*, at varying levels of organized coordination depending upon the roles they assume in the savagery. These actions may be understood as instrumental to some biological, economic, or political goals, and indeed the actors generally consider that they are acting purposefully.

There are varieties of collective violence, to be sure. The type of violence involved, its scope, its duration, and the complexity of the operational processes leading to the application of destructive, coercive control to the targeted group member vary. So, for example, numerous methods for eliminating the approximately 6 million victims of the Holocaust were explored in the interests of improving efficiency across the many years of its operation, with the German High Command eventually settling upon the use of the gas chambers. Additionally, "the high division of labor so characteristic of Adolph Eichmann's assembly line of death" (Newman & Erber, 2002, p. 341) meant that, "Even though the Nazi death machine required the active participation of thousands of executioners (as well as the passive cooperation of an even larger number of bystanders), relatively few of them were involved in the actual killing." (ibid.)

This feature of the collective violence "may have allowed many to convince themselves that they were doing something other than death work." (Newman & Erber, 2002, p. 341), conferring a social psychological advantage for the perpetrators that may make this collective violence different in terms of its dynamics than, say the Massacre at El Mazote. There, on one day in December, 1991, in a tiny, remote town in El Salvador, around 800 civilians were shot, beheaded by machete, or bayoneted to death by the Atlacatl Battalion of the Salvadorian Army under the command of Colonel Domingo Monterossa Barrios (Danner, 1994). In this case, there were fewer victims and their appalling fate was concealed to all but the perpetrators who completed the atrocities without any "division of labor" in its accomplishment. The social dynamics involved in such a small, short, sharp episode of collective violence are bound to differ in some respects from those like the Holocaust or the Holodomor, Russia's systematic starvation of seven million Ukrainians in 1932–1933, extensive, long-lasting, diffuse, and mostly bloodless. Nonetheless, the violence in all cases is collective, and engages common cultural considerations (Dutton, Boyanowsky, & Bond, 2005).

In the course of inflicting the savagery, personal motivations other than normative compliance may be met, at least for some perpetrators, and these idiosyncratic needs help sustain and augment the brutality targeted against the enemy by the group as a whole. Individuals with cruel, sadistic and sociopathic dispositions flourish in parlous times, because they are regarded as acting for their group and are therefore tolerated, encouraged, even idolized. But, they need their collective backing them to legitimize, to support and sustain their violence. The group in times of war provides an incubator for these persons, whose acts in times of peace and directed towards in-group members would result in ostracism, imprisonment, or execution. "Cry havoc, and let slip the dogs of war!" as Shakespeare (1949) phrased this sanctioned release of dark forces in *Julius Caesar*. Once released, these "dogs" become part of a collective dynamic involving many persons, each of whom has a range of motivations engaged.

The Scope of Collective Violence

Rummel has performed a monumental service to our educational agenda for the twenty first century by cataloguing the extent of collective savagery in the twentieth century. He refers to mass killing as democide, defined as, "The murder of any person or people by a government, including genocide, politicide, and mass murder." (http://www.hawaii.edu/powerkills/DBG.CHAP2.HTM) Democide is thus the umbrella term, incorporating other forms of organized destruction of human life by political groups, i.e., governments.

By "government killed" is meant any direct or indirect killing by government officials, or government acquiescence in the killing by others, of more than 1,000 people, except execution for what are conventionally considered criminal acts (murder, rape, spying, treason, and the like). This killing is apart from the pursuit of any ongoing military action or campaign, or as part of any conflict event.
(http://www.hawaii.edu/powerkills/WSJ.ART.HTM)

War, of course is part of this definition. As Rummel notes:

"Our century is noted for its absolute and bloody wars. World War I saw nine-million people killed in battle, an incredible record that was far surpassed within a few decades by the 15 million battle deaths of World War II. Even the number killed in twentieth century revolutions and civil wars have set historical records. In total, this century's battle killed in all its international and domestic wars, revolutions, and violent conflicts is so far about 35,654,000." (ibid.)

Staggering as this body count may seem, it is beggared by figures summarizing internal political annihilation by governments against their own citizens. (see Table 1 below)

In explaining these numbers and their "fearful symmetry", Rummel points out that,

The totals in the table are based on a nation-by-nation assessment and are absolute minimal figures that may under estimate the true total by ten percent or more. Moreover, these figures do not even include the 1921–1922 and 1958–1961 famines in the Soviet

TABLE 2.1. Twentieth century killed or dead by cause[a].

Cause	Totals (000)	Averages per 10,000 Population
Government	119,394	349
Non-Free	115,423	494
Communist	95,154	477
Other Non-Free	20,270	495
Partially Free	3,140	48
Free	831	22
War	35,654	22
International	29,683	17
Civil	5,970	26

a. All figures in the table are rounded; therefore the totals of subcategories may be slightly off.

Union and China causing about 4 million and 27 million dead, respectively . . . However, Table 1 does include the Soviet government's planned and administered starvation of the Ukraine begun in 1932 as a way of breaking peasant opposition to collectivization and destroying Ukrainian nationalism. As many as ten million may have been starved to death or succumbed to famine related diseases; I estimate eight million died. Had these people all been shot, the Soviet government's moral responsibility could be no greater. (ibid.)

Of course, one could dispute the approximate numbers involved, but their magnitude is daunting, however imprecise the details may be. We must remember, too, that Rummel has confined his assessment to twentieth century democide, where records are more reliable and methods more lethal. What would the figures reveal for the ninetieth century, a fragment of which provided the Spanish painter, Goya, with the painful inspiration to depict the arresting images that so powerfully embody the ugliness of war? Descending further back into the bloody history of our species, one could recount the savagery of subjugation, warfare and conquest perpetrated by the forces of Tamerlane, Genghis Khan, Julius Caesar, Vlad the Impaler, Alexander the Great, Montezuma, Muhammad Shah, the Sultan of Kulbarga and other storied characters from history. A sobering web page recounts this body count: (http://users.erols.com/mwhite28/warstat0.htm0), pointing out that the absolute numbers must be interpreted proportionally in light of a diminishing world population, as we recede further into time. Such accounts of humanity's staggering legacy led Becker to conclude that, "Creation is a nightmare spectacular, taking place on a planet that has been soaked for hundreds of million years in the blood of all its creatures." (1973, p. 283)

The absolute numbers in this litany of death are appalling enough; the proportions of the populations destroyed are sobering in their social implications. Such high proportions indicate just how widespread the complicity of the fellow citizens, active or passive, must have been to sustain these large-scale acts of sustained savagery against their fellow humans. Of course, these acts of brutality were rationalized by the agencies of state, city-state, duchy, tribe, clan, or village policy, but we must marvel at our human capacity to accept these legitimations, to endorse their animus towards the targeted group, and be mobilized to cooperate in the execution of their fearsome design.

The Costs of Collective Violence

A large part of what we as a species have come to tolerate is the loss of human life chronicled above. Such "war" is, indeed, hell. It brings in its wake "dislocation of populations; the destruction of social networks and ecosystems; insecurity affecting civilians and others not engaged in the fighting; [and] abuses of human rights" (WHO, 2002, p. 215). Furthermore, there are additional deaths due to disease flourishing as a result of the destruction to medical and other infrastructural supports for life, such the water supply and sewage disposal systems. The WHO

Report on Health and violence lists the range of additional costs in terms of mortality, morbidity and disability:

Examples of the direct impact of conflict on health

Health impact	*Causes*
Increased mortality	Deaths due to external causes, mainly related to weapons
	Deaths due to infectious diseases (such as measles, poliomyelitis, tetanus and malaria)
	Deaths due to non-communicable diseases, as well as deaths otherwise avoidable through medical care (including asthma, diabetes and emergency surgery)
Increased morbidity	Injuries from external causes, such as those from weapons, mutilation, anti-personnel landmines, burns, and poisoning
	Morbidity associated with other external causes, including sexual violence
	Infectious diseases:
	— water-related (such as cholera, typhoid and dysentery due to *Shigella* spp.)
	— vector-borne (such as malaria and onchocerciasis)
	— other communicable diseases (such as tuberculosis, acute respiratory infections, HIV infection and other sexually transmitted diseases)
	Reproductive health:
	— a greater number of stillbirths and premature births, more cases of low birth weight and more delivery complications
	— longer-term genetic impact of exposure to chemicals and radiation
	Nutrition:
	— acute and chronic malnutrition and a variety of deficiency disorders
	Mental health:
	— anxiety
	— depression
	— post-traumatic stress disorder
	— suicidal behaviour
Increased disability	Physical
	Psychological
	Social (WHO, 2002, Table 8:2)

This table catalogues an arresting sweep of suffering. Despite its range, it does not include the lost opportunities – psychological, interpersonal, economic, social, and political – that trail in the wake of collective violence. These foregone opportunities, carefully imagined, make our considerations of collective violence doubly excruciating.

The psychological costs of collective violence will be considered in various contexts and from different perspectives throughout the other chapters in this edited volume. My remit is to assess the role of culture in fomenting collective violence, and possibly in transmuting the potential for collective violence into harmonious solutions to our group interdependencies.

Becoming Encultured to Violence

Without culture, there is no collective violence. Collective violence is a group orchestration, relying for its expression and unfolding on how each cultural group has socialized its members to meet the basic concerns addressed by all cultures everywhere, anytime. As argued by Schwartz (1994), there are " . . . three universal requirements of human existence to which all individuals and societies must be responsive: needs of individuals as biological organisms, requirements of coordinated social action, and survival and welfare needs of groups" (p. 88). Each cultural system is a particular solution to these requirements, arising out of the interplay between its historical legacy, including traditions, and its current ecological-historical niche.

A culture's members are socialized to be functioning members of this solution. Within the limits imposed by each their genetic endowments, each cultural group member assumes some of the available roles on offer within his or her culture, observing the norms by which the cultural group ensures its integrity, and over time develops the psychological software necessary to function within that cultural system. Psychologists study these outputs of this life-long socialization in the form of personality dispositions and identities, along with values, beliefs, and attitudes, including political attitudes and ideologies specific to their cultural group (see Bond, 2004, for an elaboration of this argument). It is individuals, socialized into their group and orchestrated by its cultural system, who become galvanized by events to wreak collective violence upon legitimized targets. Or, who practice collective negotiation using non-coercive means . . .

Culture's Functions

"Our way of life" is our culture, and every group has a culture. It is simultaneously a *modus vivendi*, a *modus operandi*, and a *modus sustandi*, a solution to the pan-cultural human challenges of surviving biologically as organisms, of coordinating projects with one another, and of maintaining the very group upon which we are dependent for our continuing capacity to live, work, and play, and be persons. Our culture has material embodiments, in the form of tools and built environments, and also subjective realizations in the psychological repertoire of its members, moving through their individual life cycles and coordinating their enactments with those of other group members at various stages in their life cycles.

For the purpose of this essay, a cultural situation for a given group may be examined "as a lattice-work of constraints and affordances which shape the behavioural development of its members into similar patterns." (Bond, 2004, p. 62) This particular ecological-historical niche includes the social institutions that have been developed across time and across the lives of its contributing members to cope with the group's current situation. A group's institutions play a key role in this process, " . . . as the formulative agency of individual consciousness." (Berger, 1967a, p. 15) The resultant socialization process for a group's members produces the subjective realization of each cultural solution as,

A shared system of beliefs (what is true), values (what is important), expectations, especially about scripted behavioural sequences, and behaviour meanings (what is implied by engaging in a given action) developed by a group over time to provide the requirements of living (food and water, protection against the elements, security, social belonging, appreciation and respect from others, and the exercise of one's skills in realizing one's life purpose) in a particular geographical niche. This shared system enhances communication of meaning and coordination of actions among a culture's members by reducing uncertainty and anxiety through making its member's behaviour predictable, understandable, and valued. (Bond, 2004, p. 62)

Internalization of the culture is achieved, a process described by Berger (1967a, p.17) as, " . . . the reabsorption into consciousness of the objectivated world in such a way that the structures of this world come to determine the subjective structures of consciousness itself." In consequence, "The institutional programs set up by society (become) subjectively real as attitudes, motives and life projects." (p. 17, brackets added) Thereby, "Every social action implies that that individual meaning is directed towards others, and ongoing social interaction implies that the several meanings of the actors are integrated into an order of common meaning." (p. 19) Given the sharedness in such socialized output, the "subjective" realization of culture becomes objective, in the sense that most of the group's members are in public accord on many aspects of this common system.

A functioning cultural system does not require psychologically identical members, similar in every respect. Such templated outputs would be impossible, of course, given each person's distinctive genetic profile (Pinker, 2002). What is necessary is that group members play by the same set of rules for coordinating the activities necessary in meeting the pan-cultural challenges of living. These rules include a division of labor across the genders and the life span, a logic of resource distribution, and procedural norms for integrating members' inputs in meeting the various tasks of life. Thereby, "Every social action implies that that individual meaning is directed towards others and ongoing social interaction implies that the several meanings of the actors are integrated into an order of common meaning." (Berger, 1967a, p. 19)

Cultural systems evolve over time to meet these challenges and the vicissitudes of change more effectively. This evolution focuses upon "functionally specific" components of the system necessary to ensure a viable adaptation to changing external conditions, including inter-group relations (Yang, 1988); other features of the cultural system are retained, since they still work well enough. To the extent that the evolving system meets the challenges of living, a culture survives and socializes its members to appreciate and laud their heritage, its "way of life".

Some Universal Processes Potentiating Collective Violence

Each person is born into a family located in a setting that includes other families governed by a set of rules for ensuring their survival as families and for coordinating daily activities with other families and their members. This set of rules is followed as an alternative to struggling for survival separately in a Hob besian jungle Through socialization, members of this grouping come to share the tools, knowledge, language and organizational-enforcement structure necessary for the survival of the group and the extension of its members' interests.

A huge investment of human and material resources is contributed by members over their lifetimes to their system and to one another as group members. This investment is sustained by conferring status upon group heroes who contribute to the group's survival and welfare, and by ostracizing in various ways those who undermine the system. This investment is rationalized through identification with the group by its members, the development of group loyalty, and a commitment to conserve the group's "way of life". "Groupism" underpins all viable systems.

In-groupism. Just as "No man is an island, entire unto itself' " (Donne, 1950), no group, however defined, is alone, occupying its territory without interacting with other groups and that group's members. Throughout human history, groups have been brought into contact as they foraged, hunted for prey, relocated because of natural disasters and epidemics, or attempted to extend their animal, vegetable and mineral holdings by acquiring those controlled by other groups.

Our evolutionary history has thus alerted every person to the resource implications of group membership, the survival needs served by continuing group membership, and the potential threat posed by members of other groups (Suedfield & Schaller, 2002). So, "For most of the history of our species . . . it would have been quite reasonable and adaptive to (identify outsiders accurately), to mistrust outsiders and seek to minimize encounters with them." (Newman & Erber, 2002, p. 329–330, brackets added) A trans-temporal and trans-cultural inculcation into the us-them, same-other, insider-outsider distinction seems to be basic to all social groups, and to become part of the socialization processes required for continuing membership and avoidance of being ostracised by "us-same-insiders". After an exhaustive review of the historical evidence, Jahoda (2002, pp. 5–7) concludes,

"An historical perspective serves to highlight . . . the enormous power and remarkable persistence of sentiments of attachment to one's own group and of potential hostility directed against 'the *Other*'. They can be suppressed, but this does not necessarily eradicate them . . . Antagonisms between human groups have been the rule throughout history and have taken similar forms . . . The sentiments mobilized are often not only strong, but also long-enduring, and usually hard to eliminate".

In-group identification thus appears readily available to us as a social species, and mobilizable as a rallying lodestone in times of threat. The stronger the loyalty to one's group, the stronger the disposition to out-group violence (Cohen, Montoya, & Insko, 2006).

Predation. Nell (2006) has argued that another vestige of our evolutionary past is our human capacity for savagery against one another in the form of cruelty. "Cruelty is the deliberate infliction of physical or psychological pain on other living creatures, sometimes indifferently, but often with delight." (abstract) He explores the puzzle that, "Though cruelty is an overwhelming presence in the world, there is no neurobiological or psychological explanation for its ubiquity and reward value." (abstract) Nell describes three stages in the development of cruelty:

Stage 1 is the development of the predatory adaptation from the Palaeozoic to the ethology of predation in canids, felids, and primates. *Stage 2,* through palaeontological and anthropological evidence, traces the emergence of the hunting adaptation in the Pliocene, its development in early hominids and its emotional loading in surviving forager societies. This adaptation provides an explanation for the powerful emotions—high arousal and strong affect—evoked by the pain-blood-death complex. *Stage 3* is the emergence of cruelty about 1.5 million years ago as a hominid behavioural repertoire that promoted fitness through the maintenance of personal and social power. The resulting cultural elaborations of cruelty in war, in sacrificial rites, and as entertainment are examined to show the historical and cross-cultural stability of the uses of cruelty for punishment, amusement, and social control. (abstract)

Nell uses his analysis of "cruelty's rewards" to "provide a heuristic for understanding . . . why, despite the human capacity for compassion, atrocities continue." (p. 2)

The reward value of inflicting cruelty derives from "competitive aggression, which confers fitness by solving an animal's problems in relation to self-preservation, protection of the young, and resource competition." (p. 4) Components of cruelty – the sights, sounds, smells, frantic movements and taste of living creatures being killed and consumed in a successful hunt – become secondary reinforcers as part of the "pain-blood-death complex".

Predatory behaviour may thus have been stamped into our species.

Nell (2006) then describes the social use of cruelty as a tool for binding an individual to his or her social group by inflicting exemplary pain on a disloyal member or on one who refuses to serve as an instrument of state control, e.g., as a military conscript. Onlookers attending these disciplinary dramas, as in the feeding of the Christians to the lions in the Rome of the Emperor Commodus, were riveted to these cruel spectacles, and simultaneously socialized into a fearful compliance with state policies. Of additional importance for an understanding of collective violence, however, is Nell's contention that,

War may be the most significant social product of the predatory adaptation. The . . . emotional state of the warrior in combat mimics that of predators and hunters, with high arousal, positive affect, and heightened libido, which in turn raises the possibility that in the transition from predation to intraspecific, non-nutritional killing, the reinforcers of the pain-blood-death complex have become attached to combat and warfare. (p. 20)

Part of what sustains warfare in its manifold forms of violence against the enemy then is "cruelty's rewards". As Nell speculates, "It is possible that in combat and in cruel acts, the intensity of wounding and killing activity is escalated by pain, just as the dopaminergic biochemistry of predation, in itself powerfully rewarding, may be augmented by endorphin release in response to exertion and pain." (p. 20)

Of course, no society can survive if cruelty is allowed to run rampant. Its displays must be regulated and focused. Paraphrasing Elias, Nell (2006) argues that, " . . . centralised state power created pacified social spaces, the restraint of aggressive instincts was internalised, and "an automatic, blindly functioning apparatus of self-control [was] established . . . [protected] by a wall of deep-rooted fears" (p. 368). So, human nature, "red in tooth and claw", was brought to heel, in the interests of in-group stability. But, " . . . these barriers are permeable and crumble as opportunity and situation allow." (p. 22) I consider those opportunities and situations below, under the heading, "Culture as culprit".

The male role. Killing is disproportionately the work of men. Until recently, only men served as combatants in armies, paramilitaries and other state or political agencies of lethal control. Their primary role in enactments of mob violence, torture, rape, razing and pillage is obvious. Consistent with this generality, males engage in more individual acts of homicide in all countries where perpetrator gender is recorded, and are found cross-culturally to show greater levels of any externalizing disorder, such as truancy, delinquency, and vandalism, than women (Verhulst et al., 2003).

In explaining gender differences in human behaviour, Wood and Eagly (2002, p. 699) conclude that the cross-cultural data supports a biosocial analysis, such that:

. . . sex differences derive from the interaction between the physical specialization of the sexes, especially female reproductive capacity, and the economic and social structural aspects of societies. This biosocial approach treats the psychological attributes of women and men as emergent given the evolved characteristics of the sexes, their developmental experiences, and their situated activity in society.

In part, then, male predominance in destructive activity may be explained by biological gender roles, universally predicated on women's unique capacity for childbirth and male's physical advantage in hunting and foraging. Stereotypes have developed, crystallized around role specialization derived from roles associated with nurturance of children and provision of food, such that men are pan-culturally regarded as more active and as more potent (Williams & Best, 1990), using Osgood's basic three factors of affective meaning (Osgood, Suci, & Tannenbaum, 1957). These three components of meaning may be used to show that pan-culturally, the profile of men as stronger and more vigorous is closer to the associations given pan-culturally to concepts allied with violence, such as aggression, anger, argument, army, battle, competition, conflict, crime, danger, murder and pain (Osgood, May, & Miron, 1975).

Males are then socialized to adopt roles requiring greater activity and potency, and are rewarded for instantiating them ably. Endorsement of these "gender definitions" has been shown by Heimer and De Coster (1999) to explain the differential rates of delinquency between men and women. Consistent with this observation is Ember and Ember's (1994) conclusion, "that the rated level of homicide/assault across 186 societies was predicted most strongly by the socialization for aggression of males in late childhood in those societies." (quoted in Bond, 2004, p. 67) That men are raised and socialized to engage in more destructive social activities than women is clear; the size of this difference may be culturally moderated, as Archer (2006) has shown by comparing the national ratios of domestic violence by male and female partners. How this difference moderates across different social structures, and the associated socialization practices required to effect this moderation of difference and overall level of destructiveness need to be examined (Bond, 2004), since both effects are relevant to our consideration of collective violence.

Culture as Culprit

The evolutionary legacies considered above seem to predispose us as a species towards violence as a probable response to resource interdependencies. There is a ready supply of group members, usually male, socialized to act aggressively towards others who threaten their group's welfare. At least for some, there will be a delight in the predation that may be involved, and their delight may release other co-actors to join in the sustained savagery frequently evidenced during massacres (Dutton, Boyanowsky, & Bond, 2005). These evolutionary predispositions must, however, be mobilized and orchestrated. This is the role of culture, *par excellence*.

Circumstances Favouring Collective Violence

It is impossible to disentangle culture from the circumstances in which that culture functions because a cultural system is a negotiated response to those very circumstances. However, a cultural system develops slowly and cumulatively in response to routine challenges posed by its ambient conditions of life. Its previous adequacy in meeting these challenges results in a cultural conservatism that gives cultural systems inertia, sustained by the socialization for the endorsement of "our way of life" that all such systems inculcate.

The socialized logic of this cultural system will shape its response to circumstances that predispose towards collective violence. These circumstances have been identified by historically analyzing episodes of collective violence to extract common features informing these episodes. So, the WHO report on collective violence concludes that,

The risk factors for violent
conflicts include:
Political factors:
            — a lack of democratic processes;
            — unequal access to power.

Economic factors:
— grossly unequal distribution of resources;
— unequal access to resources;
— control over key natural resources;
— control over drug production or trading.

Societal and community
factors:
— inequality between groups;
— the fuelling of group fanaticism along ethnic, national or religious lines;
— the ready availability of small arms and other weapons.

Demographic factors:
— rapid demographic change. (WHO, 2002, p. 220)

As a social psychologist, Staub (2002, pp. 12–13) translates these risk factors psychologically by claiming that they constitute,

" . . . the primary activators of basic needs, which demand fulfillment . . . These include needs for security, for a positive identity, for effectiveness and control over important events in one's life, for positive connection to other people, and for a meaningful understanding of the world or comprehension of reality."

These human needs are frustrated and seemingly impossible to achieve in these threatening and anomic circumstances. Unmet, they generate, "psychological processes in individuals and social process in (their) groups . . . that turn the group against others as they offer destructive fulfillment of these needs." (Staub, 2002, p. 13, brackets added) This edited collection considers the price for both perpetrators and their victims of meeting our human needs through these acts of destruction.

What is missing from this analysis, however, is the multitude of cases throughout history when cultural systems faced the same circumstances, but did not engage in collective violence. When they consider a fuller range of cultural responses to similar sets of circumstances, social scientists conclude that, " . . . there is no universal set of necessary or sufficient conditions that will trigger a crisis." (Newman & Erber, 2002, p. 329) Difficult circumstances potentiate but do not generate collective violence (see also Suedfeld, 2001). So, what must exist in a cultural system to generate collective violence? Newman and Erber (2002, p. 329) conclude that, "Local values, attitudes and expectations will determine the degree of subjective distress associated with specific objective conditions." This is a position of cultural relativism, according culture a moderating role in exacerbating its members' degree of perceived distress.

Culture and the Perceived Distress Arising from Difficult Circumstances

Engaging in collective violence demands high levels of sustained contributions by large numbers of individuals cooperating in the messy, resource-sapping and often dangerous work of harming and destroying other human beings. High levels of distress among the population constituting a cultural group can provide fuel for such savagery. If cultural systems amplify the distress generated by difficult life circumstances, then a powerful psychological force can be recruited to mobilize collective violence. Conversely, if cultural systems moderate the distress generated by difficult life circumstances, then less psychological force can be recruited to mobilize collective violence.

Certainly individual members of a given culture vary in the degree to which they are distressed by the circumstances of life that they face as members of that culture. There is a whole literature on life dissatisfaction, negative affect, and social cynicism as psychological outcomes showing that such measures of distress are moderated or amplified by culturally related, psychological dispositions (Diener & Tov, 2007; Smith, Bond, & Kagitcibasi, 2006, Chapter 4). So, if the average level of these key psychological dispositions were greater or lesser in some cultural systems compared to others, then they might act as buffers or as amplifiers of external circumstances and their effect on levels of distress. For example, if members of a given culture were higher in their belief about the role of fate in human affairs (see e.g., Leung & Bond, 2004), then perhaps they would react with less distress to difficult circumstances because they have been socialized to believe that life is full of inevitable, unchangeable difficulties anyway. So, a sensible reaction under this cultural logic is detachment. On the other hand, if members of a given culture were higher in the value they attach to human rights and equality (e.g., Schwartz's, 1994, value domain of egalitarian commitment), then perhaps they would react with greater distress to difficult circumstances because they have been socialized to value just and humane outcomes for all.

Higher general distress of individuals is not, however, action; it certainly does not constitute organized social violence against members of another social group. Beyond a certain threshold level, it may provide a facilitating background condition, but is certainly not a sufficient condition for collective violence to occur.

Culture and Mobilizing Collective Violence

Having a large number of distressed group members is not enough to foment collective violence. A group's members must be marshaled, organized and focused.

All persons are socialized not to physically harm their in-group members. This fundamental injunction will generalize to other conspecifics, but can be overcome with the perception of in-group support for violence against the out-group and its members. This support will include direct socialization *for* aggression (Ember & Ember, 1994), and will involve providing specialized organizations and venues for its training. Historical evidence shows that most "ordinary" persons can be brought to kill and maim others (Browning, 1993), though the role is usually assigned to men, and both social pressure and specific training is required (Grossman, 1995) to overcome their initial squeamishness socialized from childhood to protect the in-group from internal disruption and harm.

Socialization that facilitates collective violence must include training other group members to support those who perpetrate the actual violence. This support comes in the form of voiced approval of their heinous acts, usually rationalized as loyal service to the in-group, a protection of the in-group against malicious others who would destroy it and its way of life. This support can even extend to accepting as "inevitable" the loss of life and suffering from "collateral damage" to non-combatants and to children of the other group ("war is hell"). The destruction of non-combatants is often rationalized during atrocities by reminding perpetrators that these others may well one day become warriors with revenge in their hearts (Dutton et al., 2005).

A group's members must also be willing to accept the costs that engaging in collective violence will always entail – the rationing, the limitations on personal freedom, the re-deployment of services to support the military, the decline in civilian health, and the destruction of the environment. They must be willing to endure these privations, and to support other group members in doing so. At the very least, group members must be socialized not to object, to interfere or to intervene in the carnage or destruction of the identified enemy. This passivity is usually easy to ensure, as strong norms of ostracism and even execution of dissenters (quislings) will be salient during times of heightened threat to one's personal and group existence (Jost & Hunyady, 2005). Any such resistance is dangerous, as it undercuts the perception of unanimity that is essential for maintaining group members' resolve to fight and to support the fighting (see Fein, 1979; Staub, 2002 on the importance of bystander intervention), and so must be vigorously suppressed. As the Russian proverb puts it, "When you run with the pack, you don't have to bark, but at least you must wag your tail."

These considerations relate to the marshaling and the orchestration of collective violence. The issue here is ensuring a broad-based participation in the collective group effort required to enact extensive, sustained destruction of other human beings. There are different social roles to be meshed in achieving this "final solution", but they all require that individuals in the group embrace the group agenda of destroying out-group members, with each playing his or her role.

Some cultural systems are more effective at socializing their members to comply in perpetrating violence against other groups. "All societies teach some respect for and obedience to authority, but there is great variation in degree." (Staub, 1999, p. 204) Considerable support for Staub's contention has emerged from cross-cultural studies of conformity – variations in agreement in the Asch line-judgment paradigm (Bond & Smith, 1996) and variations in acquiescent response bias (Smith, 2004), both showing effects across cultures corresponding to greater degrees of hierarchy, power distance or societal cynicism of that cultural grouping. Compliance-proneness is a crucial feature of more collectivist cultural groups that makes them more mobilizable for perpetrating collective violence (Oyserman & Lauffer, 2002). For, as Staub (1999, p. 204) argues,

"In strongly authority-orientated societies, people will be more affected by difficult life conditions, when the capacity of their leaders, the authorities, to provide security and effective leadership breaks down. They will have more difficulty dealing with conditions of uncertainty (Soeters, 1996). They will yearn for new leaders who offer hopeful visions of the future. They will be more likely to blame other groups for life problems, they will also be less likely to speak out against their leaders as their leaders begin to move them along a continuum of destruction. Finally, they may be more easily directed by leaders to engage in immoral and violent acts."

In-groupism is a related feature of collectivist cultural systems that predisposes them to move faster and with more deadly force along "the continuum of destruction" characterizing collective violence. The boundary between in-group and out-group members is more sharply drawn in such cultures (Gudykunst & Bond, 1997; Oyserman & Lauffer, 2002), making it easier to de-humanize out-group members, thereby legitimating their extermination (Dutton et al., 2005). This process of boundary-drawing is usually reinforced by historical animosities towards the other group and motives of revenge perpetuated by inadequate attempts at reconciliation and provision of reparations to the aggrieved group that can now regard itself as embarking on a mission of retributive justice.

Group Ideologies

Ideologies are organized explanations about reality, especially about how the social world functions and what must be done to create a just social system. Within that social system and whether promulgated as sacred or self-evident or usually both, these group-defining ideologies become undeniable. All groups develop ideologies to rationalize, legitimate and ennoble its history and to shape its future; they are necessary human adaptations to meet the basic human needs for order, interpersonal coordination and meaning.

A group's ideologies are inculcated by the group's institutions – familial, educational, occupational and religious – becoming shared and helping to define what an acceptable member of that group believes and should endorse. These institutions legitimize the social order and produce a group consensus around both what is true and what is good. As Berger (1967b, pp. 29–30) puts it, "Legitimations . . . can be both cognitive and normative in character. They do not only tell people what *ought to be*. Often they merely propose what *is*."

These legitimations are reinforced with varying degrees of unanimity by the totality of socialization processes that constitute what Berger (1967a, p. 52) calls the "plausibility structure" for the ideology. "When we add up all these factors – social definitions of reality, social relations that take these [definitions of reality] for granted, as well as the supporting therapies and legitimations – we have the total plausibility structure of the conception in question."

The plausibility structures supporting these ideologies result in "Internalization . . . into consciousness of the objectivated world in such a way that the structures of this world come to determine the subjective structures of consciousness itself." (Berger, 1967a, p. 14–15) This internalization of ideologies is content-general and arises from a powerful human motivation to embrace social order. As posited by Jost and Hunyady (2005, p. 260),

" . . . people are motivated to justify and rationalize the way things are, so that existing social, economic, and political arrangements tend to be perceived as fair and legitimate. We postulate that there is, as with virtually all other psychological motives (e.g., self-enhancement, cognitive consistency), both (a) a general motivational tendency to rationalize the status quo and (b) substantial variation in the expression of that tendency due to situational and dispositional factors".

The combined force of a group's plausibility structures plus the motivation posited above to endorse the status quo, results in the adoption of a group's ideologies by its members. So, "The institutional programs set up by society [become] subjectively real as attitudes, motives and life projects." (Berger, 1967b, p. 17, brackets added) However, " . . . the social world (with its appropriate institutions, roles, and identities) is not passively absorbed by the individual, but actively *appropriated* by him." (p. 18) The degree of this appropriation will vary along Kelman's (1961) continuum ranging from compliance to internalization, but regardless of its level of endorsement by an individual member, that ideology will be regarded as consensually embraced by members of the group and will help to define that group's identity by its members and by members of other groups interacting with that group and its members.

Ideologies of Antagonism and Violence

Staub (1988) has identified "ideologies of antagonism" as a crucial social component in focusing collective animosity and targeting an out-group for violent acts. An ideology of antagonism is "an especially intense form of devaluation . . . a perception of the other as an enemy and a group identity in which enmity to the other is an integral component . . . it often remains part of the deep structure of the culture and can reemerge when instigating conditions for violence are present." (Staub, 1999, p. 183) These ideologies provide an explanation for the difficult life circumstances being faced by a group and identify other groups and its members as causes of those adversities. They facilitate "moral disengagement" from the sanctioned act of killing others (Bandura, 1999).

As part of this ideology, an out-group is perceived as malevolent and unchangeable, indifferent to the plight of one's group, thereby justifying defensive and retaliatory violence against that group (Gudykunst & Bond, 1997; Stephan, 1985). Descendants of these out-group members are expected to engage in retaliatory acts themselves against one's group for its violence, thereby inciting and justifying one's group to exterminate men, women and children, civilians as well as combatants lest they fulfill these prophecies of doom (Dutton et al., 2005). Through the reinterpretive agency of these ideologies, in-group members come to regard themselves as doing good as they perform bad deeds in order to protect the in-group and its way of life.

In their work on system justification theory, Jost and Hunyady (2005) provide evidence that the tendency to defend and justify the status quo is strengthened by experimentally manipulated threats to the system. However, these laboratory-based threats are trivial compared to Staub's "difficult life circumstances" that confront cultural groups provoked to collective violence. Mortality salience in the form of potential death from untoward events or attack by another hostile group further enhances the endorsement of one's group and its ideology. This unification around the ideology that helps define one's system is crucially important in mobilizing members of the system to begin acting against the scapegoated out-group. Perception of this in-group consensus combines with one's own sharpened resolve to believe that one's hostile acts towards out-group members will be accepted, even lauded, by one's group members.

The Role of Religion

Religion is fundamentally implicated in some episodes of collective violence, such as the Crusades, but in others it plays an auxiliary role by supporting political agendas, as in current Sri Lankan violence, or none at all, as in Ghengis Khan's wars of conquest in the thirteenth century or Vlad the Impaler's savagery against the populace of Transylvania in the fifteenth century. Religion is ideology that includes explicit commentary on the origin and nature of the manifest world of daily affairs, a person's relationship to this mundane reality and to any imminent or transcendent forces that underpin the observable flux of mundane reality. Liht and Conway (2005, p. 3) assess the psychological purposes of religion by claiming that it serves a "meta-narrative function in which personal situations are incorporated into an over-arching sense of order and coherence that conveys a sense of meaning, control, and optimism." These are powerful human motives that can find realization and expression in religious commitment by members of a cultural system. Many cultural systems are centrally defined by their "cultures of religion", and these religious ideologies command considerable following. Their credibility in the minds of individual believers is sustained by all the "plausibility structures" (Berger, 1967b) that surround religious practices in that cultural system.

For present purposes, religious ideology addresses three crucial issues, also addressed by secular political ideologies, with varying degrees of scriptural explicitness: "Who is my brother and sister (Mao's question), and how should he or she and non-brothers or non-sisters be treated?"; "Is there an afterlife, and how does one's behaviour in this life affect one's state in that afterlife?"; and "Who is the source of authority in interpreting the religious ideology?" The answers provided to the first question define the boundary, if any, between in-group and out-group, and identifies the behaviours towards those two types of persons that will be rewarded, ignored, or punished. If non-believers are non-brothers or non-sisters, and if non-brothers or non-sisters may be treated less humanely than believers, then the groundwork for an ideology of antagonism with a basis in religion is in place and available for deployment as the occasion requires. A socially supported sense of rightness then develops around these behavioural prescriptions for dealing with non-believers.

The second issue of an afterlife and prescriptions for its attainment has become salient in light of recent acts of suicidal terrorism. Movements supporting suicidal terrorism enjoy an extended human history, and do not require ideological support from religion to motivate their destructive acts against other groups (Hazani, 1993). Nonetheless, religious ideology can be used to justify a personal disregard for this life, i.e., rejection of the quotidian world (Liht & Conway, 2005) and to promise a fulfilling afterlife whose attainment typically depends upon one's actions in this life. If those actions include the elimination of non-believers, then the logic sustaining religiously-inspired collective violence is in position.

That logic can be utilized by religious authorities if the religious ideology has historically been interpreted by individuals specially qualified for this role. This issue of authority is the third question addressed by every religion. Such theocratic traditions can invest religious leaders with interpretive legitimacy and the power to inspire followers, mobilizing them to act against non-believers. This potential for authoritarian targeting of non-believers is enhanced when the support for such animus is not explicitly contradicted by the scriptures of the religion in question and when the founding of the religion involved warfare and subjugation, as in Islam.

The Catalyst of Leadership

Staub (1999) points out that Hutu leaders in Rwanda used their control of radio broadcasts, the major form of mass communication in a poor agrarian society, to terrify their Hutu population with stories of rebel Tutsi armies mobilizing to inflict savagery upon them. Already primed by difficult life circumstances and a historically based ideology of antagonism against Tutsis, the Hutus began forming paramilitary units to engage in pre-emptive strikes against Tutsis. These acts became "group-fulfilling prophecies" with Tutsis arming and attacking Hutus in an escalating cycle of retaliatory and defensive strikes against one another. Local leaders, already identified through agencies of socialization during peaceful times, arose during these parlous times to orchestrate local acts of savagery. They acted as diligent lieutenants, executing the terrible logic unleashed by the alarmist pronouncements of the central authorities.

As illustrated in the Rwandan genocide, the crucial leadership role in collective violence is that of the politician-ideologue who galvanizes a disaffected population with credible and unchallenged visions of a malevolent other group. He (almost always a "he") is able to do so because the political-social structure has effectively muted any contrary voices. In consequence, the in-group may be mobilized and focused with no apparent internal resistance. This assessment of how leadership functions within a receptive social and institutional setting to foment and target collective violence is consistent with Andrew Nathan's assessment of Mao's role in the litany of twentieth century Chinese democide:

A caricature Mao is too easy a solution to the puzzle of modern China's history. What we learn from this history is that there are some very bad people: it would have been more useful, as well as closer to the truth, had we been shown that there are some very bad institutions and some very bad situations, both of which can make bad people even worse, and give them the incentive and the opportunity to do terrible things. (Nathan, 2005, p. 1)

The leader in collective violence does not cause the savagery; he midwives the savagery, crystallizing a group's resolve to mobilize itself in defense of its interests, to attack and eliminate those who threaten its survival and advancement.

Individual Differences in the Social Processes Sustaining Collective Violence

In analyzing predatory savagery, Nell (2006, p. 22) acknowledges that there exist "large individual differences in cruelty's eliciting triggers and behavioural expressions on the one hand, and an understanding of the needs and gratifications of perpetrators on the other." The reward value of cruelty-elicited stimuli varies unequally across a population, such that most group members find inflicting pain on other humans repugnant. However, a crucial few in any large group will be predisposed through as yet-unspecified genetic endowment (Nell, 2006), early nutritional deficiencies leading to inadequate pre-frontal development (Raine, Mellingen, Liu, Venables, & Mednick, 2003), or socialization processes leading to the development of sadistic sociopathy (Murphy &Vess, 2003) to revel in the opportunity to brutalize others in a socially sanctioning environment.

For them, predation is arousing, and now the circumstances are right. The normative structure of group life changes during periods of collective violence, and violence against non-group members becomes both justifiable and justified. Normally suppressed acts of savagery are now ennobled, and those readier and more able to enact them become group heroes, rewarded for their skills (Dutton et al., 2005). They inspire ambivalent others to participate, and there is evidence to suggest that victim-elicited pain responses become gratifying to some of these group members now inspired by the core sociopaths to brutalize the enemy. They become addicted to the rush of the carnage through the same opponent-process model of learning that is hypothesized to render any initially repelling act pleasurable, as in many addictions (Baumeister & Campbell, 1999). Acts of collective violence thereby become self-reinforcing, as many normally persons are transformed into predatory beasts (Browning, 1998). The number of "willing executioners" reaches a critical mass (Ball, 2004), and sustains the fighting group's destructive momentum. A social tipping point may be reached (Gladwell, 2000), and, given sufficiently frequent encounters with the enemy, the frenzy can continue unabated. This is exactly what happened during the Japanese occupation of China from 1937–1945 – the Nanjing massacre was the apogee of concentrated carnage, but episodic massacres occurred routinely until the Japanese were defeated. (Rummel, 1991).

These frenzies may generate reprisals from the now mobilized out-group, if it has the capacity and the will to resist. The level of retaliatory savagery spawned often involves counter-brutalization of the enemy, further justifying and mobilizing attacks by the original attackers. This cycle of brutality is common in war, but is also characteristic of episodic terrorism. The latest atrocity experienced legitimizes the next atrocity inflicted, provoking each group to counter-attack in its turn. Having been unleashed, The Furies may only be stopped by the capitulation of one group or the intervention of a superior power to enforce a cessation of hostilities.

Culture as Solution

The preceding part of this essay has analyzed how difficult life circumstances confronting groups can combine with the ideologies of antagonism socialized by threatened groups to mobilize their members for group protection and to target members of other groups for destruction. Basically, if the group on which each of us depends for our survival and flourishing socializes us for violence against another group and circumstances motivate our group mobilization, enough of us will act destructively and be supported by most of the other group members to sustain collective violence.

We humans have a deep-seated capacity for intra-species violence and an extensive historical record of its collective perpetration and fearsome *sequelae*. Despite this depressing evolutionary legacy, Wilson (1975, p. 554), the founding father of sociobiology wrote,

"Human societies have effloresced to levels of extreme complexity because their members have the intelligence and flexibility to play roles of virtually any degree of specification, and to switch them as the occasion demands. Modern man is an actor of many parts who may well be stretched to his limit by the constantly shifting demands of the environment."

Has our twenty first century environment shifted to the point that non-violent solutions to inter-group conflict become more demanding than their primitive alternatives? Recently it has been pointed out that war is on the decline in the last part of the twentieth century. As reported by the Human Security Report, 2005, (http://www.humansecurityreport.info/index.php?option=content&task=view&id=196)

The number of conflicts rose steadily from the early 1950s until about 1992, then dropped sharply, today, 20 to 30 armed conflicts are under way worldwide, depending on the definition. That's down from 50 to 60 in 1992, none pits developed countries against one another, although several are "asymmetric" conflicts between industrialized countries and relatively primitive enemies (e.g., America in Iraq) ... Instances of genocide and mass killings of ideological foes are also down from 10 a year in the early 1990s to one in 2004 (i.e., Arab militias killing Black Africans in Darfur, Sudan)

Wilson (1975, p. 569) himself seemed optimistic in this regard when he wrote, "Aggressiveness was constrained and the old forms of primate dominance replaced by complex social skills." What has been happening worldwide to promote this reduction in savagery? What "complex social skills" are being socialized and institutionalized to support this new *modus operandi*? What insights can our examination of culture as culprit suggest for proposing culture as a solution?

The Growth of Democracies

In his assessment of twentieth century democide, Rummel (1988) concluded that, democratic political systems are less likely to engage in war. By democracy, Rummel means,

" . . . liberal democracy, where those who hold power are elected in competitive elections with a secret ballot and wide franchise (loosely understood as including at least 2/3rds of adult males); where there is freedom of speech, religion, and organization; and a constitutional framework of law to which the government is subordinate and that guarantees equal rights." (http://en.wikipedia.org/wiki/R._J._Rummel)

From his historical analysis, Rummel concludes that,

"There is a consistent and significant, but low, negative correlation between democracies and collective violence", and further, " . . . that when two nations are stable democracies, no wars occur between them." (p. 9) Even more important in light of the numbers of human beings killed, "There is no case of democracies killing en masse their own citizens." (p. 2) (quoted in Bond, 1994, p. 68)

Rummel (1988) believes that democracies suppress the collective will to mobilize violence against another group:

"[a democracy] promotes a social field, cross-pressures, and political responsibility; it promotes pluralism, diversity, and groups that have a stake in peace."(p. 6) These institutional, social and psychological components of democratic political systems make it more difficult for leaders to mobilize the necessary public support required to undertake large-scale forms of coercive social control (see also Olmo, 1975; Sullivan & Transue, 1999). " . . . the normal working of a democratically free society in all its diversity is to restrain the growth across the community of that consuming singleness of view and purpose that leads, if frustrated, to wide-scale social and political violence. (Rummel, 1988, p. 4) (quoted from Bond, 1994, p. 68)

Are democracies on the rise? In the Human Security Report quoted above it was also reported that, "In 1946, 20 nations in the world were democracies, according to the Maryland Institute's Peace and Conflict 2005 report. Today, 88 countries are." Is the *spiritus mundi* embracing democracy, and is that quest one core feature of globalization, with its giving voice to the voiceless and reducing of economic and social inequalities (Smith et al., 2006, Chapter 12)?

If so, increasing democratization may depress levels of collective violence further. Democratic polities are characterized by numerous institutional provisions that counter collective mobilization against fellow citizens:

A nation's degree of democracy is strongly associated with its provision of freedom and its observance of human rights, as Rummel (1988) maintained and as Lim & Bond (2003) have shown empirically. The percentage of its national wealth spent on military expenditure is also lower, as would be expected given its lesser pre-occupation with war (Lim et al., 2003). Its legal culture will also be different, with guarantees of due process in place, availability of legal aid, political independence of the judiciary, and so forth (see e.g., Feest & Blankenburg, 1997). (quoted from Bond, 2004, p. 68)

This last consideration concerning legal culture is crucial. Democracies can create oppressive regimes in multi-ethnic polities where one ethnic group enjoys a numerical majority. If citizens of such political units vote along ethnic lines, then a tyranny of the majority can be legitimized unless there are restraining institutions in place. These include a constitution guaranteeing equality before the law, but also a judicial system independent of political interference and intimidation. Enforcement of judicial decisions must also be carried out by authorities serving the law, not the party in power.

Many former colonies have thrown off their shackles in post-WW2 wars of liberation that accounted for much of the collective violence before 1992. In many of these post-colonial regimes, however democratic they may claim to be, the judiciary and its enforcement agencies are subservient to the majority ethnic group in political power, as in contemporary Zimbabwe. The incendiary potential for internal repression and violence is obvious, as Muller and Weede (1990) have argued.

In this regard, cultural collectivism may well provide a dampening influence on the widespread provision of political freedoms. Conway, Sexton, and Tweed (2006, p. 38) provide evidence to show that, " . . . cultural collectivism predicted future political restriction across nations, but not vice versa . . . an explicitly cultural dimension does causally predict which cultures will become, and remain, politically free." How a lifting of such political restrictiveness will emerge in the cultural systems that most need them in considering the potential for collective violence, viz., collectivist cultures, is an open question. As Clague, Gleason, and Knack (2001, p. 19) warn,

"Attempts to introduce foreign institutions such as elections, legislatures, and judicially enforced rule of law may succeed in one society and fail in another because of deep-seated cultural attitudes and expectations about how political authority should and will be used."

Other group characteristics may be required to promote the development of the institutional checks and balances that make democracies protective of all their citizens. After all, collectivist Japan showed a dramatic about-face following the imposition of democracy and an independent judiciary in 1945. These change processes may be cultural, albeit different from the collectivism of Conway et al. (2006), and relate to prior national experience, such as being founded as a nation by immigrants, as was Australia; losing a conflict to a democracy, as did Panama in 1989; or installing a post-revolutionary egalitarian to head its government, as the South Africans did with Nelson Mandela in 1994.

Psychological Concomitants

Citizens in democracies are socialized differently, as Sullivan and Transue (1999) have shown. In particular, public education is more widely available, especially across genders, and a greater proportion of national wealth is invested into education. The educational curriculum is broader, with liberal arts and social sciences given greater attention. History is taught less ethnocentrically, and multi-cultural perspectives are presented. Educational practices encourage greater initiative and participation by students, providing opportunities for skill training in non-violent modes of dispute resolution (Hofstede, 1986). All these educational features of many democracies are believed to conduce towards greater unity intra-state (Bond, 1999) by legitimizing and encouraging public dialogue. As Staub (1999, p. 204) points out, "The public dialogue makes scapegoating, the wide-spread adoption of destructive ideologies, and progression along a continuum of violence less likely."

The next generation is given voice by these institutional provisions, taught that there are many legitimate voices, each of which is protected, and taught the discipline to tolerate differences of beliefs and the skills to harmonize these voices as much as possible without reverting to repression or violence. Such socialization combined with parenting practices that promote caring for others (Staub, 1988) has crucial psychological consequences for the members of such social systems:

Persons in more democratic nations place a greater value on social integration relative to cultural inwardness (Lim et al., 2003), a finding consistent with Rummel's (1988) assertion that those socialized into democratic systems are motivated to engage themselves positively with diverse others. Higher levels of trust (Wilkinson, Kawachi, & Kennedy, 1998) and collective efficacy (Bandura, 2001) probably also characterize the citizens of such social units. Levels of intolerance against out-groups (Berry & Kalin, 1995), authoritarianism (Altemeyer, 1988), ideologies of antagonism (Staub, 1988), and other divisive attitude constellations should likewise be weaker in citizens of democracies. (Bond, 2004, p. 68–69)

Given Nell's (2006) analysis of the predatory potential derived from our evolutionary heritage, one might add revulsion at another's pain to this list of socialized outputs from democratic polities. The value attached to human life is sustained by the legal institutions arising from the cultural endorsement of human rights (Humana, 1992), and is a feature of democracies and wealthier social systems. There is no direct measure of this personality variable, but it seems an integral component to any consideration of mobilizing a group to engage in collective violence. Part of educating this revulsion probably involves exposing members of the system to the dark side of human history in a moralistic setting that affirms the group's aspiration to avoid hurting others. This unsettling input will generate resistance from some quarters, but those who object might well be reminded of Santayana's (1905) warning,

Progress, far from consisting in change, depends on retentiveness . . . when experience is not retained, as among savages, infancy is perpetual. Those who cannot remember the past are condemned to repeat it.

Given the costs of collective violence documented earlier, socializing for this and the other psychological resources counteracting inter-group aggression creates valuable, perhaps even necessary, social capital (Bourdieu, 1986).

Counter-Ideologies

Crucial in this educational process is the inculcation of ideologies, systems of beliefs, norms, values and injunctions that oppose strong and rigid hierarchy, vilification of identifiable groups, and the legitimacy of using destructive means for social control. We know much more about their ideological opposites, such as social dominance orientation (Sidanius & Pratto, 1999) or hierarchic self-interest (Hagan, Rippl, Boehnke, & Merkens, 1999) and ethnocentrism (Altemeyer, 1988) along with specific scales designed to measure animus towards a specific target group, and the tendency to justifiy aggression more generally (Caprara, Barbaranelli, & Zimbardo, 1996). Nonetheless, there are worldviews that counteract ideologies of antagonism, like worldmindedness, defined by Sampson and Smith (1957, p. 105) as, "a frame of reference, or a value orientation favouring a world-view of the problem of humanity, with mankind, rather than the nationals of a particular country, as the primary reference group", but rarely studied since (cf., Der-Karabetian, 1992). Likewise, a number of personality orientations, like tolerance (Berry & Kalin, 1995) or Schwartz's (1992) value domain of universalism, are also relevant and probably fall under the Big Five dimension of openness to experience (Trapnell, 1994). These counter-ideologies are discussed at length in Bond (1999), but should probably be expanded to include training that runs counter to a belief in fate (Leung & Bond, 2004) as a controlling factor in human affairs.

Third-Party Intervention

Responsible parents intervene when their children fight, so as to protect them from physical damage. They impose a truce, and begin training their children about justice and developing the procedural routines for ensuring peace and re-enabling productive exchanges among their charges. Numerous commentators have argued that a parallel process should be instituted when collective violence breaks out within or between nations (Robertson, 2002). A number of institutional provisions would be required to effect these interventions successfully. As argued by Genocide Watch (see e.g., Stanton, 2004), they would include: a standing, volunteer, professional response force under the UN; early-warning systems independent of the United Nations Security Council; and an internationally supported International Criminal Court. As Power (2002) has repeatedly pointed out, no single nation can intervene unilaterally because its citizens will not tolerate the costs, especially in lives of their own people. Also, their independent intervention will be regarded as motivated by national interest pursued at the expense of other nations, and invite retaliatory actions or resistance to the initiative by these other nations.

Some supra-national authorities, not subject to diplomatic maneuvering for national advantage (Robertson, 2002), must be installed to suppress on-going violence, ensuring that its perpetrators will be brought to account, and that alternative means can be deployed to resolve the conflict and impose its provisions if need be. A supra-national authority, operating to protect the basic human right to a natural span of life, would have a better chance to be perceived as just and its actions as legitimate and therefore supported. Every group's culture would then be modified with respect to this qualification of its right to independent assertion.

What forces are available to goad nations into renouncing some of their sovereignty so that these safeguards may be emplaced? Perhaps it is only an emerging sense of our shared humanity, of our common fate as members of this imperiled globe and of revulsion at our evolutionary legacy of viciousness, domination and annihilation. The alternative is continuing savagery.

Conclusion

Each person is born into a family that nurtures the child, socializing that individual into the norms, beliefs, values and way of life that family and the group of which it is a unit has fashioned in its ecological-temporal niche to survive and flourish. Within the individual's genetic constraints, he or she is encultured and becomes an adequately functioning member of that group. That process results in a sense of loyalty and investment in the group and its way of living.

Groups intersect with other groups, and use their group's logic for managing interdependencies to resolve the competition for resources and dominance that emerge. Collective violence of one group against another is the occasional result of these intergroup struggles, often with horrific consequences. A group's members are mobilized to support and participate in this struggle for collective dominance by the group's legitimation processes that deem the targeted outgroup and its members as dangerous, immoral, or sub-human, and hence killable. These legitimation processes and the ideologies that underpin them are quintessentially cultural, responsive to the group's history and current life circumstances.

A different culture for inter-group relations may be emerging in the twenty first century, one informed by an understanding of the human propensity to group savagery, the enormous costs arising from collective violence, and a commitment to human equality. This diffusing culture will render individual members of specific groups less mobilizable for violence by their groups, more resistant to chauvinistic appeals for self-sacrifice. With sufficient supra-group institutional supports in place, the expected value of engaging in collective violence will be reduced; nonviolent solutions to the issues of resource distribution and group identity can be developed.

" . . . how much more suffering and ruin must be experienced by our race before we wholeheartedly accept the spiritual nature that makes us a single people, and garner the courage to plan our future in the light of what has been so painfully learned."

(Baha'i International Community, *Who is writing the future?* 1999, p. 15)

Epilogue: Writing about Collective Violence. Academic writing is always difficult for me, requiring as it does the discipline of my sprawling, poetic style and a mastery of an extensive literature. But, writing about collective violence is more than difficult; it is deeply disturbing. For, in order to do this work, I must encounter the basest forms of human behaviour, at its most repugnant and appalling. Writing about collective violence across history and across cultural groups constantly reminds me that the specter of savage mass violence is lurking in our midst, ever ready to burst forth.

This awareness scares me. But, I often shudder in realizing that the Beast also lurks within me. In Golding's (1962) *Lord of the flies*, Simon hears a voice taunting him: "Fancy thinking the Beast was something you could hunt and kill! You knew, didn't you? I'm part of you." This intuition that violence is in here as well as out there is constantly surfacing, as I do the reading and thinking necessary to do this writing.

I live an ordered life made possible by doing an intellectual's work at a sheltered university managed by reasonable people, all of us sustained in our daily rounds by a peaceful and prosperous society. I do not directly encounter the harrowing realities that form the *explicandum* that we call "collective violence". For this mercy, I am grateful. If I had been born into some of the circumstances I have described in the chapter above, there is no doubt in my mind that I would be a deeply wounded and a profoundly different person. As Conrad (1900) describes this present danger in *Lord Jim*, "It had the power to drive me out of my conception of existence, out of that shelter each of us makes for himself to creep under in moments of danger, as a tortoise withdraws within its shell." This is a terrifying prospect, and yet it is a daily reality coursing through the life-veins of too many fellow human beings. And through the life-veins of those who try to help those confronting such terror . . .

I grieve for them and for those innumerable millions whose possibilities have been cut down, whose lives have been demeaned and whose raw pain has encompassed their every living hour. I protest this manifest injustice! The only viable alternative I can imagine to the despair and madness it draws in its wake is to write for understanding. That understanding is for doing our social life differently, so that our species is not cursed by Santayana's (1905) warning that, "Those who cannot remember the past are condemned to repeat it." We must remember our past and consider it carefully, so that we can re-fashion our future together on this imperiled planet. I hope that we can discover what makes the difference between war and peace, so that we can train ourselves to wage peace rather than suffer war. As Berger reminds us, " . . . all human societies and their institutions are, at their root, a barrier against naked terror." (1967b, p. 95) Let us build such barriers with the fruits of our understanding!

References

Altemeyer, B. (1988). *Enemies of freedom: Understanding right-wing authoritarianism.* San Francisco, CA: Jossey-Bass.

Archer, J. (2006). Cross-cultural differences in physical aggression between partners: A social-structural analysis. *Personality and Social Psychology Review, 10,* 133–153.

Baha'i International Community (1999). *Who is writing the future? Reflections on the twentieth century*. Haifa, Israel: Baha'i International Community.

Ball, P. (2004). *Critical mass: How one thing leads to another*. London: Random House.

Bandura, A. (1999). Moral disengagement in the perpetration of inhumanities [Special issue]. *Personality and Social Psychology Review, 3*, 193–209.

Bandura, A. (2001). *Self-efficacy: The exercise of control*. New York: Freeman.

Baumeister, R. F., & Campbell, W. K. (1999). The intrinsic appeal of evil: Sadism, sensational thrills, and threatened egotism. *Personality and Social Psychology Review 3*, 210–221.

Becker, E. (1973). *The denial of death*. New York: Free Press.

Berger, P. L. (1967a). *The sacred canopy: Elements of a sociological theory of religion*. New York: Anchor.

Berger, P. L. (1967b). *A rumour of angels*. Harmondsworth: Penguin

Berger, P. L., & Luckmann, T. (1966). *The social construction of reality: A treatise in the sociology of knowledge*. New York: Doubleday.

Berry, J. W., & Kalin, R. (1995). Multicultural and ethnic attitudes in Canada: An overview of the 1991 national survey. *Canadian Journal of Behavioral Science, 27*, 301–320.

Bond, M. H. (1999). Unity in diversity: Orientations and strategies for building a harmonious, multicultural society. In J. Adamopoulos & Y. Kashima (Eds.), *Social psychology and cultural context* (pp. 17–39). Thousand Oaks, CA: Sage.

Bond, M. H. (2004). Culture and aggression – from context to coercion. *Personality and Social Psychology Review, 8*, 62–78.

Bond, R., & Smith, P. B. (1996). Culture and conformity: A meta-analysis of studies using Asch's (1952b, 1956) line judgment task. *Psychological Bulletin, 119*, 111–137.

Bourdieu, P. (1986). The forms of capital. In J. E. Richardson (Ed.), *Handbook of theory of research for the sociology of education* (pp. 241–258). New York: Greenwood.

Browning, C. R. (1993). *Ordinary men*. New York: Harper Collins.

Caprara, G.-V., Barbaranelli, C., & Zimbardo, P. G. (1996). Understanding the complexity of human aggression: Affective, cognitive, and social dimensions of individual differences in propensity toward aggression. *European Journal of Personality, 10*, 133–155.

Clague, C., Gleason, S., & Knack, S. (2001). Determinants of lasting democracies in poor countries: Culture, development and institutions. *The Annals of the American Academy of Political and Social Science, 573*, 16–41.

Cohen, T. R., Montoya, M. R., & Insko, C. A. (2006). *Group morality and intergroup relations: Experimental and cross-cultural evidence*. Manuscript submitted for publication.

Conrad, J. (1900). *Lord Jim: A romance*. Garden City, NY: Doubleday.

Conway, L. G., Sexton, S. M., & Tweed, R. G. (2006). Collectivism and governmentally initiated restrictions: A cross-sectional and longitudinal analysis across nations and within a nation. *Journal of Cross-Cultural Psychology, 37*, 20-41.

Danner, M. (1994). *The massacre at El Mazote*. New York: Vintage Books.

Der-Karabetian, A. (1992). World-mindedness and the nuclear threat: A multinational study. *Journal of Social Behavior and Personality, 7*, 293–308.

Diener, E., & Tov, W. (2007). Culture and subjective well-being. In S. Kitayama & D. Cohen (Eds.), *Handbook of cultural psychology*. New York, NY: Guilford Publications, Inc.

Donne, J. (1950). *John Donne: A selection of his poetry*. Harmondsworth, Eng.: Penguin.

Dutton, D. G., Boyanowsky, E. O., & Bond, M. H. (2005). Extreme mass homicide: From military massacre to genocide. *Aggression and Violent Behavior, 10*, 437–473.

Ember, C. R., & Ember, M. (1994). War, socialization, and interpersonal violence: A cross-cultural study. *Journal of Conflict Resolution, 38*, 620–646.

Feest, J., & Blankenburg, E. (Eds.) (1997). *Changing legal cultures*. Onati, Spain: International Institute for the Sociology of Law.

Fein, H. (1979). *Accounting for genocide: National responses and Jewish victimization during the holocaust*. New York: Free Press.

Garner, R. (1997). *Social movement theory and research: An annotated bibliographic guide*. Lanham, MD: Scarecrow Press.

Gladwell, M. (2000). *The tipping point: How little things can make a big difference*. London: Little, Brown and Co.

Golding, W. (1962). *Lord of the flies*. London: Faber and Faber.

Grossman, D. (1995). *On killing: The psychological cost of learning to kill in war and society*. New York: Little Brown and Co.

Gudykunst, W. B., & Bond, M. H. (1997). Intergroup relations across cultures. In J. Berry, M. Segall, & C. Kagitcibasi (Eds.), *Handbook of cross-cultural psychology* (Vol. 3, pp. 119–161). Needham Heights, MA: Allyn & Bacon.

Hagan, J., Rippl. S., Boehnke, K., & Merkens, H. (1999). The interest in evil: Hierarchic self-interest and right-wing extremism among East and West German youth. *Social Science Research*, 28, 162–183.

Hazani, M. (1993). Sacrificial immortality: Toward a theory of suicidal terrorism and related phenomena. In L. B. Boyer, R. M. Boyer, & S. M. Sonnenberg (Eds.), *The psychoanalytic study of society* (pp. 415–442). Hillsdale, NJ: The Analytic Press.

Heimer, K., & De Coster, S. (1999). The gendering of violent delinquency. *Criminology, 37*, 277–317.

Hofstede, G. (1986). Cultural differences in teaching and learning. *International Journal of Intercultural Relations, 10*, 301–320.

Human Security Center, Human Security Report, 2005 (available from http://www.humansecurityreport.info/index.php?option=content&task=view&id=19)

Humana, C. (1992) *World human rights guide* (3rd ed.). New York: Oxford University Press.

Jahoda, G. (2002). On the origins of antagonism towards "The Others". *Zeitschrift fur Ethnologie, 127*, 1–16.

Jost, J. T., & Hunyady, O. (2005). Antecedents and consequences of system-justifying ideologies. *Current Directions in Psychological Science, 14*, 260–265.

Kelman, H. C. (1961). Processes of opinion change. *Public Opinion Quarterly, 25*, 57–78.

Leung, K., & Bond, M. H. (2004). Social axioms: A model for social beliefs in multicultural perspective. *Advances in Experimental Social Psychology* (Vol. 36, pp. 119–197). San Diego, CA: Elsevier Academic Press.

Liht, J., & Conway, L. G. (2005). *Religious fundamentalism: An empirically derived construct and multi-religion measurement scale*. Paper presented at the 28th Meeting of the International Society of Political Psychology, Toronto, Canada, July.

Lim, F., & Bond, M. H. (2003). *The gender ratio in the perpetration of homicide: Explaining differences across 70 nations*. Unpublished manuscript, Chinese University of Hong Kong.

Mao, Z. (1960). *Selected works of Mao Tse-Tung* (Vol. 1). Peking: Foreign Language Press.

Muller, E. N., & Weede, E. (1990). Cross-national variation in plitical violence: A rational action approach. *Journal of Conflict Resolution, 34*, 624–651.

Murphy, C., & Vess, J. (2003). Subtypes of psychopathy: Proposed differences between narcissistic, borderline, sadistic and antisocial psychopaths. *Psychiatric Quarterly, 74*, 11–29.

Nathan, A. (2005). Plastic and jade: A review of *Mao: The Unknown Story* by Jung Chang and Jon Halliday. *London Review of Books*, November 17.

Nell, V. (2006). Cruelty's rewards: The gratifications of perpetrators and spectators. *Behavioral and Brain Sciences, 29,* 211–257.

Newman, L. S., & Erber, R. (2002). Epilogue: Social psychologists confront the holocaust. In L. S. Newman & R. Erber (Eds.), *Understanding genocide: The social psychology of the Holocaust* (pp. 325–345). New York: Oxford University Press.

Olmo, del R. (1975). Limitations for the prevention of violence: The Latin American reality and its criminological theory. *Crime and Social Justice, 3,* 21-29.

Osgood, C. E., May, W. H., & Miron, M. S. (1975). *Cross-cultural universals of affective meaning.* Urbana, IL: University of Illinois Press.

Osgood, C. E., Suci, G. J., & Tannenbaum, P. H. (1957). *The measurement of meaning.* Urbana, IL: University of Illinois Press.

Oyserman, D., & Lauffer, A. (2002). Examining the implications of cultural frames on social movements and group action. In L. S. Newman & R. Erber (Eds.), *Understanding genocide: The social psychology of the Holocaust* (pp. 162–187). New York: Oxford University Press.

Pinker, S. (2002). *The blank slate: The modern denial of human nature.* New York: Penguin.

Power, S. (2002). Genocide and U.S. foreign policy: A conversation with Samantha Power by Henry Kreisler, April 29.
(http://globetrotter.berkeley.edu/people2/Power/power-con0.html)

Raine, A., Mellingen, K., Liu, J., Venables, P., & Mednick, S. A. (2003). Effects of environmental enrichment at ages 3–5 years on schizotypal personality and antisocial behavior at ages 17 and 23 years. *American Journal of Psychiatry, 160,* 1627–1635.

Robertson, G. (2002). *Crimes against humanity: The struggle for global justice* (2nd ed.). London: Penguin.

Rummel, R. J. (1988). *Political systems, violence, and war.* Paper presented at the United States Institute of Peace Conference, Airlie House, Airlie, Virginia, June. (available on the web: http://www.shadeslanding.com/firearms/rummel.war.html)

Rummel, R. J. (1991). *China's bloody century: Genocide and mass murder since 1900.* New Brunswick, NJ: Transaction Publishers.

Sampson, D. L., & Smith, H. P. (1957). A scale to measure world-minded attitudes. *Journal of Social Psychology, 45,* 99–106.

Santayana, G. (1905). *The life of reason* (Vol. 1). New York: Scribners.

Schwartz, S. H. (1992). The universal content and structure of values: Theoretical advances and empirical tests in 20 countries. In M. Zanna (Ed.), *Advances in Experimental Social Psychology* (vol. 25, pp. 1-65). New York: Academic Press.

Schwartz, S. H. (1994). Beyond individualism and collectivism: New cultural dimensions of values. In U. Kim, H. C. Triandis, Ç. KaShakespeare, W. (1949). *Julius Caesar.* Cambridge, UK: Cambridge university Press.

Sidanius, J., & Pratto, F. (1999). *Social dominance: An intergroup theory of social hierarchy and oppression.* Cambridge, UK: Cambridge University Press.

Smith, P. B. (2004). Acquiescent response bias as an aspect of cultural communication style. *Journal of Cross-Cultural Psychology, 35,* 50–61.

Smith, P. B., Bond, M. H., & Kagitcibasi, C. (2006). *Understanding social psychology across cultures.* London: Sage.

Soeters, J. L. (1996). Culture and conflict: An application of Hofstede's theory to the conflict in the former Yugoslavia. *Peace and Conflict: Journal of Peace Psychology, 2,* 233-244.

Stanton, G. (2004). Twelve ways to deny a genocide. Speech available from http://www.genocidewatch.org/SudanTwelveWaysToDenyAGenocidebyGregStanton.htm

Staub, E. (1988). The evolution of caring and nonaggressive persons and societies. *Journal of Social Issues, 44*, 81–100.

Staub, E. (1999). Predicting collective violence: The psychological and cultural roots of turning against others. In C. Summers & E. Markusen, (Eds.), *Collective violence: Harmful behavior in groups and governments* (pp. 195–209). New York: Rowman & Littlefield Publishers.

Staub, E. (2002). The psychology of bystanders, perpetrators, and heroic helpers. In L. S. Newman & R. Erber (Eds.), *Understanding genocide: The social psychology of the Holocaust* (pp. 11–42). New York: Oxford University Press.

Stephan, W. G. (1985). Intergroup relations. In G. Lindzey & E. Aronson (Eds.), *Handbook of social psychology* (3rd ed., Vol. 2, pp. XX–UU). New York: Random House.

Suedfeld, P. (2001). Theories of the Holocaust: Trying to explain the unimaginable In D. Chirot & M. E. Seligman (Eds.), *Ethnopolitical warfare: Causes, consequences and possible solutions* (pp. 51–70). Washington, DC: APA Press.

Suedfield, P., & Schaller, M. (2002). Authoritarianism and the Holocaust: Some cognitive and affective implications. In L. S. Newman & R. Erber (Eds.), *Understanding genocide: The social psychology of the Holocaust* (pp. 68–90). New York: Oxford University Press.

Sullivan, J. L., & Transue, J. E. (1999). The psychological underpinnings of democracy: A selected review of research on political tolerance, interpersonal trust, and social capital. *Annual Review of Psychology, 50*, 625-650.

Trapnell, P. D. (1994). Openness versus intellect: A lexical left turn. *European Journal of Personality, 8*, 273–290.

Verhulst, F. C., Achenbach, T. M., Ende, J. V. D., Lambert, M. C., Leung, P. W. L., Silva, M. A., et al. (2003). Comparisons of problems reported by youths from seven countries. *American Journal of Psychiatry, 160*, 1479–1485.

Wilkinson, R. G., Kawachi, I., & Kennedy, B. P. (1998). Mortality, the social environment, crime and violence. *Sociology of Health and Illness, 20*, 578 - 597.

Williams, J., & Best, D. (1990). *Sex and psyche: Gender and self viewed cross-culturally.* Newbury Park, CA: Sage.

Wilson, E. O. (1975). *Sociobiology: The new synthesis.* Cambridge, MA: Harvard University Press.

Wood, W., & Eagly, A. H. (2002). A cross-cultural analysis of the behavior of women and men: Implications for the origins of sex differences. *Psychological Bulletin, 128*, 699-727.

World Health Organization (2002). *World report on violence and health.* Geneva, Switzerland: WHO Publications (available on line at: http://www.who.int/violence_injury_prevention/violence/world_report/en/index.html)

Yang, K. S. (1988). Will societal modernization eventually eliminate cross-cultural psychological differences? In M. H. Bond (Ed.), *The cross-cultural challenge to social psychology* (pp. 67–85). Newbury Park, CA: Sage.

3
Destroying the World to Save It

Robert Jay Lifton

Introduction

On March 20, 1995, Aum Shinrikyō, a fanatical Japanese religious cult, released sarin, a deadly nerve gas, on five subway trains during Tokyo's early-morning rush hour. A male cult member boarded each of the trains carrying two or three small plastic bags covered with newspaper and, at an agreed-upon time, removed the newspaper and punctured the bags with a sharpened umbrella tip. On the trains, in the stations where they stopped, and at the station exits, people coughed, choked, experienced convulsions, and collapsed. Eleven were killed and up to five thousand injured. Had Aum succeeded in producing a purer form of the gas, the deaths could have been in the thousands or hundreds of thousands. For sarin, produced originally by the Nazis, is among the most lethal of chemical weapons. Those releasing it on the trains understood themselves to be acting on behalf of their guru Shōkō Asahara and his vast plan for human salvation. The world had to be destroyed in order to be saved.

One-Eyed Child

Shōkō Asahara's childhood brings to mind Erasmus's aphorism "In the country of the blind the one-eyed man is king." But this particular one-eyed child was apparently an odd and uneasy king. Born in 1955 into the impoverished family of a tatami craftsman in a provincial area of Kyūshū, the southernmost of Japan's main islands, he was the sixth of seven children and the fourth of five boys. Chizuo Matsumoto (Asahara's birth name), afflicted with congenital glaucoma,

Excerpt adapted from DESTROYING THE WORLD TO SAVE IT by Robert Jay Lifton. Copyright © 1999, 2000 by Robert Jay Lifton.
Originally published in *Destroying the World to Save It*
Reprinted by permission of the author.

was without sight in one eye and had severely impaired vision in the other. Because he did have some vision he was eligible to attend an ordinary school, but his parents chose to send him to a special school for the blind. It had the advantage of providing free tuition and board, and a completely sightless older brother was already enrolled there.

Having some vision while his fellow students had none, and being bigger and stronger than most of them, he could be a dominating, manipulative, bullying, and sometimes violent figure in the school, where he would remain until he was twenty years old. He would, for instance, force his roommates to strike one another in a contest he called "pro wrestling," and when he found their efforts unsatisfactory he would himself demonstrate how it should be done. He could be rebellious to the point of threatening teachers but, if challenged, would back down and deny any provocation. He always had a few completely blind followers toward whom he could at times exhibit great kindness, and his teachers observed that he was also capable of tenderness toward his older brother and a younger brother who later became a student at the school. But he was generally coercive, gave evidence of resentment over having been forced to attend this special school, and was prone to quick changes in attitude and demands.

In his early ventures into proto-guruism, this one-eyed "king" did not command wide allegiance. He unsuccessfully ran for class head on several occasions, and each failure left him dejected. Once, after being voted down by fellow students despite an attempt to bribe them with sweets, he accused a teacher of influencing the election by saying bad things about him, but the teacher pointed out to him that the other students were simply afraid of him.

While his actual background was humble enough, there were rumors of a further taint—that his family came from the outcast group known by the euphemism *burakumin* (literally "village people") or that they were Korean, also a victimized group in Japan. These rumors, though false, suggest something of others' attitudes toward him. Yet later he would sometimes himself imply that he was *burakumin*, in order to identify himself with a despised and victimized group and so to claim extraordinary triumph over adversity.

Most accounts of Asahara's early years emphasize his preoccupation with money. He would charge other students for favors his partial sight allowed him to accomplish and insist upon being treated by them when he took them to food shops or restaurants. He is said to have accumulated a considerable sum of money this way by the time of his graduation. But whatever the complexities of his school life, he apparently obtained rather good grades as a student and achieved a black-belt ranking in judo.

One aspect of Asahara's childhood is not frequently mentioned. He was attracted to drama of all kinds. From an early age, he loved to watch melodramas on television; later he acted in various school plays and as a high school senior wrote a play of his own about Prince Genji, a great romantic figure, taking the exalted leading role for himself. His stated ambition was to become prime minister of Japan. One teacher remembered him avidly absorbing a biography of Kakuei Tanaka, the new prime minister in 1972. He even reportedly said in those years that he wished to be "the head of a robot kingdom" (although in the context of the popular science-fiction culture of his adolescence, this fantasy might not have been as strange as it may now sound). His teachers generally came to think of him as someone who wished to "extend his own image into someone strong or heroic." A former classmate made the interesting observation that as the school for the blind was a closed society, so in Aum Asahara would try "to create the same kind of closed society in which he could be the head."

Asahara's childhood undoubtedly contributed to his sense of alienation, of otherness, to his generalized hatred of the world, to his tendency toward paranoia, to what was to become a habit of violence, to his cultivation of the art of performance, and to his aspirations toward the heroic and transcendent. Overall, he developed in childhood an inclination toward controlling and manipulating other people, and perhaps the beginnings of an identity as a "blind seer."

The Guru Myth: Beginnings

After graduating from a special extension course at the high school for the blind in 1975, he moved to the Kyūshū city of Kumamoto, where he became, at the age of twenty, an acupuncturist and masseur (the latter a traditional occupation for the blind in Japan). But in 1976 he was convicted by a Kyūshū court of causing bodily injury to another person (one report suggests that he misused the judo he had studied) and was fined 15,000 yen ($150). In 1977 he moved to Tokyo, largely because of that incident. He was said to have at times expressed an ambition to enter either the law or the medical school of Tokyo University, Japan's most elite educational institution. According to the narrative of his life (largely supplied by him), an important reason for his move was to attend a preparatory, or "cram," school in order to take that university's extremely difficult entrance examinations, which he then failed. Since there are no clear records connecting him with either the examinations or a "cram" school, it is possible, as some observers have speculated, that Asahara invented that sequence of events as part of his mythic tale.

In any case, in Tokyo he resumed his work as an acupuncturist and masseur, while at the same time immersing himself in the revolutionary writings of Mao Zedong. In 1978, he met, impregnated, and married Tomoko Ishii, who gave birth to a daughter and would eventually bear their five other children. That same year, with the financial support of his wife's family, he opened a Chinese herbal-medicine pharmacy, which made a great deal of money. But in 1982, at the age of twenty-seven, he was arrested for selling fake Chinese medicines, convicted, fined 200,000 yen (about $2,000), and given a brief jail sentence. He went into bankrupcy, experienced a profound sense of humiliation, and plunged more deeply into studies he had already begun of various forms of traditional fortune-telling, Taoist medicine, and related expressions of divination and mysticism.

This pre-Aum experience suggests that Asahara (then still going by the name of Matsumoto) wavered between fantasies of mainstream power (entering Tokyo law school or becoming prime minister) and radical rebelliousness (lawbreaking and a fascination with Mao). He did the same in his preoccupation with healing: the vision of Tokyo University medical college giving way to fringe expressions of spiritual healing that relied on con-man tactics. His trajectory went from grandiose plans to conquer society from within to embittered failure to idiosyncratic healing enterprises.

He would later place all of his experience within a guru myth. He described himself as having been "mentally unstable" and full of "doubts about my life." In connection with such doubts, he described "a conflict between self-confidence and an inferiority complex." Then came his heroic spiritual quest: "One day I stopped fooling myself altogether and thought: "What am I living for? Is there anything absolute, does true happiness really exist in this world? If so, can I get it?" I did not realize at this point that what my soul was looking for was enlightenment. But I couldn't sit still. Urged by such restlessness, I started a blind search. It was an intense feeling; it was a faith."

Many people in such situations, he further explained, would simply change jobs or "just disappear." In him, however, there "awoke . . . the desire to seek after the ultimate, the unchanging, and I began groping for an answer." His spiritual journey, he tells us, meant "discarding everything . . . everything that I had" and required "great courage and faith, and great resolution." The emerging guru had found a way to heal himself and could embark on "a long and arduous eight years of practice" on the road to enlightenment.

In 1981, at age twenty-six, during his troubled Tokyo days, he joined Agonshū, one of the most successful of Japan's "new religions." The term refers to religious sects that have arisen since the late nineteenth century, often beginning with the vision of an ordinary person who becomes the sect's founder and borrowing eclectically from various religious traditions. Although he was later to disparage Agonshū and even claim that it had been spiritually harmful to him during his three years of membership, there is every evidence that he derived from it many of his subsequent religious principles. Indeed, he found there a powerful guru model, sixty-year-old Seiyū Kiriyama, a highly charismatic figure. Kiriyama claimed, as the British scholar Ian Reader (1996) tells us, "miraculous and extraordinary happenings, visitations, and other occurrences that created a sense of dramatic vigor and expectation around the religion and its leader, endow[ed] them with a legitimacy and suggested that they possess[ed] a special, chosen nature." In those three years Asahara was in effect apprenticing for joining the ranks of the "dynamic, charismatically powerful . . . religious figures" who, Reader (1996) says, "have frequently, by their very natures, upset or challenged [Japanese] social harmony and norms."

From Kiriyama and Agonshū, Asahara also drew upon a variety of ideas and practices that would become important in Aum: expressions of esoteric Buddhism, mystical forms of yoga, and forms of self-purification aimed at freeing oneself from bad karma. He was also much influenced by Agonshū's use of American New Age elements from the human-potential movement, individual psychology, and applied neurology. It was here as well that he first encountered the writings of Nostradamus, the sixteenth-century French astrologer and physician who predicted the end of the world with the coming of the year 2000. Asahara, who was to radically alter, supplement, and totalize these influences, soon became a fledgling guru, acquiring a few disciples by the time he left Agonshū.

The emerging guru may have a number of visions, but one in particular usually serves as a crucial illumination and a sacred mandate for a special spiritual mission. This should not be seen as simply a matter of calculation or fakery: intense personal conviction is essential to the guru's success. But that conviction can be helped considerably by grandiose ambitions and manipulative inclinations, which themselves can be enhanced by impressive demonstrations of superhuman powers. Prior to his main vision, Asahara claimed to have experienced during his early period in Agonshū an "awakening of Kundalini"—a concept of mystical yoga in which one gains access to the cosmic energy that ordinarily lies "sleeping" at the base of the spine. An accomplished practitioner, he opened a yoga school in Tokyo at about this time and was to gain many early converts through the skills he demonstrated.

In 1984 Asahara founded Aum Shinsen no Kai. Aum (often rendered in English as Om or Ohm), a Sanskrit word that represents the most primal powers of creation and destruction in the universe, is often chanted in Buddhism as part of a mantra or personal incantation. Shinsen no Kai means "circle of divine hermits" or "wizards" and has a strong suggestion of esoteric supernatural power. Asahara also created a commercial enterprise, the Aum Corporation. It was to have the important function of publishing his books.

In 1985 Asahara became famous when a photograph of him "levitating" appeared in a popular occult magazine, *Twilight Zone*, identifying him as the "Aum Society representative." The ability to levitate is considered to reflect extraordinarily high spiritual attainment. In his case it was apparently simulated by means of an upward leap from the lotus position along with a bit of trick photography. The placing of the picture in such a visible outlet was an early example of Asahara's strong sense of the importance of the media.

That same year, at the age of thirty, Asahara experienced his central, self-defining vision. While he was wandering as a "homeless monk" near the ocean in northern Japan, a deity appeared before him and ordained him as Abiraketsu no Mikoto, "the god of light who leads the armies of the gods" in an ultimate war to destroy darkness and bring about the kingdom of Shambhala—in Tibetan and other Buddhist traditions, a utopian society of spiritually realized people. The vision was announced to the world in a Japanese New Age magazine in the form of an interview with Asahara.

In the original report of the vision, the god who manifested himself was nameless, but in later versions of it Asahara identified the god as Shiva, the Hindu deity who by then had become his ultimate spiritual authority (or his guru, as he sometimes put it). It was somewhat odd for Asahara to invoke a Hindu god in the creation of an essentially Buddhist group, even if the esoteric Buddhism he drew upon stayed close to its Hindu roots. His choice of Shiva (as opposed to Vishnu or Brahma, the other great Hindu gods) probably had two important determinants. First, Shiva is specifically identified as the god of yoga. Second, while all Hindu gods have destructive as well as beneficent tendencies, Shiva is specifically associated with salvation through world destruction. Asahara was later to claim that Aum Shinrikyō emerged directly from this vision, but he was rewriting history a bit since he had formed Aum Shinsen no Kai the previous year. In 1987, two years after his vision, he renamed the group Aum Shinrikyō, the Shinrikyō meaning "teaching of the supreme truth." Very likely the change reflected his desire for a name that was less obscure, more accessible, and more absolute.

The context in which Asahara placed the vision set the tone for what could be called Aum's New Age Buddhism. Aum did not employ traditional Japanese Buddhist terms, which originated in China and are expressed in Chinese characters, but instead used early Buddhist terms from Sanskrit, Tibetan, and Pali and expressed them in katakana, a Japanese phonetic system employed for retained foreign words. These terms were combined with American New Age ones like *empowerment* (rendered in katakana as *empawahmento*). This application of a New Age sensibility to ancient Buddhist and Hindu mysticism was to have great appeal for many young people.

In 1986 Asahara claimed another transcendent religious experience, a "final enlightenment," achieved while meditating in the Himalayas—perhaps the world's ideal place for such visions. A New Delhi holy man whom Asahara sometimes referred to as his master and a "great saint" later told a Japanese reporter that he referred a supplicant Asahara to monks in the Himalayas and was "surprised" when he reappeared four or five days later with a claim to enlightenment, as the master had always assumed that such spiritual achievement required a lifetime. Yet Asahara seems to have been convinced, in at least a part of his mind, that he had indeed become enlightened and that his spiritual achievement entitled—even required—him to be a great guru or perhaps a deity.

Asahara would soon combine such spiritual grandiosity and his organizational and financial skills with endless self-promotion. He would make a point of meeting with prominent Buddhist figures in various parts of the world—most notably the Dalai Lama in India—and of having photographs taken with them, which would then be displayed in Aum publications together with his hosts' lavish expressions of praise for him and his spiritual quest. Here the emerging guru undoubtedly took liberties in converting spiritual hospitality into self-advertisement.

The Emergence of Aum Shinrikyō

By the mid-1980s, Chizuo Matsumoto, a name suggesting nothing but ordinariness, had become Shōkō Asahara, a much more striking and unusual name (Shōkō means "bright light," and the characters he chose for Asahara suggest a field of hemp, a plant associated with the Buddhist idea of connection.). The respected yoga practitioner and teacher (or *sensei*) became the charismatic guru with long, flowing hair and beard. As time went on, he would also begin to dress in the flowing purple robes that suggested a Hindu holy man. Asahara was skillful in his eclecticism, enlarging his teachings to include the Mahyâna Buddhist theme of the salvation of all beings—salvation here suggesting happiness, welfare, emancipation, and enlightenment—and developing a "Shambhala plan" for the peaceful salvation of all of Japan by means of Aum communes to be set up everywhere.

In his pre-Aum days, Asahara had focused on nonreligious ways of attaining supernatural power, advocating the exploitation of sexual partners along with frequent masturbation as means of achieving transcendence and enlightenment. In Aum he instead preached sexual abstinence while continuing to emphasize that superhuman powers could be achieved, though now by spiritual means. He used his own "levitation" as proof of this, claiming as well that advanced Aum practitioners were capable of remaining underwater up to fifteen minutes or in an airtight box immersed in water for twelve hours. As guru, moreover, Asahara retained his own sexual privileges in what was in principle an otherwise celibate community, continuing to live with his wife and family, taking on long-term mistresses from among Aum disciples, and offering Tantric sexual initiations, or "transfers of energy" to various female followers.

Even in its early years, Aum Shinrikyō showed signs of extreme guruism, intense apocalypticism, and the violent potential in both. Asahara was spoken of and addressed as *Sonshi*, meaning "revered master" or "exalted one," a highly worshipful term not ordinarily used in Japanese Buddhism. A disciple came to understand that without the guru nothing was possible, but with him there opened up a path to perfection and to reincarnations in higher realms. It was expected that the disciple would not only surrender himself to the guru but "merge" or "fuse" with him. He was to become what Asahara in one of his sermons spoke of as a "clone" of the guru. As early as 1986, Asahara declared in another sermon that Japan would sink into the ocean, there would be a third great war, and the world would end. He initially claimed that by creating thirty thousand enlightened beings Aum could prevent Armageddon, but he came to emphasize its inevitability and Aum's role in the final battle.

Asahara recruited scientists more actively than did any other group. His enthusiasm about science undoubtedly was connected with his lust for murderous weapons. But the guru also wished to consider himself a scientist and once declared, "A religion which cannot be scientifically proven is fake." He was especially interested in brain waves and claimed that by studying them Aum could establish a scientific basis for the stages of spiritual attainment described by past Buddhist saints. With the help of Hideo Murai, his chief scientist, Aum introduced the use of a headset that purportedly contained the guru's brain waves, which it transmitted to the disciple in a procedure known as the "perfect salvation initiation" (or PSI). The PSI, much revered in Aum, was meant to bring about the desired "cloning" of the guru by means of technology and science. In this way science readily became pseudoscience, or simply fantasy. There was also a strong element of science fiction in the PSI and other Aum projects, much of it actively fed by television. What took shape in Aum was a blending of science, occultism, and science fiction, with little distinction between the fictional and the actual.

Among Asahara's most crucial early decisions was the creation of *shukke*, or renunciants. *Shukke* means "leaving home" and is a traditional term for monks or nuns who give up the world. Aum's message was that if one really wished to follow the guru and join in his full spiritual project, one had to become a *shukke*, removing oneself completely from one's family and one's prior work or study and turning all one's resources—money, property, and self—over to Aum and its guru. Even one's name was to be abandoned, replaced by a Sanskrit one. Such a renunciation of the world in favor of life in a small, closed society is the antithesis of the this-worldly emphasis of most Japanese religious practice and a repudiation of the still powerful hold the Japanese family has over its members. As a family-like alternative to an actual family's conflicts and confusions, however, it proved a definite attraction to many young people.

Living together in Aum facilities, *shukke* underwent severe forms of ascetic practice, including celibacy and a prohibition against ejaculation, fasting, long hours of meditation, intense breathing exercises, and vigorous sequences of prostration combined with demanding work assignments and irregular sleep (often only a few hours a night). Their existence was a spartan one—two meals a day of extremely simple "Aum food" (rice and vegetables), tiny sleeping spaces, and no personal possessions. The fervent atmosphere was further heightened by Aum's gradual adoption of a series of initiations.

Killing the World: Poa for Everyone

No truth was more central to Aum than the principle that world salvation could be achieved only by bringing about the deaths of just about everyone on this earth. Disciples described their embrace of this vision and their understanding of its evolution from Hindu, Buddhist, and Christian doctrine, but they always assumed that the world ending violence would be initiated by others, not by the cult itself. Yet Asahara's idiosyncratic version of these traditions came to focus on the Buddhist concept of *poa*, which, in his distorted use, meant killing for the sake of your victims: that is, to provide them with a favorable rebirth. One can speak, then, of a weapons-hungry cult with a doctrine of altruistic murder—murder ostensibly intended to enhance a victim's immortality. Aum's violence could be said to begin with a dispensing of suffering: not only was killing a person with a great accumulation of bad karma a way of "transforming" his life, but under the right circumstances, it could be considered "an act of love."

The Totalistic Community

Aum's environment became one of intense *ideological totalism*, in which everything had to be experienced on an all-or-nothing basis. A number of psychological patterns characterize such an environment. Most basic is *milieu control*, in which all communication, including even an individual's inner communication, is monopolized and orchestrated, so that reality becomes the group's exclusive possession. Aum's closed subculture of guru and renunciants lent itself to an all-encompassing form of milieu control, though no such control can ever be complete or foolproof. Another pattern of the totalistic environment is *mystical manipulation*, systematic hidden maneuvers legitimating all sorts of deceptions and lies in the service of higher mystical truths. Aum had a hierarchy of mystical manipulators, each disciple being under another's authority, reaching up to the guru himself.

In such a closed world, there is often a *demand for purity*, an insistence upon an absolute separation of the pure and the impure, good and evil, in the world in general and inside each person. In Aum, only the guru could be said to be completely pure. Disciples, even the highest ones, engaged in a perpetual, Sisyphean struggle for purity, their guilt and shame mechanisms taken over by the cult if not by the guru himself. An *ethos of confession* can provide a continuing mechanism for negative self-evaluation. In Aum, abject confession became a form of shared group arrogance in the name of humility—so that each member (and Aum as a whole) would, in Albert Camus's words, "practice the profession of penitence, to be able to end up as a judge," since "the more I accuse myself, the more I have the right to judge you."

Contemporary totalistic communities like Aum claim special access to a *sacred science*, so that what are understood to be ultimate spiritual truths also become part of an ultimate science of human behavior. There is a *loading* of *the language*, in which words become limited to those that affirm the prevailing ideological claims (Aum "truth" versus outside "defilement"). At the same time a principle of *doctrine over person* requires all private perceptions to be subordinated to those ideological claims. In Aum, that meant that doubts of any kind about the guru, or about his or Aum's beliefs or actions, were attributed to a disciple's residual defilement.

Finally, in their most draconian manifestation, totalistic environments tend to press toward the *dispensing of existence*, an absolute division between those who have a right to exist and those who possess no such right. That division can remain merely judgmental or ideological, but it can also become murderous, as in Aum, which rendered such a "dispensation" altruistic by offering a "higher existence" to those it killed. Aum ultimately became convinced that no one outside the cult had the right to exist because all others, unrelated as they were to the guru, remained hopelessly defiled.

Within that totalism Aum disciples could thrive. They could embrace the extremity of the cult's asceticism as a proud discipline that gave new meaning to their lives. Above all, they could repeatedly experience altered states of consciousness, what in Aum were known as "mystical experiences." These too had a characteristic pattern: light-headedness followed by a sense of the mind leaving the body, the appearance of white or colored lights, and sometimes images either of the Buddha or of the guru. Such altered states resulted from intense forms of religious practice—especially from the oxygen deprivation brought about by yogic rapid-breathing exercises—and, later on, from the use of drugs like LSD.

But they were all attributed to the guru's unique spiritual power and so were considered indicators of one's own spiritual progress.

There was considerable violence even in the training procedures to which disciples could be subjected: protracted immersion in extremely hot or cold water, hanging by one's feet for hours at a time, or solitary confinement for days in a tiny cell-like room that had no facilities and could become unbearably hot. Though the distinction between training and punishment often blurred, these procedures were justified by the need of the disciple to overcome the bad karma he brought to Aum or, in the phrase commonly used in the cult, to "drop karma."

Asahara's tendencies toward megalomania required, and were fed by, his disciples' infinite adulation. Over the years that the interaction was sustained, one can speak of the guru's *functional megalomania*. He presented himself to the world as civilization's greatest spiritual figure—an embodiment of Shiva, the Buddha, and Christ—and as a genius in virtually every field of human endeavor. In addition, there were claims that he possessed nirvana-like brain waves, blood with special properties that could be transmitted to disciples who drank it, and a unique and distinctive form of DNA. Within the cult his megalomania was made manifest through his claim to spiritual omniscience and to control over everyone's bad karma. The megalomania also drew Asahara to weapons of ultimate destruction, the possession of which in turn fed and enhanced that mental state.

The High Disciples

Though many Aum members were middle-aged and not particularly well educated, the cult had a higher percentage of university students and young university graduates than any of the other new religions in Japan, of which there are thousands. Noting that many of Aum's crimes were committed by young people from leading universities, some Japanese journalists spoke of its disciples as "the best and the brightest." But that characterization is somewhat misleading. While a few Aum leaders were highly trained professionals, most high disciples were bright people with university backgrounds who were nonetheless only half-educated, uncertain of the meaning of what they had learned or, unsure of the value of what they were doing when they first encountered Aum Shinrikyō. The people I interviewed (who were in less exalted positions in Aum) tended to be alienated from their society, somewhat isolated from others, drawn to occult forms of religious experience, and struggling to extricate themselves from strong feelings of dependency toward their families. They were often at a confusing point of transition in their lives.

Within Aum there was a strict spiritual hierarchy. Simply joining the group made one a *zaike*, or lay member; then the pressure was immediately on to become a *shukke*. As Aum's founder and guru who had achieved final enlightenment, Asahara of course was at the top. Only he was considered what in Aum was called a "victor of truth" (from the Buddhist concept of "one who on the way of truth has attained supreme enlightenment"). The next-highest spiritual level was that of "great master" (or *seitaishi*), a category that included among others Asahara's wife, Tomoko Matsumoto, and his third daughter, Ācharii. The rank just below that was the one of the "truly enlightened master" (or *seigoshi*). These spiritual categories, decided upon by the guru himself, were taken very seriously in Aum. The prospect of moving up a category could motivate a disciple to do almost anything.

Aum Shinrikyō's leaders also took seriously its extraordinary division into "ministries" and "agencies," as though it were a vast governmental structure. These divisions were ostensibly a form of preparation for the post-Armageddon world. A number of people have commented, however, on the broad resemblance of Aum's structure to that of Japan's World War II – era government and emperor system, including a version of the imperial household. While each of Asahara's ministries and agencies had specific functions, they can be understood psychologically as grandiose projections of an individual and collective megalomania.

Another expression of that megalomania was Aum's expansion into a corporate empire. It made enormous amounts of money from the business of religion, not in itself unusual for Japanese new religions, but with particular mercenary ferocity. Through the Aum Publishing Company and its printing presses, located at the Fujinomiya headquarters, the cult churned out and sold vast numbers of books, magazines, pamphlets, videotapes, *manga* (comic strips or graphic novels, an extremely popular form in Japan), and religious pictures and objects. Religious experience did not come cheap. A *shaktipat* by the guru cost $500 for everyone but a renunciant (who would already have given Aum all his money and holdings); a liter of the guru's bathwater, which one could drink for its special effects, was $1,000; a month's rental of a Perfect Salvation Initiation headset was $10,000; for a "blood initiation" (drinking the guru's blood), one also paid $10,000.

Aum soon extended its corporate interests in highly secular directions. One of its most lucrative enterprises was the assembling and marketing of computers; the cult's negligible labor costs enabled it to undersell competitors throughout Japan. Its far-flung business activities included noodle shops and other restaurants in many Japanese cities, a fitness club, baby-sitting and dating services, travel agencies, and real estate interests.

Aum's enormous accumulation of money made possible its outrageous actions. Its assets by early 1995 were said to be as high as a billion dollars. Whether or not that figure is accurate, the full Story of Aum's finances has not yet been told. For instance, rumors have circulated about Aum's selling its illegally produced drugs on the black market with the help of the Japanese mafia, an endeavor that would have brought in huge amounts of money.

Over time Asahara and his closest disciples came to think of Aum as a military organization. They sought to acquire weapons of every variety on behalf of the guru's visions of either a triumphant Armageddon or a this-worldly political and military coup d'état that would enable him to take over Japan. In early 1990 Aum began working on its first weapons of mass destruction, which were biological. In April of that year, the cult attempted to release botulinus toxin from trucks first in central Tokyo, then near American naval installations at Yokohama and Yoko-suka, and finally at Narita Airport, the largest in Japan. But biological weapons are easier to produce than to release; repeated technical problems interfered with the viability of the released toxin and nothing much happened. Three years later, there was another effort to release botulinus toxin, this one near the imperial palace at the time of the royal wedding of the crown prince. Again nothing happened. Three weeks after, Aum released anthrax spores from the roof of its Tokyo headquarters; once more no one was killed or as far as is known, injured. In March 1995 Aum made one more attempt to release botulinus toxin, this time in a large Tokyo subway station by means of briefcases containing dispensers. It turned out that no botulinus toxin had been put in the brief cases.

And then, in March 1995 the sarin attack in the Tokyo subway took place.

Megalomania

Aum's danger to the world—and its greatest significance—lay in its joining of megalomania to ultimate weapons. That combination found quintessential expression in the guru's reception of his high disciples upon their return from carrying out the subway attack. First the guru invoked his all-encompassing authority to render mass murder altruistic and absorb it into a mantra of spiritual practice. Then, all the accounts agree, Asahara rewarded his returning murderers with praise and juice and cookies and ordered them to repeat one thousand or ten thousand times or more sentences like, "It was good to be given *poa* by the great god Shiva and all the victors of truth" or "It was good to be *poa'd* by the grace of the guru and the great god Shiva and all the victors of truth." The only disputed point is whether Asahara was saying that the act was ultimately sanctioned only by the god Shiva or that he, the guru, shared sufficient status to join Shiva in granting the *poa*. Probably the guru hedged a bit on this point.

At this postsarin ritual, guru and disciples alike displayed a certain unease. Both were involved in the completion of a murderous melodrama staged in concordance with an extravagant world-destroying vision. But even as that vision held sway, the guru and his disciples seemed to retain portions of their selves that doubted its truth or rightness and felt anxiety about the destructive act that could not be entirely quelled by the declaration of ennobling *poa*. Even Asahara slipped into something close to psychotic denial when he said to one of his disciples at a separate meeting, "They claimed it was Aum who spread the sarin." Either he was insisting, even as he gave his *poa* blessing to the disciples who carried out the act, that the incident was an attack on Aum by outside forces or he was expressing surprise and concern that the authorities suspected Aum as its perpetrator. It is likely that he embraced both of these stances. His megalomanic self enabled him to view any event—in fact, all of history—according to his own narrative needs. Thus he could declare in a radio talk three days after the attack that the police were "Lucifer" and that not only the attack but the police raid represented "a step in the expansion of the Aum Shinrikyō plan of salvation."

Functional Megalomania

The guru brought to the amassing of ultimate weapons what I have called a functional megalomania. Within megalomanic function, self becomes world. The megalomanic self lacks limits and boundaries; it resists or denies restraints of any sort. Hence the self envelops the world; the world dissolves into the self. Or put another way, the totalized self replaces the external world.

Contemporary ultimate weapons can hold a special lure for the megalomanic guru because they enable him to feel that he alone—or perhaps with a few disciples—is capable of destroying the world. He can claim a kind of world-controlling as well as world-ending power. Indeed, as the Cold War suggests, megalomanic feelings can be experienced by just about anyone who becomes involved with such weaponry and can play a part in attracting strategists as well as scientists to the weapons in the first place.

As a clinical phenomenon, megalomania is generally encountered in advanced paranoid schizophrenia. In that condition, the patient usually is alone with his delusions and hallucinations, his totalized self condemning him to radical isolation from the external world it replaces. In contrast, a guru like Asahara had disciples who interacted with his megalomanic self in ways that reinforced it, rendering it functional. The arrangement offered seductive rewards—mutual ecstasy and a shared sense of absolute truth—that could sustain it for long periods of time as disciples became more and more immersed in the guru's megalomania, both endorsing it and realizing their own megalomanic potential. The extreme cultic process, in other words, became a version of collective megalomania. The arrangement, however, was inherently unstable, subject to the breakout of suppressed antagonisms between guru and disciples and, more dangerously, apt to result in violent attacks on the external world by guru and disciples whenever they felt their bond with one another, or anything else in the arrangement, to be threatened.

Megalomania contributed greatly to Asahara's attempts to actualize his world-ending visions. The idea of vast destruction in the service of spiritual renewal became something more—and less—than a metaphor or mythic truth. The megalomanic self, in fact, insists upon the breakdown of such distinctions, claiming dominion over myth and metaphor no less than over actual events. The ultimate power of the weapons themselves, their promise of destroying humankind or even the planet, contributes greatly to the breakdown of those distinctions. In our time, the wildest fantasy of total annihilation holds the all too evident possibility of becoming an engine for the literal destruction of the world.

The Oxford English Dictionary (1989) defines megalomania as "insanity of self-exaltation." As characterized in the *Psychiatric Dictionary* (1960), the megalomanic person considers himself "possessed of greatness" and may "believe himself to be Christ, God, Napoleon" or "everybody and everything." Asahara epitomized this sense of multiform omnipotence in every way. That genius was extended to his physiology with the claim that he possessed nirvana-like brain waves and uniquely distinctive DNA. When Asahara spoke of himself as a catalyst for "chemical changes that we cannot imagine in the usual sense" but that would lead to "a new form of matter" he was offering further proof of his bodily genius.

The guru's most insistent megalomanic claim was to deity. In addition to declaring himself an avatar of Shiva, he professed to have achieved "the state of a Buddha who has attained mirror-like wisdom" and to be the "divine emperor" of Japan and of the world; the declared Christ, who will "disclose the meaning of Jesus' gospel"; the "last twentieth-century savior"; the "holiest holy man," one "beyond the Bible"; and the being who will inaugurate the Age of Aquarius and preside over a "new era of supreme truth." For disciples transfixed by guruism, he could indeed be all these things.

An external manifestation of the megalomanic self was Aum's organization into "ministries" and "agencies" suggestive of a huge governmental structure. Much of Aum's spiritual project dealt with preparing for the next life, the transfer of consciousness to a higher dimension—Asahara's "great *poa*." An indication of Asahara's megalomania was his manipulation of *poa* from a concept of ideal spiritual transformation to a euphemism for murder.

Asahara was never more megalomanic than in his recitation of his past lives. These included that of an absolutely loyal disciple (who killed at the order of his guru), a guru to many of his Aum followers ("Most of my close disciples were also my disciples in their former lives"), and the king of various upper realms of rebirth. He also claimed to have had previous existences in America, including one as Benjamin Franklin, a charter member of the first American Freemasons' lodge. Reflecting on past lives, he once commented, "It becomes very difficult to tell who is a friend and who is an enemy." And in a sermon he declared that there would eventually be a union of Aum Shinrikyō and the Freemasons in which the latter would come to revere the former: "This is all related to one of my former lives, so I can say that the two are certain to unite."

Asahara's most expansive past-life claim concerned the very origins of civilization. Visiting Egypt and observing its oldest pyramid, he was struck by the realization not only that he had seen it before but that "I designed it myself a long time ago." In his "current" life, Asahara was attracted to such world-destroying figures as Hitler, Stalin, and Mao, both identifying himself with the omnipotence of mass murderers and incorporating them into his megalomanic self.

It was essential for Asahara to be distinguished absolutely from all other human beings. He alone was completely free of "defilement," of any need for further spiritual quest, of desire itself. Since he was, of course, free of none of these, the claims can be understood as compensatory, as an extreme psychological reversal of his actual "defilement" (cruelty and murderousness), his radical spiritual insecurity (inner doubts about his exorbitant claims), and his insistent desires (for power over other human beings, sex, and forbidden food). The megalomanic claim to have no desire meant, in practice, the presence of unlimited self-aggrandizing desire.

Even after the sarin incident Asahara continued to convey to his disciples the message that his capture was to be avoided at any cost and that continuous terror

was to be employed to prevent it. A collective Aum megalomania was still opera-
tive in the bizarre assumption that terrorism (letter bombs, additional releases of
lethal chemicals, and assassinations) would so divert or intimidate the police that
the guru would be left alone.

His actual arrest was in fact delayed by the police until they could be sure that
his most prominent followers were in custody and could not attempt violent retali-
ation. Two months after the sarin attack, the police found Shōkō Asahara in a small
hidden cubicle in Aum headquarters dressed in his purple priestly robes, lying in
his urine, and surrounded by piles of Japanese currency totaling about ten million
yen, or a hundred thousand dollars. The guru's inability to leave the cubicle probably accounted for the urine, though it might also have reflected his psychological
deterioration. The money could have been placed there for the guru's use, should
he have decided to flee. Whatever the case, the symbolism of useless money and
humiliating urine could not have been more apt. A kind of de-guruizing process—
and the subversion of whatever functional megalomania remained—began when
the police gave him orders that he had to obey and ignored his insistence that "no
one is allowed to touch the guru's body." To the last, though, he invoked his con-
man self: told he was being arrested for murdering eleven people in the subway
attack, he replied, "Could a blind man like me possibly do such a thing?"

During his first months in prison he tried to sustain his guru self by holding to
a routine of meditation and fasting. He also sought to maintain control over his
disciples, though, given his isolation, he could do so only partially and temporarily. The one continuing disciple I interviewed, a slight woman in her twenties who
worked in an Aum bookstore, told me ten months after Asahara's imprisonment
that, while on the "phenomenal level" he was of course not with her, "on the astral
level we are in close touch with each other. I still feel his presence." When she and
other disciples were in the vicinity of the prison, she added, they could "feel his
energy, the wonderful vibrations that come out from him."

Divided Selves

Most striking to me was the extreme inner division that former disciples displayed—
one part of their minds angrily condemning Aum and its guru, another still feeling
profoundly connected to him and to the group. This existence of two relatively separate, even warring selves within the same psyche was a version of the doubling that
was part of cult life. There was now the self of the bitter survivor and opponent of
Asahara, Aum, and guruism in general and the self of the disciple still merged with
the guru and still experiencing, through memory, guru dispensed ecstasy. The Aum
self, retaining ties to Asahara in this life and others, was painfully at odds with the
post-Aum self struggling to confront the guru's violence and extricate itself from
him and cult life. The greatest difficulty the former members I interviewed faced was
leaving behind the perceptions of transcendent experience that the Aum self retained
(even as the post-Aum self was experiencing extreme loss, bewilderment, or a sense
of disintegration, of falling apart). Although the two selves, of course, were never

completely autonomous, it proved a daunting task for any former disciple to integrate them into what was, after all, a single psyche.

Thoughtful disciples could also criticize Asahara and Aum for their distortions of reality and for their psychological aberrations . . . to achieve critical perspective on Aum and spiritual resolution, many former disciples sought to embrace various forms of Buddhism.

When present Aum members defended Aum more directly, speaking of the guru's violent actions as "beyond the understanding of ordinary beings," part of a higher purpose, unknowable to others, they too were struggling with their confusion while suppressing their moral and psychological conflicts. But former members who . . . were intent upon separating themselves from Aum interpreted the guru's collapse in the courtroom as a form of ultimate judgment. Stunned by the guru's sudden fall from seemingly untouchable omniscience into mumbling incoherence, one of them found himself wondering "if he has a sense of shame." For them, the guru had become "a naked king"—that is, the emperor had no clothes.

Discussing Aum in Its Context: Sociopsychological, Historical, and Political Dimensions

The "Aum Aftershocks"

Japan was profoundly shaken and confused by the Aum debacle. Whatever else was said about the cult in an endless stream of articles, books, and media probes, Japanese could not avoid the realization that Aum had emerged from their society, that it in some way represented them. People spoke of "Aum shocks" and "Aum aftershocks"—as if the cult's activities had been the social equivalent of the Kobe earthquake—and sometimes of an "Aum syndrome" of general malaise and fear. Intellectuals expressed concern that social agitation over the cult might intensify Japanese nationalism or lead to the implementation of draconian social controls, as in the past. There was also a new suspiciousness of introspection, so that a person who raised ethical and spiritual questions of any kind might quickly be told "Don't be so *Aum!*"

We should not be surprised that Aum, so immersed in global conspiracy theories, provoked a wave of them as it collapsed. In one typical instance, it was claimed that the cult was part of a sustained program to "destabilize Japan" run by a British "Occult Bureau" working through "its agent, the Dalai Lama, who met with Aum leader Shōkō Asahara, in India." While such wild theories appeared mostly at the fringes of society or on obscure web pages, they were at times published in widely circulated magazines.

Historians have spoken of the "free security" two great oceans have provided the United States and of Americans' nuclear-age anxiety over losing their sense of that safety. Japan's "free security," only decades old, lay in its perception of itself as a well-ordered and therefore safe country. Aum destroyed that. A diffuse

Aum-related anxiety now became part of a larger constellation of fears about earthquakes, economic recession or depression, weakening family ties, and increasing domestic and social violence. Certainly, there is now a feeling in Japan of its deteriorating as a nation and a society while its leaders stand by helplessly, leaving ordinary people unprotected.

Psychohistorical Dislocation

Aum is in many ways a product of Japanese history and of a society that may have experienced in the last century and a half more wrenching historical and psychological upheaval than any other on earth. In Japan's extraordinarily rapid journey from a feudal to a modern (and then postmodern) culture, the two overwhelming events were the Meiji Restoration that began in 1868 and the annihilating defeat of World War II. Out of feudal society the Meiji-era leaders created the beginnings of a powerful, modern, emperor-centered state that expanded into a vast Asian empire, only to be crushed in war. By September 1945, Japan was in ruins, its people starving and rudderless.

When exposed to such extremes of social, political, and cultural transformation and collapse in such a short period of time, people experience what I call psychohistorical dislocation, a breakdown of the social and institutional arrangements that ordinarily anchor human lives. What are impaired are the symbol systems having to do with family, religion, social and political authority, sexuality, birth and death, and the overall ordering of the life cycle. Symbols and rituals by no means disappear but, because less effectively internalized, come to feel less natural and more coercive. People experience a profound gap between what they feel themselves to be and what a society or a culture expects them to be.

One Japanese observer has referred to the Meiji Restoration period, with its stunning array of Western-modeled reforms in every area of society, as a time of "thunderboltism." As the historian Carol Gluck (1985) points out, the elaborate construction of emperor worship—an ideology melding religion, myth, nationalism, and political need—was, to a significant degree, an effort to contain that thunderboltism, to manage the intense conflicts and confusions accompanying what many experienced as the "disturbing demands of social change." But the new emperor-centered system turned out to have its own thunderboltism. Created artificially but attributed to an ancient past, it had a tenuous claim on national unity that all too often required large-scale social suppression and escalating levels of violence abroad. Psychohistorical dislocation, a "surfeit of change," can give rise to proteanism, a pattern characterized by psychological experiment, individual and collective shape-shifting, and a struggle to retain a sense of continuity in the midst of that change. But such dislocation can also lead people into forms of "restorationism," or what we now call fundamentalism. The Japanese political genius of the Meiji era was to combine the proteanism of a social revolution with a fundamentalist-like plunge into a sacred imperial restoration.

There was, however, a psychological price to be paid: Japan's formidable modern accomplishments have coexisted with an unusual degree of psychological turmoil. In the grip of such turmoil, some people may seek extreme remedies.

The novelist Kenzaburō Ōe (1995), in his 1994 Nobel Prize acceptance speech, described Japan as "split between two opposite poles of ambiguity." He pointed to a long-standing psychological division between Western-inspired modernization and traditional cultural influences, emphasizing as well the painful sense of ambiguous identity that exists on both sides of this inner dividing line. "The modernization of Japan," he explained, "was oriented toward learning from and imitating the West, yet the country is situated in Asia and has firmly retained its traditional culture. The ambiguous orientation of Japan drove the country into the position of an invader in Asia, and resulted in its isolation from other Asian countries not only politically but also socially and culturally. The Second World War came right out of the middle of the process of modernization, a war that was brought about by the very aberration of that process itself." Ōe (1995) was telling us that such ambiguity can be lethal and that it pervades both national behavior and the individual Japanese psyche as "a kind of chronic disease that has been prevalent throughout the modern age," one that he himself as a writer experiences as "a deep-felt scar." In his use of the term *ambiguity*, he evoked Japan's particularly troubled version of psychohistorical dislocation and suggested that it could lead either to violent behavior or toward the country's becoming "invisible," without any dear ethical presence among other peoples. Such ethical "invisibility" within Japanese society was undoubtedly a factor in the Aum phenomenon.

Japanese Roots

Asahara's spiritual—and violent—urges were nonetheless largely shaped within his own society and culture. The eminent sociologist of religion Susumu Shimazono (1997) calls Aum the "potential nightmare" of Japanese religious experience, and, however unpalatable the idea, Aum was indeed its creature.

The question of Japanese religiosity is a confusing one to outsiders, and often to the Japanese themselves. They are frequently described as a highly secular people, focused on the pragmatic details of everyday life, and there is much truth in this description. But it is no less true that they have deep-seated spiritual inclinations with respect to the infinitely powerful forces of nature and to the question of individual fate, or karma. Perhaps the confusion lies in failing to see that Japanese can be secular *and* religious, that they can bring to religious rituals highly pragmatic purposes (visiting a Shinto shrine, for instance, to ask for success in a business venture), and to everyday life a rather casual religiosity (keeping a small Buddhist family altar in the home in order to stay connected with dead parents). There is a saying to the effect that Japanese are born as Shintoists, marry as Christians, die as Buddhists—and in between believe in new religions. In fact, their cultural tendency toward a multifaceted religious life fits quite well with the contemporary development of the many-sided, protean self.

Religious pluralism began early in Japan: Shinto and Buddhism have coexisted there for almost two thousand years with much overlapping of religious practice—including Shinto-style shrines in Buddhist temples and Buddhist-style altars in Shinto shrines. Generally speaking, Buddhism has been concerned with family and ancestors, Shinto with village and community.

For its guru-centered example, Aum had in some sense to look no further than state-manipulated Shinto. Until the Meiji Restoration an amorphous, village-based, nature-oriented religion, Shinto was consciously and somewhat artificially converted into a systematic state religion by the new regime. Drawing on Western imperial models, Meiji leaders rendered the emperor divine and placed him at the center of that state religion. The concept of the emperor as a god, as a descendent of the ancestor goddess Amaterasu, had long existed but mostly in connection with ritual acts surrounding an essentially marginal figure. Now this idea of divinity was strongly emphasized and embedded in an elaborate national ideology. The emperor became both symbol and actor in a mystical *kokutai*, or national polity, providing the Japanese with a sense of national identity in a sacralized state. Distinctions between Shinto and Buddhism were newly insisted upon. Buddhism was controlled or suppressed (temples and texts were destroyed and celibate priests pressured to marry in order to weaken the Buddhist tradition) until it, too, allied itself with the new emperor cult. Even local Shinto shrines were destroyed or closed: to maintain close control over its new emperor-centered state religion, the regime wanted only a single shrine in each village.

The Shadow of World War II

However striking these various antecedents and influences, none is as powerful in accounting for Aum as Japan's annihilation in World War II and its aftermath. The more I studied Aum, in fact, the more I became convinced that it could be understood only in relation to the impact of that war on Japan.

What could not be faced then or since, however, was the criminal nature of what the soldiers and civilian officials of that sacralized, emperor-worshiping state did in East and Southeast Asia. There were the policies that we might now call "ethnic cleansing"—the creating of "people-free zones" in China; there was the Nanking massacre in which hundreds of thousands of Chinese civilians were murdered in gruesome fashion and tens of thousands of women raped. There was the enslaving of three million people, mostly Chinese and Korean, for labor projects. In addition to the large-scale efforts to carry out biological warfare, there were the grotesque experiments on Asian and Western prisoners, using typhus, tetanus, anthrax, smallpox, and salmonella materials. There was the seizure of 100,000 to 200,000 "comfort women," mostly from Korea but also from other parts of Asia, forced to serve as prostitutes for the military and civilian personnel of Japan's new imperium. There was the systematic bombing of civilians in China's cities from 1931 on, a forerunner of the massive Allied "strategic bombing" campaign against German and Japanese cities.

During the early occupation years, these atrocities were exposed in war-crimes trials. Many Japanese were shocked, but the trials had only limited impact. For one thing, the prosecution of accused war criminals proceeded erratically, and some of them, released from custody, were quickly rehabilitated. For another, there was a high-level American decision against prosecuting the emperor in whose name the crimes had been committed. Most Japanese, moreover, were preoccupied with their own survival. Both authorities and ordinary people, sometimes with American encouragement, colluded in creating what the historian Gavin McCormack (1996) calls a "milieu of willful forgetting." But that does not mean that these mass atrocities did not permeate the Japanese psychological experience. They did so in ways that were powerful, lasting, and yet seldom publicly acknowledged. . . . But the subject was largely suppressed, and when it did begin to reappear in popular culture it often took the form of *manga* renditions of exciting battles, Japanese heroism, and ultimate Japanese victory in the war.

Yet the lack of public discussion of the subject after the American occupation ended neither erased it from consciousness nor eliminated the need of members of the wartime generation to find a way to address the acts they had committed and the war they had prosecuted for their emperor. In order to deal with that war and undergo a process of mourning, thereby acquiring a measure of survivor meaning from a terrible defeat, many assumed a stance of simple victimization. They emphasized not the suffering of other Asians at Japanese hands but Japanese suffering in the atomic bombings of Hiroshima and Nagasaki and the strategic bombing of Japanese cities, as well as at the hands of the Russian armies during the war's last days. That suffering was real, but by embracing a victim role they avoided a sense of responsibility or of guilt, an avoidance that also became part of the structure of the postwar self. "Victim consciousness" influenced, and was reinforced by, representations of wartime history that further encouraged numbing and forgetting.

In Japan, there was far less confrontation with wartime evil than in Germany. Important here was the American decision to grant immunity to the emperor, the result of which, as McCormack (1996) points out, was a "devolution of responsibility downward onto the lower ranks . . . which led, in due course, to denial of responsibility altogether." To which I would add that the imperial system lent itself to such denial because the only responsibility of every Japanese was to serve the emperor, who, as a deity, could not be held to so profane a concept as responsibility, even when he participated in policies associated with atrocities. Instead, under the protection of Japan's occupiers, the wartime deity was rendered a postwar symbol of peace and democracy. While there has been much critical acknowledgment in Japan of the extremity of wartime emperor worship and of the love felt for his symbolic person (in some ways he was the psychological equivalent of the Führer), the process of individual psychological separation from him was for many extremely difficult until his death in 1989. Since the emperor system provided, as McCormack (1996) observes, "the kernel of Japanese identity in the modern era," confronting the emperor's culpability in the war threatened the sense of individual psychological integration of many Japanese.

As a result, there was an even greater tendency than in Germany to gloss over wartime crimes and excesses. By the mid-1950s, initial economic successes were already encouraging people to look forward toward a brighter future, not back at the painful horrors of a lost war. Conservative politicians, some of whom were themselves war criminals, did much to prevent serious discussion of the war, often distorting or falsifying wartime events. All this heightened cultural tendencies to avoid confrontations with the past, to compartmentalize psychological experience, and to adapt to whatever group arrangements presented themselves. But such cultural predilections are far from absolute and such a situation far from purely Japanese. The United States, for instance, has faced a similar dilemma in examining its conduct of its own lost war in Vietnam. Without an emperor to restrain them, at least a minority of Vietnam veterans, if not the public at large, have insisted on confronting unpleasant truths about the atrocities American troops committed, truths that have became necessary to their own integration of suffering and loss, while importantly influencing the country's overall historical understanding of that war.

No nation ever fully confronts its own behavior, especially when that behavior is widely perceived as destructive or evil. But in Japan the failure of any such confrontation to occur—the degree of unfinished psychological business in connection with World War II—has been unusually stark. Avoidance and denial have not only angered former victims throughout Asia but prevented significant transmission of disturbing wartime truths across the generations.

New New Religions

In the wake of the war, many Japanese found their spiritual state to be as much in rubble as their cities. With the emperor's radio speech of surrender on August 14, 1945 (shocking not only in its message but also in permitting the divine voice to be heard by ordinary ears), and an American-inspired Imperial Rescript of January 1, 1946, which officially denied his divinity, the ideology of state Shinto collapsed. In the confusion of occupied Japan, there was what was called a "rush hour of the gods," as literally thousands of new religions emerged. That explosion of spirituality continued throughout the postwar era, spurred by the country's radical urbanization, which caused large numbers of its citizens to lose contact with their local gods and communities. New religions could respond to such dislocations by offering improvised sets of borrowings, flexible ways of worshiping gods from a distance, and active grassroots leadership and involvement. Their founders were generally parental and nurturing and could project a certain comforting androgyny as well, as when a female founder claimed to have merged with a male god.

Aum members were the cultural inheritors of every form of spiritual confusion, including the dislocations caused by Western influences, the dramatic, almost world-ending collapse of imperial megalomania, and the painful contradictions and corruptions of a deeply flawed postwar democracy and a decade-long economic boom. No wonder that young people could be attracted to a syncretic religion that seemed to combine ancient truths with the latest spiritual trends in Japan, the United States, and elsewhere. New religions like Aum, moreover, had a substantial prewar Japanese tradition to build on.

In combining New Age currents and post-Hiroshima apocalypticism with a wide variety of Japanese and world religious traditions, Asahara shaped a cult that was both protean and totalistic. He brought to bear on every aspect of the cult's function two seemingly contradictory qualities: the openness of a rash innovator in a tradition-damaged world and the closed mentality of a dictatorial fundamentalist. Aum also brought both proteanism and totalism to bear on a very Japanese preoccupation with technicism and technology and with profit-centered corporate power. Aum's claim to technical and scientific precision enabled it to anchor fantastic other-worldly visions in highly active this-worldly concerns. Even its exalted spiritual mission was described as providing "good data" for remaking human beings, computerese that echoed the intense technical and technological focus of much of Japanese society.

Young Rebels

It was from young adults in rebellion against their society that Aum took much of its energy. These are the people who in any society bring a special passion to articulating, and acting upon, the kinds of dislocation I have been discussing. I have been talking to young Japanese for more than four decades, and in our many dialogues they have conveyed their complex struggles with extraordinarily disparate belief systems pertaining to family, society, religion, and career. Often they have exhibited rapid shifts in convictions, attitudes, and ideals. Whatever their ambivalences and confusions, though, I have invariably been impressed with the way many of them integrate such disparate elements, generally by making use of the various groups so important in Japanese life.

At the same time I have encountered among them a strong potential for totalism, for all-or-nothing belief systems and moral precepts that can be expressed through absolutized forms of group behavior. A version of this was exemplified by Marxist student leaders. One of them told me, for example, that "to change the present society we must somehow destroy its foundation. This is our task now, and the society which will be created in the future—well, I do not think that we ourselves will be able to see it in its magnificence." There is more than a suggestion here of Aum's brand of mysticism—especially when one learns that the same activist's dreams and associations revealed a deep nostalgia for an idealized past as well as a yearning for a visionary, blissful future. Also striking were similar yearnings among the far smaller numbers of students who expressed an urge to return to some form of emperor-centered totalism. One such student spoke to me in 1961 of ancient prophecies of an Armageddon-like "time of purification (before) a birth pain, which is the coming of the Third World War," after which the whole world would exist as one family headed by the emperor.

In the late 1970s and the early 1980s, Japanese youth became politically far more quiescent, but inner rebelliousness and dissatisfaction with society did not disappear. Rather they were rerouted to such outlets as new religions, cultic groups, personal expressions of taste in music and literature, or forms of hostile demeanor and confrontational styles. This generation—sometimes called the Aum generation—is usually seen as having been preceded by an immediate post-war generation that embraced democracy and worked extremely hard to rebuild Japan, a radically rebellious generation of the sixties, characterized by idealism and commitment (if later giving way to violence), and a "withdrawn generation" that passively accepted Japan's stunning new affluence. The Aum generation gave indications of a deep uneasiness with Japan's materialism (or "economism"), a hunger for meaning, and disillusionment with American legacies: a democracy seen as corrupt and a "peace constitution" that had not prevented Japan from building a vast military "defense" force. More than that, many young Japanese shared in a broadly cultural, in fact worldwide, disillusionment with modernity—with the ostensible benefits of science, technology, and rational thought—an attitude inseparable from ambivalence toward Western cultural influences. While any statement about a generation must overgeneralize, many in the Aum generation seemed to experience a malaise that covered over potentially explosive impulses, a listlessness, and a longing for the kind of energy promised and largely delivered by Shōkō Asahara and Aum.

The intensity of Japanese group formation has been remarked on by most observers, myself included. In earlier work with young people, I stressed the psychological power of groups, which attracted them but also triggered resentments and an urge for greater individual autonomy. I often found that they attempted to resolve such conflict by seeking realization of the self via the group. But when it became too severe, it tended to contribute to hermetic group formation, that is, to groups' sealing themselves off from much of the outside world in order to further their own principles and interests. Young people's efforts to break out of groups perceived as suffocating (family, school, company), moreover sometimes led to their joining new groups more closed and totalistic than those they had left. Group totalism, as in the example of Aum, can radically impair perceptions of realities within as well as outside the group and help spur both hostility toward outside forces and feelings of persecution by them. Resentments toward one's own group, on the other hand, must be suppressed, blamed either on oneself or on the outside world. For what one most fears is expulsion or ostracism, a threat that can be equated psychologically with death.

Death-centered macho—the calling forth when confronting death of extreme energies that in themselves can be bound up with killing—has a long history in Japan. The literature of Bushidō (Lifton, 1979), the traditional code of the warrior (influenced originally by Buddhism), is essentially a meditation on death: "The essence of Bushidō lies in the act of dying." "Every morning make up thy mind to die. Every evening freshen thy mind in the thought of death." The "great man" must be willing to "sacrifice body for the sake of spirit . . . [so that] his spirit will be alive eternally even if his body perishes." Dying, then, is equated with the experience of transcendence and with the achievement of immortality. A noble failure in battle can be even more immortalizing than success, so long as one achieves a heroic death. The model of the samurai contemplating and achieving his heroic death was extended to Japanese soldiers in World War II and especially to kamikaze pilots late in the war. Many of the latter (but not all, as some were fearful and felt coerced) were said to undergo a temporary "rebirth" prior to their deaths, becoming calm, proud, and exemplary in behavior as if having already become (in the language of the time) "gods without earthly desires."

Major military decisions not infrequently hinge on death-centered macho. Just before ordering the attack on Pearl Harbor and initiating war with the United States, a country the Japanese had no possibility of defeating, Admiral Hideki Tōjō, the prime minister, observed to one of his leading advisers that there are times when a man must close his eyes and jump from the veranda of Kiyomizu-dera, a famous temple outside of Kyoto, into the ravine below. "Jumping off Kiyomizu" is, in fact, an old saying that suggests taking a desperate plunge, embarking on an overwhelming task even if there is little prospect of success, because it is the right or necessary or "sincere" thing to do (Butow, 1961). As in the case of the samurai seeking his death, there could have been a suicidal dimension in Tōjō's use of the phrase: the idea, in some part of his mind, that he was leading Japan to glorious destruction.

Aum's destructive expression of group totalism and death-centered macho may have lacked the cultural structuring and conscious ideological awareness that characterize samurai and kamikaze actions, but the Kiyomizu that Asahara jumped from was a high mountain and below it was not a ravine but an abyss, for he was initiating a war not against a stronger nation but against all humankind.

Contemporary Japanese commentators are quite right, then, in recognizing their own selves in Aum. But that recognition only tells us that apocalyptic violence must take the form of the particular culture in which it occurs. Destructive expressions of the Japanese apocalyptic turn out to have much in common with versions of our own. Aum is a Japanese phenomenon but a more general one as well. To begin to explain its emergence we must look at various psychological and historical currents in contemporary and modern Japan, which are replete with violence, national guruism, and apocalyptic temptation. But we are, of course, only dealing with a Japanese expression of our universal psychological repertoire, with feelings now being experienced everywhere, perhaps most strongly in the United States. We all have to face Aum's significance for the human future and to ponder.

Conclusions-Characteristics of a World-Destroying Cult

The first characteristic of Aum was *totalized guruism*, which became *paranoid guruism* and *megalomanic guruism*. Instead of awakening the potential of his disciples, Shōkō Asahara himself became his cult's only source of "energy" or infinite life-power and its only source of the new self that each Aum disciple was expected to acquire (as epitomized by the religious name every disciple took as a renunciant). For disciples there was no deity beyond the guru, no ethical code beyond his demands and imposed ordeals, or mahâmudrâs. When the guru invoked a higher deity it was only in order to incorporate the god's omnipotence into his own. Guru and disciples were both energized and entrapped by their claim to ultimate existential truth and virtue.

This desymbolization became bound up with a second Aum characteristic: *a vision of an apocalyptic event or series of events that would destroy the world in the service of renewal.* All great religions contain variations of that vision, ordinarily causing followers to struggle largely with symbolic meanings.

A third Aum characteristic was its *ideology of killing to heal, of altruistic murder and altruistic world destruction.* Such a stance readily evoked an "attack guruism" and an "action prophecy" directed toward forcing the end. The concept of *poa,* as manipulated by Asahara, epitomized this stance, encouraging as it did the killing of a spiritually inferior person by a spiritually superior one for the sake of improving the prospects of immortality for both. Similar ideologies (or theologies) have been embraced by others. Some Christians held much the same conviction with respect to the killing of Jews at the time of the Inquisition or during the Middle Ages. The Thugs of India, a Hindu sect that killed and robbed in a ritual fashion from the thirteenth to the nineteenth century, viewed their victims as sacrifices to the goddess Kali, who was associated with disease, death, and destruction; the victims' reward was entrance to paradise. In Aum, however, the principle of killing to heal went much further. It extended into a vision of altruistic omnicide.

Altruistic mass murder depended, in turn, on a fourth characteristic: *the relentless impulse toward world-rejecting purification.* Here Aum drew upon its version of karma as ubiquitous defilement. Asahara was once quoted as saying that "the essence of the devil is matter," suggesting that what Aum had to "purify" was physical existence itself. Such an unrealizable purification goal kept Aum disciples on a spiritual treadmill in the service of the guru and of a process that was envisioned as transhistorical. Asahara sought, or claimed to seek, a level of eternal perfection that defied the petty external standards of any particular era; yet he didn't hesitate to apply his standards of purification to the most immediate social and political behavior. For Asahara, the people of this world were so hopelessly defiled that their inevitable fate was the lowest of reincarnations, the closest to Buddhist hell and therefore dominated by death and suffering.

A fifth characteristic of Aum was *the lure of ultimate weapons.* If Asahara's consciousness of nuclear weapons was initially related to Hiroshima and Nagasaki, ultimate weapons in general became bound up with his action prophecy in pressing toward Armageddon. For Asahara it was an easy and natural path from nuclearism to dreams of mass killing via chemical and biological devices. Crucial to his pursuit of mass murder was the fact that he was a "floating guru," unencumbered by a restraining god, by a restraining code of traditional values, or even, as a state might be, by the interests of an entrenched bureaucracy. As they did for the United States and the Soviet Union during the Cold War, weapons of mass death increasingly took their place at the center of Aum's structure and function. Aum was the first nongovernmental religious or political cult to achieve this kind of weapons involvement, but it is unlikely to be the last. For such weapons have come to affect human consciousness everywhere and are bound to remain a powerful lure to totalistically inclined, paranoid, and megalomanic gurus.

Essential to success in Aum's killing project was a sixth characteristic: *a shared state of aggressive numbing*. That mental state began with a disciple's merger with the guru, with the ideal of becoming his clone and of thinking and feeling as he did. . . . Such dedication was a form of numbing, which one enhanced by an absolute focus on the violent attack immediately at hand, on one's efficacy in carrying it out; a focus that could sweep away past scruples as well as any empathy for potential victims. The principle of viewing the guru's most outrageous demands as an appropriate form of personal ordeal or "test" reinforced the numbing process and resulted in a mental state similar to that cultivated among Japanese soldiers during World War II. . . . Asahara and his disciples moved in and out of a state of total ideological conviction: from immersion in an ideological vision of *poa*, to cynical killing of ostensible enemies with a rationalizing invocation of *poa*, to various in-between states in which both stances were present.

A seventh characteristic of Aum was its *extreme technocratic manipulation*, coupled with its *claim* to *absolute scientific truth*. Aum held to a computer theory of the mind: the principles of replacing "bad data" from the culture with "good data" from the guru. The cult's entire effort at spiritual self-transformation was, in fact, reduced to systematic techniques, whether in the form of breathing exercises, drug-centered initiations, or endless repetitions of the guru's words or his assigned mantras. Practitioners were given specific technical functions to perform—running businesses, doing translations, making publishing arrangements, creating artwork, composing or playing music, working in Aum "factories," preparing chemical or biological weapons, drawing up legal contracts—always as cogs in a larger machine of "salvation."

Aum also demonstrated the bizarre consequences of the fanatical conversion of scientists to totalistic guruism, of what might be called megalomanic science. Despite its scientific and technological bungling, one cannot ignore the extent of Aum's success with its weaponry or the deadly consequences of turning scientific energies to the service of religious fanaticism. In merging the two, Aum made a grotesque pioneering foray into the most dangerous of all contemporary imaginative combinations.

I carry away from my work with Aum Shinrikyō a stronger conviction that, even as we insist upon holding people responsible for their actions, we desperately need to explore ways in which to alter the psychological and historical conditions so conducive to the kinds of destructiveness and evil in which Aum engaged.

References

Butow, R. J. C. (1961). *Tojo and the coming of the war* (p. 267). Princeton: Princeton University Press.

Gluck, C. (1985). *Japan's modern myths: Ideology in the late Meiji* (pp. 17–41). Princeton: Princeton University Press.

Lifton, R. J. (1979). *The broken connection: on death and the continuity of life* (p. 102) Washington DC: American Psychiatric Press.

McCormack, G. (1996). *The emptiness of Japanese affluence* (pp. 229–234). Armonk, NY: M.E.Sharpe.

Ōe, K. (1995). *Japan, the ambiguous, and myself* (pp. 105–128). Tokyo: Kodansha International.

Psychiatric Dictionary. (1960). (pp. 448–449). New York: Oxford University Press.

Reader, I. (1996). *A poisonous cocktail? Aum Shinrikyō's path to violence* (p. 14). Copenhagen: Nordic Institute of Asian Studies.

Shimazono, S. (1997). *Gendai Shukyo no Kanosei: Oumu Shinrikyō to boryoku*. Tokyo: Iwanami Shoten. **SHI**

Simpson, J., & Weiner, E. (Eds.). (1989). *Oxford English Dictionary* (2nd ed.). Wotton: Clarendon Press.

4
Reversing Cultures: The Wounded Teaching the Healers

John P. Wilson

Introduction

In terms of mental health care, cultures provide many alternative pathways to healing and integration of extreme stress experiences which can be provided by shamans, medicine men and women, traditional healers, culture-specific rituals, conventional medical practices and community-based practices that offer forms of social and emotional support for the person suffering the adverse, maladaptive aspects of a trauma (Moodley & West, 2005). But how does culture influence an individual's reaction to trauma? How do they make sense of their experiences in situations of extreme stress? This chapter will describe "reverse learning," how a Western PTSD specialist was taught culture-specific forms of ritualistic healing by Native Americans.

To illustrate how culture shapes belief systems and influences the perception of traumatic events and their subsequent processing and integration into cognitive structures of meaning and attribution, let us consider the following case example.

Dancing with Wolves

In 1985 I attended an intertribal "pow wow" on the Lakota Sioux Indian reservation in South Dakota (Sisseton-Whapeton). A pow wow is a ceremonial gathering during which there is traditional dancing, arts and crafts, exchanges of gifts (i.e., the pot latch), and various types of rituals. The pow wow was a four-day event for Vietnam War veterans and their families. The event contained Native American ceremonies and rituals to honor the veterans for their military service and sacrifices. These ceremonies included sweat lodge purification (Lakota Warrior "sweat" for healing), the Red Feather induction ceremony, traditional communal singing and dancing, pot latch sharing of gifts and ceremonial fires with "talking circles" and communal dinner with the eating of traditional native American foods.

During this pow wow, I had the opportunity to meet Lakota Sioux Vietnam combat veterans. Among them was a veteran who I will refer to as Tommy Roundtree (not his real name). Tommy was a two-tour combat veteran who had been highly decorated for his valor and courage in combat with the 101st Airborne Brigade between 1967–1969. Tommy grew up on the Rosebud reservation of the Sioux Nation in South Dakota. He was an athletic, tall, handsome man with black hair and ruddy dark skin. In many respects, he had a "Hollywood" character that resembled the famous actor, Erroll Flynn.

When I met Tommy, he was dressed in traditional tribal clothing and had his face painted in traditional Lakota ways for warriors. Visibly noticeable were the scars on his chest and back from when he had participated in Sun Dance ceremonies in which the participants were skewered with straps to a pole located in the center of a pow wow arena. The pow wow arena is similar to a football stadium in Europe or America. The straps are skewered into pectoral and upper back muscles by small bones or sticks. At the climax of the Sun Dance ceremony, which involves dancing and blowing through a small bone, the celebrant, at the critical time, leans back and releases himself from the straps which link him to the pole. The skewers tear the skin and cause bleeding. The Sun Dance ceremony is a physically arduous process and requires stamina, mental concentration and preparation, including a Sweat Lodge purification event prior to the actual Sun Dance itself. In traditional ways, it is thought that the ritual aids in the development of spiritual strength. When I observed Tommy's scars, he immediately told me that he had done three Sun Dances during his life, two prior to deployment to Vietnam. I told him that I had read about the ceremony and others that were part of Lakota culture. It was at this point that he said, "You know, John, I would like to talk with you about my Vietnam War experiences, but I am afraid that you will think I am crazy or psychotic if I tell you how I understand what happened to me there and since coming home from the war." I responded that I have great respect for traditional Native American culture, especially Lakotan, and would like to hear his story. He smiled nervously at me as I looked at him straight in the eyes and said, "Well, okay, let's talk."

We found a quiet spot in the pow wow grounds and began to talk. In the background, the pulsating beat of the tom tom drums could be heard along with the singing of traditional songs. Tommy explained that prior to his deployment to Vietnam, the tribal elders prepared him in various ways for going to war. He was taught his "death song" to sing if fatally wounded. He was instructed as to how to use his Native American cosmology and natural connection to the earth and its creatures to help him stay alert and knowledgeable about danger and threats. Tommy said, "In Vietnam, I would ask the insects to be my eyes while I slept to look for the enemy; I asked the trees to signal me if the enemy is creeping towards me." He continued by saying that during active combat with his M-16 automatic rifle, he would sometimes see a blue protective shield surrounding him that deflected enemy bullets away. Tommy said that at other times during combat he could hear his grandmother speaking to him, saying not to worry and that he was going to live and be free from injuries or death. He added that his grandmothers' voice told him that if he did get shot, to sing his "death song" so that ancestral spirits would be with him to join him and provide care and assistance to the other world (Heaven).

Tommy asked me if I thought he was psychotic or delusional. I replied that I did not believe that he was "crazy" or psychotic. I felt that he was testing me and being defensive. Later, we would talk and he would detail how he survived Vietnam and his post-war coping with traumatic memories. However, I asked him how he dealt with his war trauma after coming home from Vietnam. Tommy said, "John, I will show you our way of healing" and arranged for me to participate in a Lakota Sweat Lodge with a sacred pipe carrier of the Sioux Nation. He also arranged for me to observe and participate in several other rituals and ceremonies for healing and psychological well being. Afterwards, he explained to me that his perspective of the Vietnam War was diffeΔrent than that of the white Anglo-American culture, that he volunteered for military service to honor agreements his ancestral grandfathers made about fighting for their "land and way of life." He continued by saying that by keeping to the traditional ways, abstaining from alcohol, and working to help others who had adverse residual traumatic war injuries, he could live with harmony and balance in life in all his affairs. This he explained, was part of the Lakota way, the great circle of life.

The Sweat Lodge Ceremony

After Tommy and I talked, he and some of the other pow wow organizers invited me to a Sweat Lodge to be held late in the afternoon. I had no idea or understanding at that time what a Sweat Lodge was as a ritual. The organizers, all Vietnam War veterans, simply said to me, "don't eat or drink very much today and come back here around five o'clock." I returned later and we drove to the countryside on the Sioux Reservation. We got out of the car and walked down a hilly slope to a place where the Sweat Lodge was located. I was surprised to see a dome-shaped tent-like structure covered with canvas. In front of the lodge was a fire with a large number of rocks being heated by firewood. There were other men there, about 12 combat veterans, Native Americans, who had come to participate in the pow wow. They stood by the "ceremonial" fire and talked quietly. Then one of the men said, "Hey, here comes 'Crazy Buffalo'," the medicine man who would lead the Lakota Warrior Sweat Lodge ceremony. I looked up and saw a short, grey-haired man come down the hill carrying with him a tote bag. When he approached us he said, "Get ready." The men began undressing (naked) to prepare to enter the lodge. At the same time, Crazy Buffalo took sacred objects out of his bag – a wing of an eagle, the sacred pipe of the Sioux Nation and other objects. He created an alter in front of the dome-shaped tent on which to place the sacred pipe, which he would smoke after the ceremony was concluded. I felt scared and curious at the same time as this was a strange cultural event for a Caucasian, middleclass male university professor.

The medicine man, Crazy Buffalo, purified the lodge both inside and out with smoke that came from a small bowl-like object that he held in his hand. The bowl contained "sweet grass" and is a traditional way of symbolically preparing the lodge for the sacred ceremony. Once the lodge was prepared, Crazy Buffalo asked us to enter through the small opening ("door") to the interior of the lodge. One by one we crawled into the pitch black interior and once everyone was seated in a circle, the ceremony began.

I had no idea what was about to take place and felt my heart pounding in my chest. It was now early evening and the sun was growing lower in the sky against the rolling plains of South Dakota. It was a beautiful evening in May. Crazy Buffalo spoke eloquently and with focused words of information and knowledge. I remember him saying, "This lodge is our (Lakota) way of healing. Good things can happen in here if we put our minds together." He said, "Physical and mental pains can be cured if we put our minds together. We all have pain in life; pain is a part of living. You can let go of your pain in here. We all suffer in this life. We are here (sitting) on our mother earth on our (Lakota) land." He then sang a song in Lakotan, which I found soothing to my apprehensive mental state. I felt nervous as I was the only person who was not of native blood. Most of the men were pure-blooded Native Americans who resembled the true native actors in Kevin Costner's movie, *Dances with Wolves*.

The ceremony continued as Crazy Buffalo asked for the heated rocks to be brought into the lodge. The "fire keeper" used antlers and brought in the red-hot rocks, which were then placed into a small pit located in the middle of the lodge. Finally, a bucket of water containing tree branches (pine boughs) was handed to the medicine man. Crazy Buffalo closed the flap covering the entrance to the lodge. It was now totally dark. Crazy Buffalo, one of the few sacred pipe carriers of the Sioux Nation, then splashed water onto the rocks four times to formally begin the ceremony. He sang as he splashed the red-hot rocks with water. Steam poured forth from the rocks. It was incredibly hot – hotter than any "sauna" or "steam bath" I had experienced during my life. My heart was pounding very fast and I felt fearful. The hairs in my nose burned. I started sweating profusely. I wanted to leave the lodge and felt tense all throughout my body. I carefully felt the edge of the "tent" to see if I could find a way to escape as I found it hard to breathe. The veteran seated next to me (cross-legged) passed out and fell onto me unconscious. He let out a moan. At that point, Crazy Buffalo said, "Death is a part of life. If it is your time to die, you will die. If it is not your time to die, you must will to live." I propped up the veteran and thought, "You must will to live," and wondered if he would die that night. He later regained consciousness and confessed during the ritual that he had an addiction to drugs. However, as the first of four rounds of the ritual proceeded, I continued to have fears and anxiety, painful muscle tension, and wondered if I would survive the experience. I remember thinking, "You have to go way inside and find the strength to get through this steam and high heat." My hair was now totally soaked with sweat and I felt pain all over my body. It was at this point, in the total darkness, that Crazy Buffalo said, "If you hold onto your pain and fight it, you will have more pain. You must learn to let go." His voice was calm and soothing, but at that point, I just wanted relief, a drink of water and fresh air to breathe. To make matters worse, the first veteran was about to begin the ritual in which each person speaks of their pain and suffering for as long as necessary. Since I knew nothing of the ritual or its 'rules' and procedures, I felt uncertain as to what would happen in this traditional purification and healing ritual. But, I clearly recall that the first combat veteran said, "Ah, Grandmother and Grandfather, Vietnam was so hard." He went on to speak of being wounded in battle several times and how he suffers to this day from bad memories and dreams. As I sat and listened, it seemed like he had spoken for one hour, and I knew that were 11 others to follow. Once again, I wondered if I was going to survive the experience and felt panic and fear. Finally, the first veteran, in the traditional way, concluded his disclosures about his Vietnam combat experience by saying, "All my relations," which was the cue for the next person to speak.

The heat was overwhelming and seemed to penetrate my body. I began to notice that the more that I would concentrate on the words of others, to focus on their war-related pain and suffering, the less pain I had. In this sense, it was one of many lessons I would learn about myself, others, and living life with compassion. Eventually, the first round of the Sweat Lodge came to an end. Because I had no personal knowledge of the ritual, I thought the ceremony had concluded. I felt relief when Crazy Buffalo called out to the "fire keeper" to open the entrance to the lodge. As the flap was opened, cool air rushed in and I felt good that I had "made it" through the ritual. Little did I know there were three more rounds to follow. The "fire keeper" replenished the bucket of water and handed it to Crazy Buffalo. I desperately wanted a drink of water and hoped that the bucket would be passed around for all of us to rehydrate our bodies. But, that was not to be. Crazy Buffalo then said, "Every time I open the door to this lodge, you will see more of what is out there (pointing to the hills of the plains and setting sun) and more of what is in here (spiritual space)." I was struck profoundly by those words, as this wise medicine man had just metaphorically juxtaposed the concept of knowing external reality clearly and balancing it with spiritual groundedness. He then said to the "fire-keeper," "Twenty-four more stones," signaling the start of the second round. I was in disbelief that we would repeat that which we had just endured. The Lakota warriors entered a new phase and once again I wondered if I would survive what was to come.

As the second round began, Crazy Buffalo spoke, "You may see visions in here. You may hear the elders speak to you. It is ok if these things happen. You may hear from dead Grandmothers and Grandfathers. This is our way. Don't be afraid." I wondered what he meant by visions, hearing ancestral voices and those of the elders. In this setting it felt perfectly natural and little did I know that before the fourth and final round of the lodge was concluded, that I would have "visions" of two different types which Crazy Buffalo asked me about after the lodge while smoking the sacred pipe with him. It was at that time he looked at me directly in the eye and said, "John, did you 'see' anything during your lodge?"

I remember at this point thinking of the Sweat Lodge ritual and its four rounds in which more stones were added to the pit in the center of the lodge, having different functions, such as purification (emotional release), thanksgiving, atonement, and more. During the second round, I continued to perspire profusely but experienced less bodily tension. I was starting to get a sense of the ritual and its protocol, so to speak. To clarify, there are no discussions or conversations during the ritual. Each person speaks in turn around the inner circle of the lodge. However, the medicine man (or woman) may say words of reflection (e.g., "life involves pain and suffering," "we can release it if we choose to." etc.). The medicine person may sing songs to aid in the release of emotions or grief. Further, when a lodge participant says something of deep personal importance or has a powerful disclosure or cathartic release, he may acknowledge by saying in Lakota, "Ho!" which roughly translates as "that was a good thing."

In the second round, the intensity of the heat inside the lodge was more powerful than in the first round. By now, I was dehydrated and the sweating began to diminish and then, eventually, stop, as if I were "baked" dry. My physical tension reduced and my heart stopped pounding so quickly. I noticed my body beginning to feel "light" in weight and my ability to concentrate on the painful stories of the participants seemed to sharpen in focus. I noticed that as I let myself listen freely without "clinical or psychological mindfulness," that I had more energy and an increasing sense of well being. My state of fear, panic and anxiety in the first round was seemingly being transformed as the ritual unfolded. While initially reticent to disclose my personal concerns in the first round, I suddenly felt myself more comfortable in sharing my stories of a painful nature without fear of judgment in the solemnity of the lodge and its darkness. I spoke of my sadness about my friends who committed suicide as they could not put the horrors of Vietnam to rest. By the time the second round ended, I felt a sense of serenity and calmness emerging and wondered how this was occurring. Once again, the flap was opened at the end of the second round. By now the sun was about to set – an orange ball sitting on top of a distant knoll of South Dakota descending over the earth's surface. Crazy Buffalo requested more hot stones for the ceremonial fire as we all sat inside the lodge, quiet and reflective with red faces and skin form the intense heat. I noticed that the men's eyes were clear and that their faces looked healthy and clean. The steam had done its job inside and out – the body was purged from emotional toxins and posttraumatic pains. There was now present in the lodge an unspoken feeling of acceptance and understanding – one common to combat veterans after battle. Only this time the battle was spiritual in nature – to become whole in oneself again. I knew at that moment that I had a long journey ahead of me.

The ritual continued with the third round – more hot stones, water for the bucket with pine boughs and incantations from Crazy Buffalo. Strangely, I now looked forward to having more heat and steam in the lodge. How could this be? After all, I had fear and trepidation during the first two rounds and had hoped by the painful conclusion of the first round of the Lakota Warrior Sweat that the entire ceremony had ended. Now, as I sat looking outside at the Sacred Pipe on the alter and the setting sun, that this was a place of healing and unique in nature. I hoped that Crazy Buffalo would sing more songs in Lakota and talk to us at the start of the third round. He did. He disclosed parts of his history and struggles in life, including a near death experience from illness. He maintained a sense of presence that was reverent, calm and peaceful. He had wisdom and insight about alcoholism, emotional trauma, and suffering. He had a gift to share psychologically profound insights with just a few words.

As the third round began, I felt physically light in my entire body – as if I had lost 30 pounds of weight. My body seemed buoyant, flexible and loose – like that of a yogi master. As the steam emerged from the hot rocks, I breathed it in my face and nose, using my hands to pull it towards me; welcoming it as a friend. "How strange," I thought, since this same steam burned me and scared me into a state of panic during the first round. Now, I embraced it and enjoyed the warm sensation it provided my body, like a soft, pure cotton, silky blanket of comfort. My skin was totally dry and my hair was starting to dry out as the sweating had stopped. I thought, "I have gone from one state of being to another during this ritual. How is this happening?" It seemed weird, magical and wonderful at the same time.

The third round seemed to pass very quickly, the total opposite of the first round. Time had altered as did my perceptions of space and that of my body itself. At some moment, I realized in the most playful and joyous way that I was in an altered state of consciousness (ASC). I felt happy, euphoric and did not want the third round to end. Moreover, listening to the stories of the participants, I began to visualize what they were saying in three-dimensional color, almost as if I had been there at the time when the events unfolded. There was a remarkable clarity of connection to everyone, one in which I walked along with them on their life's journey. It was a psychic virtual reality. At this point in time, I did not want the lodge experience to end. But, to test my new sense of awareness and consciousness, I moved my right hand in front of my face in the blackness of the lodge and tried to reach it with my left hand. I could not find my right hand. I remember smiling at this sense of altered kinesthetic experience. Then, the third round ended, the door to the lodge opened and the sun was gone. It occurred to me at that moment that Crazy Buffalo had chosen the time of the lodge to begin as the sun was casting its rays into the opening of the lodge and now, as the fourth round was to begin, the South Dakota plains were dark and the moon was rising. How wonderful, I thought, these mythic themes. Lightness versus darkness; birth versus death; pain and transformation; individual and collective healing in a common earthy space of a long evolved tradition of healing. Where could it go from here?

The fourth, and final round, seemed to disappear in a few minutes. By now, I was fully enjoying the altered state of consciousness (ASC). We continued the ritual with individual self-disclosures related to Vietnam War experiences and its effects on our lives. Then unexpected and strange things began to happen to me (and maybe others, but I did not inquire). I had two different sets of powerful visual experiences. In the first set of experiences, I saw white lights of small balls of energy shooting across the top of the interior of the lodge. There were at least four or more of these "ghost-like" energy balls flying around the lodge. I was not frightened by them and several times tried to touch them. My sense of them was that they were not physical objects but spiritual states of consciousness emanating from the members of the lodge. In the second vision, which I have never shared with anyone before writing this chapter, I saw a large Lakota Sioux Chief dressed in a full headdress, breast plates, and formal traditional clothing who came to me and said, "John, it is your mission in life to continue what you have started and are doing. You will have a long and hard journey but it is your calling to do this. You were called to this lodge by us!" He then disappeared and I felt a sense of relief and renewal. Soon, the final round ended. We all exited the lodge and stood up in the cool clear air of the night. I felt cleansed, serene and with a peaceful mind.

After moving outside in the star-filled night, Crazy Buffalo shared the sacred pipe with us, one by one. When it was my turn, he handed the long pipe to me, packed tobacco into its bowl, lit it and I drew the smoke into my mouth. It tasted soft and fragrantly light. As I inhaled the smell of the "sweet grass" and tobacco, Crazy Buffalo looked me in the eye and asked me, "How was your lodge? Did you see things?" I felt a sense of trust and unity at that moment and told him of my visions in the fourth round. I continued smoking for a short while and said little more. When I was done, I gratefully handed him the beautiful, hand-carved sacred pipe. I asked him what the visions meant. He looked me in the eye with a strong, powerful sense and said softly and calmly, "You are a medicine man." He then turned and left, restoring the pipe, eagle wing, and sacred artifacts in his tote bag. I watched him walk away and thought what a beautiful, holy man it is who wears Levi jeans and simple clothes.

I returned to my hotel room after the Sweat Lodge. I had an incredible sense of serenity. I could not sleep. I tried watching television, but it just seemed noisy. So, I made notes about the Sweat Lodge. I did not know it, but there was a whole lot more to be revealed and taught to me by Native American medicine men over the next fifteen years. When I left the pow wow, I went to the elders to thank them for inviting me to the event. The truth was that I was not invited and that I just made my own arrangements to attend, as I had learned of the event from friends in the Pacific Northwest who were interested in traditional healing practices. I shook hands with the four ruddy-faced elders, thanking them for my experiences. They stoically looked me in the eye and said, "You were not invited. You were called to be here." I looked at each of them, felt a tingle in my spine of a moment of life-changing experience, one that did alter my life forever. However, these few days in South Dakota on the Sioux reservation were a prelude of what was to come next. I will describe this later in the chapter but before I left the pow wow, I was to learn of the Red Feather Ceremony

The Red Feather Ceremony

The Red Feather Ceremony honors "warriors" or veterans who have made sacrifices for their country and tribal community. The Red Feather Society is a prestigious society among the Sioux and plains Native Americans. The 'red feather' takes its name from the ritual itself, during which inductees are given an eagle feather with "red" blood from the existent members. The nominee is selected for membership by the society. During the communal ritual, the veteran selected has his record of valor and service acclaimed before the group in a stadium-like pow wow grounds. Then those selected for membership are eventually recognized by other members of the Red Feather Society, who draw their blood upon the sacred eagle feather, which is later given to the inductee. Following the grand, collective, honoring of the inductees who have been free of alcohol and substance abuse for at least two years, there is a sweat lodge ritual during which the medicine man affirms their commitment to abstinence and then makes a task for the inductee, which in this instance was to "take care of and look after" elder members of the tribal community. So, once officially accepted into the Red Feather Society, the combat veteran gained a new sense of respect and status within the community. He was a sober Native American combat veteran who was taking care of others, especially the elderly tribal folks. In return, he had unique respect and status amongst his peers, family and community. As long as he maintained his status as a Red Feather, the community, in turn, would take care of him and his family. In this regard, the wounded became the generative healers. The wounded who became healthy, became wise men and the teachers of the children to follow in the community. Life had come full circle. The wounded veteran now has achieved a new home and meaning in life.

Orcas, Salmon and the Olympic National Park

After the 1985 pow wow in South Dakota, I was invited one month later to another four day gathering for Vietnam War veterans at the Howling Dog ceremony in Port Angeles, Washington located in the Pacific Northwest of the United States across from Victoria, British Columbia. This ceremony was being conducted by a mental health counselor who worked closely with a traditional medicine man from tribes located in the Northwest, USA and Canada. It was there that I met Andy Callicum, medicine man and Chief of the Mawachet Tribe from Vancouver Island, Canada. The mental health counselor, Bruce Webster, was a personal friend whom I had met previously while doing consulting and training for professionals working with the department of veterans affairs for the State of Washington. Bruce lived on a beautiful property located on the ocean front in Port Angeles. From the beachfront one could see killer whales and, in the distance, Victoria Island. Bruce told me about sweat lodges and other ritual ceremonies being employed at that time to assist Vietnam War veterans suffering from PTSD and related problems. So, after the profound experience in South Dakota, I was curious to see and learn more of culture-specific rituals and practices to help individuals suffering from psychic trauma.

The four-day Howling Dog ceremony began with a sunrise sweat lodge which was constructed on the ocean front. The lodge was similar to the one in South Dakota but different in the sense that the winds blew inland off the Strait of Juan

Defuca, bringing the smells of sea salt, fish, kelp and the richness of the waters teeming with salmon, trout, halibut, octopus and crabs.

On the first day, everyone gathered at the ocean front before sunrise. The "fire keeper" had prepared the stones for the sunrise sweat lodge and the war veterans anxiously awaited the arrival of the medicine man, Andy Callicum. Soon, as the first light of dawn emerged over the large spruce and fir trees, someone said, "Here comes Andy." I looked up at the path leading to the beach and saw a short, black-haired man in a Levi jacket and jeans walking towards the lodge. A veteran familiar with Andy said, "Watch, his bald eagle will soon fly over him." I was skeptical and said to myself, "If an eagle does come by, it will be random chance." Andy continued walking and as he got closer to the beachfront sweat lodge, a magnificent bald eagle swooped down out of the mountains of the Olympic National Forest and flew over his left shoulder and over the lodge itself. I thought, "Well, that was interesting, I wonder how many times that has occurred." To "fast forward" the story, over the next 14 years, I had many encounters and experiences with Andy, and every time he came to do healing work, the bald eagle was present and flew over him before making a return flight to the wilderness of the Olympic National Forest. I stopped my scientific, Western, rational, deductive logic after that and just accepted what I had witnessed. Over the years, I had the opportunity to learn from Andy and he took me "under his wing" and taught me a great deal about traditional Native American healing but from a different cultural tradition from the Lakota Sioux of the American Midwest and plains states.

During the first sunrise sweat, Andy sang many songs from his tribal past. He had a beautiful voice which he could modulate in brilliant ways to elicit sadness, grief or happiness. He sometimes would start a sweat lodge with a song that elicited crying and grief from all of us in the lodge. His singing seemed to reach everyone in a powerful way and there was usually a purging of emotions. The strangest thing for me was that time and time again I found myself singing with him and knowing the songs, without any prior knowledge of his native tribe or people. It just came natural and seemed good. Later, after many years, I directly asked him about this seemingly odd ability or occurrence and he just laughed and said that one day he would explain it to me but that I asked dumb questions for a "bright guy." I was puzzled at the time and later we had more serious talks and he explained to me what Crazy Buffalo had told and more.

I returned almost every year for 14 years to Port Angeles to be with Bruce and Andy. During that time, I was taught more about sweat lodges and other ritualistic forms of healing. For example, Andy once took me to the Elwah River to select stones for the sweat lodge. He explained to me that it was important to find the proper stones because selection of the wrong ones could result in an explosion in the heat of the lodge or a ceremonial fire. I asked him, "How do you know which ones to select?" He answered by pointing his fingers at certain rocks in the crystal clear river bed and said, "They will talk to you, John, but you must learn to listen carefully." On that day we gathered stones and took them back to the sweat lodge for introduction into the sacred fire. As we walked and talked together, Andy taught me that there were many uses and purposes of the sweat lodge: healing, purification, marriage, socializing, "power sweats" for major life decisions, peyote sweats and more. Over the years of our connection and friendship, I experienced all of these and more, as Andy shared his personal knowledge of native healing. To this day, I am eternally grateful to this gifted and beautiful man.

The Talking Circle Ritual

Among the many rituals that Andy introduced me to was the "Talking Circle," which could occur before or after a sweat lodge ritual. In the "Talking Circle," the participants of the Howling Dog ceremony gathered around an open, outdoor fire. The grounds on the beachfront at Bruce Webster's property had a special location near the ocean in which there was a circle of logs on which to sit. In the middle was a large space for a log fire which was kept alive from early morning to after midnight with a steady supply of seasoned hardwood to feed and nourish the fire, which gave off a wonderful woodsy smell in the breeze blowing inland from the ocean.

The ritual of the "Talking Circle" is a most powerful one. Andy showed me the process. First, as a medicine man, he stood up at the six o'clock position in the circle and spoke to everyone gathered together in the circle. He spoke of the importance of honesty, friendship and love. He spoke of the need for self-revelation and care for one another. Then, he moved to his left in a clockwise fashion and greeted those present, one at a time. As the participants were standing, he turned to face the individual, shook and held their hand, looked them in the eyes and spoke to them about his perceptions and feelings for them as a person. Then, one by one, he completed the circle, moving patiently from person to person. Once he returned to his original place, the next person was instructed to repeat the process. As I sat to his left (seven o'clock), I next did the same set of actions, greeting the participants and expressing my feelings and perceptions with them. At first, it was difficult and anxiety-provoking, since this is an intimate collective experience by all who witness each individual encounter. However, as I progressed around the circle and the warm fire, it became easier and much more comfortable. Eventually, I returned to my "seat" on the log and the next person got up and repeated the process. In this way then, the "Talking Circle" meant that every person encountered each other at least twice. It created deep connections of bonding and openness in a short period of time. Once the entire circle was completed, we sat around the fire to continue talking with each other. The process is informal after everyone has completed the circle of mutual greetings. It was not unusual for this "talking circle" to last for four hours or more. While there are a whole host of insights I could share about this ritual, among the most central and poignant is that persons suffering from psychic trauma could break through their isolation, detachment, avoidance, defensiveness and embrace others without fear of shame, guilt or rejection. I witnessed true human love, acceptance and the embracement of each other without judgment.

Beyond Traditional Cultural Rituals

My work with Andy Callicum, Bruce Webster and other medicine men and women led to some innovations in developing new rituals for Vietnam veterans, some of which were derivations of traditional Native American rituals. Andy was supportive of these efforts and I was cautious to solicit his opinions and criticisms as to their potential usefulness and value. In this section of the chapter, I want to share a few examples of the rituals that Bruce Webster and I created and which have been partially described elsewhere (Wilson, 1989).

In particular, Bruce and I created an intensive experimental treatment program during September of 1985. The program combined modalities of treatment during the week-long experience. There were group therapy sessions, one-to-one counseling, sweat lodges on a daily basis, special rituals, early and late involvement of spouses and family, physical exercise programs, responsibility for cooking meals and cleaning and other activities. We knew that most Vietnam combat veterans were alienated and did not trust the U.S. government program for mental health treatment in veteran administration hospitals. So, we designed the program as multimodal in nature in a wilderness area that had certain geographical features similar to Vietnam. We believed that the men would be more comfortable in this setting, being with other combat veterans. There was designed a matched set of groups, randomly selected from Bruce's client roster of over 200, who were assigned to the treatment or control group. There was pre- and post-testing on psychological questionnaires for PTSD, psychiatric symptoms as well as other psychosocial measures (e.g., marital conflict, issues of intimacy, etc.) at three month intervals for one year. The results found significant and lasting positive changes for the treatment group on nearly all of the measures. Interestingly, however, they did not find changes in capacity for intimacy with spouses or partners.

To place these descriptions into perspective, I should note that from 1973 to 1989, the major focus of my clinical and academic work concerned victims of war, especially military combat veterans. Therefore, I am going to describe six rituals that Bruce Webster and I created as "alternatives" to traditional psychotherapy.

The Ritual Homecoming Welcome and Warrior Feast

The first ceremony involved the ritual homecoming on the first day of the program. Once everyone was registered, the clients and veteran staff members were divided into two "squads." The clients wore an orange armband and the counselors a blue one. The men were taken in two pickup trucks to opposite locations in the wilderness about two miles from the Camp David resort on Lake Crescent. Once there, they were instructed to walk back to the camp as a squad in single file. The purpose of this event was to symbolically recreate the homecoming from Vietnam, i.e., to "rotate" home one by one just as they did years before after their tour of duty had ended.

At the entrance to the campsite, along the dirt road that led to the main lodge, were stationed the family, friends, and other staff members, who waited in a long line to greet the men. We believed it was important to have them present in order to provide an authentic welcome and homecoming ceremony of appreciation for the service in Vietnam. We also thought that a symbolic reenactment of walking "back home," one by one, to an extended family was an important beginning to the week-long treatment program. So as the veterans came into the camp, the children would run out to greet their "daddy" and a sentry shouted out that the veteran was home from Vietnam (e.g., "Hey, Mom, Bill is home from the war"). Then each person greeted the veteran with a handshake and a hug and said, "Welcome home – thanks for serving. I am proud of you."

After the last individual had returned, a warriors' feast was held in the main lodge. The men sat around a long table and were served smoked salmon, nuts, fruits, and other native foods of the Pacific Northwest. As they ate they were surprisingly solemn. The men were encircled by their families and friends, who later joined them in a communal dinner which honored their sacrifices in the war.

The Ritual of the Ceremonial Fire

On the last day of treatment, the families and significant others returned to the camp in the afternoon to rejoin the men and to participate in a ceremonial fire. In this ritual everyone gathered around the fire in a circle. Then one by one, in a clockwise order, each person walked up to the fire and "released" into it an object, actual or symbolic, of something negative and painful that they wished to "let go" from their life. For example, several veterans put their soft "bush" hats from Vietnam into the fire as a symbolic act of "letting go" of war trauma. After the ceremonial fire a special sweat lodge was conducted for the women. While this was in progress, the men prepared a meal to serve to their wives, children, and significant others.The dinner concluded with a traditional potlatch during which gifts were provided for the staff and participants in the program.Finally, a "talking circle" was conducted. Everyone sat around a log fire to continue conversation and dialogue about the week's activities.

The Ritual of Release and Transformation

Another Native American technique adapted for our program involved the planting of two fir trees at the conclusion of the session which addressed the issues of guilt, rage, anger, hatred, sorrow, grief, killing and destruction as related to the Vietnam experience. Each individual was given two fir saplings and instructed to find a special place to plant them. It was explained that among some Native American groups it is believed that Mother Earth receives that which is given to her in a spirit of harmony, balance, love, and the cycle of the seasons. Thus, by planting the trees one could ask Mother Earth to receive them and in the process take away pain, despair, sadness, hatred, and other negative emotions. It was said that in return, she would nurture the young trees and help them to grow in their natural way.

Alone, and at the place he had chosen, each person was instructed to put his mental focus on the part of his body where he felt tension, pain, or negative feelings. He then placed that part of his body over a hole he dug with his hands and released the negative energy into the earth. The task that followed was to plant the tree and let Mother Earth transmute the negative emotion into an object of growing beauty. Thus, a "negative" was replaced by a "positive" to complete a cycle which had as its image the act of "receiving" by "letting go."

Although it is possible to render various conceptualizations of this simple ceremony, it bears remarkable similarity as a ritual form to the psychosocial modalities that Erikson (1950, 1968) has characterized as "to get" and "to take" (oral sensory kinesthetic) and "to hold on" and "to let go" (anal muscular). These psychosocial modalities are well recognized in psychoanalytic theory as central epigenetic concerns during the first three years of ego development. Letting go of pain and symbolically transmuting it to Mother Earth contains the image of gaining personal strength by the proper release of that which blocks healthy adaptation. By letting go of the negative emotion, the cycle of adaptation can become balanced again by a positive change (the growth of the tree = self) which emanates from nurturance of the Mother Earth, the maternal symbol that gives freely of what one needs "to get" to restore psychological and physical equilibrium.

The Salmon Feast of Thanksgiving

A salmon feast of thanksgiving was held early in the week. A gift of fresh king salmon was donated to the group and provided the basis to celebrate in a meal of thanksgiving for all that is good in life with the fish that is regarded as sacred to many of the native tribes of the Pacific Northwest. There was an abundance of freshly baked salmon, and each participant was asked to fill himself with this special meal and to recognize that life contains many good things to be appreciated and shared with others.

The Mail Call Ritual

The mail call ritual involved a surprise, unexpected delivery of letters to the men each night after dinner. It was prearranged so that every veteran received a letter a day from a friend or family member during the stay at Camp David. The letters were written to encourage the men to continue their efforts to work through their stress disorder and other problems that brought them to the treatment program.

The "Unfinished Business" Ritual

Towards the end of the week, each participant was given two stamped envelopes and stationery in order to write letters to two persons, living or dead, with whom they had "unfinished business." Afterward, the letters were mailed if the individual wished to have them sent. The purpose of this ritual was to attempt to bring closure or resolution to a previous and conflicted relationship with someone important in one's life.

The Morning Ritual of Rebirth

Since all of the participants suffered from PTSD and allied conditions (e.g., depression) we wanted to start each day with physical exercise. A participant was selected by his fellow combat veterans to awaken everyone at 6:00 a.m. to go to the deep glacial lakefront. The person selected was the most senior participant who had the most years of service in Vietnam in an elite Special Operation Forces unit (US Navy Seals). Once the men were awaken and formed into a "unit," they walked to the lakefront where Bruce and I greeted them. Then with us acting as their "commanding military officers," we ordered them into the very cold (65 °F) water for a wake-up plunge and swim. Our goal was threefold: (1) decrease PTSD-related hyperarousal; (2) stimulate good appetites; and (3) increase alertness and clarity of mind. As a part of this ritual, Bruce and I alternated diving in to the cold water to "lead" the men.

The Desensitization Ritual

Since veterans suffering from PTSD are chronically hyperaroused and extraordinarily sensitive to trauma-specific stimuli, we designed a desensitization ritual conducted in a group setting. The setting for the group desensitization ritual was a small cabin located on the edge of Lake Crescent. It was remote and isolated from the main lodge. It was here that we had planned a complex procedure that involved all of the counselors and the U.S. park ranger in charge of this area of the Olympic National Park.

The men were gathered in the cabin and seated facing a wood-burning fireplace that warmed the room. The topic of the "group" session was understanding hyperarousal and hypervigilance as a part of PTSD. We asked the men to talk about what "set them off" and how it related to their war experiences. This was a two-hour session during which certain items were passed amongst the men which were designed to elicit hyperarousal. The items included JP-4 helicopter fuel soaked into cotton towels, strings of M-60 bullets, empty shells from AK-47 and M-16 automatic rifles, a Vietcong flag and U.S. Army uniforms. While the items were being distributed and passed around, Bruce Webster stood in front of me juggling a grenade in his hands, tossing it up in the air and catching it. Although the grenade was inert, it had a "firing pin" and the men did not know the weapon was not explosive.

In the next phase of this ritual, I had organized the counselors outside the cabin near the doors and windows. We had placed strings of different strength firecrackers around the cabin and towards the end of the first hour they were detonated to simulate machine gun and mortar fire. However, before that was initiated, the park ranger cooperated with us by wearing a black shirt and pants, like that worn by the Vietcong enemy in Vietnam. He also wore an Asian sampam straw hat and rode a motorbike with a bell, in front of the window of the cabin, ringing the bell as he did so. This set of stimuli was designed to further create hypervigilance amongst the men. Then, at the set time, I detonated the firecrackers, Bruce dropped the grenade and a loud set of combat-like noise filled the air. As we expected, all of the men reacted instantly with exaggerated startle response and either ran out of the cabin or fell to the floor to cover and protect themselves. Upon reaction, each participant was greeted by a counselor and for hours afterwards talked about their PTSD-related hypervigilance and hyperarousal. At the end of the session, a sweat lodge was held with a specific focus of "what happened in Vietnam." The ritual was clinically successful and facilitated recognition of cues for hyperarousal but also helped the men identify more positive coping patterns.

The Graduation Ceremony

On the last day, a graduation ceremony was held. Each man received a specially designed diploma which displayed an eagle-like jet aircraft (the Vietnam Freedom Bird) emerging from Lake Crescent and the cedar forests that surround it. After all the diplomas were distributed, a final group session was held at which time expressions of appreciation and gratitude were exchanged.

Lessons from the Sweat Lodge and Beyond

My experiences from work with Native Americans has taught me about the archetypes for healing and recovery from psychic trauma, grief, and human suffering. In many respects, it is difficult to know where to begin to share some of the wonderful gifts I have been given since 1985 to the present by Native American healers but also from others in different parts of the world. In an overly simplistic way, I would like to share what I have learned as it relates specifically to the focus of this book.

- There are wounded victims and wounded healers, as Carl Jung (1963) informed us many years ago. Wounded victims can inform wounded healers in profound ways as to the pathways of healing.
- Wounded victims have as much to teach as their primary treaters, therapists, shamans, medicine healers, traditional doctors and rehabilitation specialists.
- Western (American-Western European) traditional approaches and methods for helping psychically traumatized persons have limits and constraints.
- One to one psychotherapy is *not* the only way to have intensive and curative therapeutic processes for distressed and traumatized persons.
- Throughout the millennia, each culture has evolved mechanisms, culture-specific rituals, and other ways to assist victims of abuse, trauma, violence and war.
- Ethnocentrically based approaches to trauma, abuse and disaster are limited by their own assumptions and experiences with coping with trauma. As noted in this chapter, how could Western psychotherapists understand the elegance and brilliance of Native American rituals for recovery from trauma if they do

not understand the cosmology, traditional ethnicity of indigenous peoples and their cultural traumatization by colonial powers and political domination? Many similar analogies exist today in Angola, Sudan, the Balkans and other areas of ethnic and national conflict. So, the question emerges as to what culturally specific techniques, rituals and practices are utilitarian for these people? In this regard, the Native American tribes and natives were forced to evolve their own distinct rituals for restoring members of their community to wellness and health. Indeed, they developed elaborate and complex ritualistic practices that were not "medical treatments," but part of a way of living to maintain healthy harmony and consistency of "ideology" and religious cosmology in the tribal community. In short, they found ways to facilitate helping people: what works best for whom in our cultural traditions?

• My personal experiences with Native American practices, of which I have only highlighted a few, taught me the profound importance of community commitment to those who suffer. Sweat lodges and other traditional practices are an integral part of a way of living in which people know the ways to love and help one another. The one practical ritual that cross cuts both cultures is Alcoholics Anonymous and in that sense there are significant and profound parallels.

Conclusion

My experiences with Native American rituals helped me to face the ghosts of my past – not to just find brilliance and elegance in Native American rituals. Crazy Buffalo, the medicine man of the Sioux Nation helped open my consciousness; Andy Callicum taught me as if he were my father and opened his soul to me. He showed me aspects of reality that do not have a place in psychology textbooks. Bruce Webster became my spiritual brother for life and walked by my side in near-death experiences. I can say today that what I sought to understand about these rituals out of what I believed was purely academic and intellectual interest. But what I got in turn was a portal to living life itself – just as Crazy Buffalo said, "To see more of what is out there and in here."

References

Erikson, E. (1950). *Childhood and society*. New York: Norton.

Jung, C. G. (1963). *Memories, dreams and reflections*. New York: Vintage Books.

Moodley, R., & West, W. (2005). *Integrating traditional healing practice into counseling and psychotherapy*. Thousand Oaks, CA: Sage Productions.

Wilson, J. P. (1989) Trauma, transformation and healing: An integration approach to theory, research and posttraumatic theory. New York: Brunner/Mazel.

5
Fourteen Djinns Migrate Across the Ocean

Jaswant Guzder

He shakes his head. "It's probably nothing. Isn't it from Muridke that a holy man has been summoned by that family on Faiz Street, to come and exocise their daughter of the djinns?"

"Yes. He'll come soon," she replies. "She's not behaving appropriately towards her family and husband. Last night I found myself wondering whether that was what was wrong with our daughter, the djinns possessed her and caused her to rebel."

(Aslam, 2004)

This case study of an eight year old boy of Canadian-Egyptian origin and his family involved the interventions of a child psychiatry day treatment team, his school, and traditional healers from both Canada and the Middle East. Constructing meaningful interventions for this family involved a shifting location of illness meaning at the intersection of psychosocial, historical, and religious factors integrated in systemic formulations of trauma intervention. The treatment team positioned interventions between individual (intra-psychic, identity or personality factors), family systems (marital and child issues), and socio-cultural agendas (host Canadian culture, culture of origin, djinn possession, dynamics of culture change, religious and historical legacies) as the treatment evolved. Cultural camouflage (Friedman, 1982) with intertwining emotional and psychodynamic agendas of trauma and djinn possession states (El Khayat, 1994) placed the unraveling of cultural metaphors at the heart of the therapeutic process. Friedman has (1982) hypothesized that culture does not supply the determinants of family dynamics, but rather is the medium through which family process works its art or camouflages its emergence. Kleinman has (1991) similarly argued that healing in the realm of the psyche is enacted through symbols of the patient's cultural context. In this family, the cumulative trauma determinants included their experiences of domestic violence, marital infidelities, downward socio-economic status, culture change, family deaths, medical illnesses and sexual abuse.

Djinn possession was integral to the family mythology and is deeply rooted in ancient, medieval and modern Islamic Egyptian experience. According to Michael Dols (1992, p. 213):

"The djinns appear frequently in the early or Meccan portions of the Qur'an, as in the common expressions "djinn and mankind"(jinn wa l-ins). The Qur'an says the djinn were

105

created of smokeless flame, whereas humankind and angels-the other two classes of intelligent beings in the sublunar world-were created of clay and light, but their purpose was
also to serve and worship God. Prophets were sent to them from God, so that they may be
either believers or unbelievers. On one occasion, it is reported that some djinn became
Muslims after having heard the Qur'an recited by Muhammad. The unbelieving djinn
might go to hell, but it was not stated explicitly that the believers might go to heaven.
Furthermore, it was commonly believed that everyone had a personal djinn, like the
classical daemon, or genius. According to a late Muslim tradition, the Prophet's djinn
became a Muslim and instructed him to do only what was right."

The narratives of the family members in our case study shifted in meaning and
content, as the family processed their trauma with members of the therapy team.
The building of a therapeutic alliance was a slow process informed by previous
treatment failures and an understanding of stigma factors silencing family
discourse. In the course of treatment, we understood the central role of djinn possession in the family's post migration life in Canada. We worked with significant
family resistances, initially reflected in their hopelessness that treatment could
ever effect a change in their suffering. Our child patient, eight-year-old Abdul, was
admitted for a five-month period to our child psychiatry day treatment program
with an intensive family therapy component. On discharge from the program the
family had follow-up intermittently for a year, with ongoing family treatment,
intermittent school consultation, and a brief youth protection involvement.

While the psychiatric literature on trauma treatment emphasizes the definitions
of the DSM IV (APA, 1994) criteria for posttraumatic stress disorder and psy-
chopharmacological interventions grounded in a perspective of subjective suffering,
this story underlines that intercultural and systemic affiliations or relationships are
essential to proposing formulations of meaning and intervention. The symptom
bearer was the identified child patient while the sources of distress were uncovered
within traumatic disturbances in his family. The underlying motifs of medieval
Islamic society and a post-modern world were collaged across generations, forming the basis of identities that shifted and reframed meaning over the course of therapy. Family therapy appeared to function as a container and holding environment
(Winnicott, 1966) that allowed the family to realign their personal mythologies and
create emerging options.

Presenting Problems of the Family

The family consisted of father Ehab (49 yr), mother Naz (43 yr), 20 year old
daughter Ayisha, 18 year old son Hamid, 15 year old daughter Amina, identified
patient Abdul, 8 year old, and a youngest son aged 6 year old, Yasin. They had
never been seen together for family therapy in previous therapeutic encounters.

Since the birth of their oldest children, the parents had had an increasingly
conflicted relationship, which coincided with their departure from the network of
extended family in Egypt, with their first migration to a neighboring Middle
Eastern country, and the second one to Canada. Father had often threatened

divorce throughout his marriage to Naz. After their Canadian migration to Vancouver, he had decided to leave for Montreal alone, when Abdul was two years old and his wife had just given birth to their son Yasin. He later said he could no longer tolerate his wife who had become a "raving mad woman" under the influence of the djinns since Abdul's birth. These possession states had completely changed her character from her usual obsequious gentle nature to an "enraged" woman at home. Naz had endured years of traumatic domestic violence and the couple functioned with a virtual emotional divorce, though in the initial sessions she expressed no overt hostility towards her husband. Abdul had become the phobic companion of his dissembling mother and was highly reactive to her moods or episodes of distress from early in his life. He had had little time or opportunity to bond with his father, who openly stated he had not wanted either of his two younger children, perceiving their births as a prelude to his bad luck. Father had lost his savings in a high-risk investment venture shortly after arriving in Vancouver, so they had fallen from affluence in the Middle East to welfare subsistence in a cramped, low-cost housing complex apartment. Father was deeply ashamed of his inability to support the family and his social dislocation was also a deep source of distress for him. He disclosed once in despair, "I have three sons but cannot leave them any inheritance." He seemed to make no conscious connection or identification with his childhood predicament when his family origin in Egypt was left destitute after his father's premature death. His eruptions of rage were displaced onto Naz and his children as his shame progressively eroded his identity.

Naz initially saw herself as a victim. She was unable to work as she absorbed herself in the special needs of Abdul and suffered from her own debilitating depression. While Naz took some solace from her Islamic values and prayer, Ehab had disconnected from religious beliefs. Naz had been particularly hurt by Ehab's affair with an American flight attendant soon after their first migration and by his continuing infidelities when he traveled internationally for his Middle Eastern employers. When he had brought an impoverished older brother into his company in the Middle East and employed him as a company driver, his brother's wife had often intruded in their martial rifts. Naz believed the envy of this sister-in-law was the poisonous intent that led to her djinn possession. She commented that fortunately this curse, born of envy, could not affect the fetus or young children in the family.

Both parents had become clinically depressed since coming to Canada, as they felt mired in shame and financial loss as well as estranged by their social and cultural dislocation. They avoided the mosque and the local Egyptian community as they felt their poverty was a barrier to any comfortable interaction. Naz commented how she would discard her furniture each Eid (the annual religious holiday marking the end of the holy month of Ramadan), in the Middle East to redecorate her home and "buy completely new things", while now she worried about affording groceries and school books.

Ehab felt he could not call his older siblings in Egypt for support as he had been the only successful sibling and now he had fallen on hard times. Shame was the presiding affect in his discourse and it often erupted as rages or dysthymic moods, which he would vent in the family. In the previous years, several of his elder siblings had died of heart disease and cancer, leaving nieces and nephews who looked to him for assistance. In Egypt, Naz had a brother who looked after her parents until her father's death but now her widowed mother looked to Naz for emotional comfort. Neither Naz nor Ehab wanted to live in Egypt again as they saw no hope there for economic security. Though they agreed that the children would have a better life and educational opportunities in Canada, the couple felt guilty that they had relinquished the role of caring for family to their siblings in Egypt. They felt some apprehension as the only siblings on either side of the family to live in North America, and discomfort at their renunciation of family duties.

In Vancouver, the family had been offered both a community psychiatrist for mother and mental health home support. This team had been much appreciated by Naz as their instrumental help of a homemaker and home visiting was beneficial and reduced her social isolation. She had been told her depression had caused Abdul's regressions and separation anxiety. Though she shared her anguish about her recurrent djinn possession states with the psychiatrist privately, he had tried various antidepressants and admonished her not to dwell on her superstitions and false beliefs. Father also suffered from a severe depression in this post migration period for which he sought consultations of Middle Eastern, Vancouver and Montreal psychiatrists. He had tried many medications including anti-psychotics, antidepressants and benzodiazepines with poor results.

When Naz had returned to Egypt both for the death of her father and later her mother's deteriorating heart ailments, she had sought out traditional healers for her djinn possession. Ehab had returned in 2003 to Egypt after some "unpleasant incidents" with Hamid in Vancouver. His return visit had been an opportunity for both father and son to "reconnect with family and Islamic values." As a patriarch, Ehab was very apprehensive about his children "losing respect" for him, which he ascribed to their "becoming too Canadian." Since Ehab had always been both emotionally absent and abusive in Naz's view, he needed to invest and gain respect in his parental and spousal role. This conflict often erupted in alternately screaming quarrels or retreat into sulky withdrawals with Naz supporting the children. Though it was Naz who kept the religious traditions of Islam at the centre of family life, Ehab rejected religious traditions. However, he was more apprehensive about the sexuality and autonomy of Canadian culture as transgressive influences. Naz and the children felt more supported and autonomous in the Canadian cultural milieu, which unsettled the patriarchal homeostasis of their past Middle Eastern life with Ehab.

Scripts of Family Members

Parents

Naz, was an articulate woman who had been a librarian in Alexandria, though she had been a homemaker since her marriage to Ehab. She had a soft moon-shaped face and was somewhat obese. She dressed in sober earth colours with a headscarf and long flowing coats. She had been raised in a caring, urban, middle class family and her parents had been "progressive" by encouraging her to have an education and develop a career. Her father had been concerned about the many Egyptian woman who divorced and left without financial means for a livelihood. She had been deeply saddened by her father's sudden death from a myocardial infarct when Adbul was five years old. Naz had had an idealized relationship with her father, which made her deteriorating relationship with Ehab particularly painful, saying, "my father would never have treated his family like this." She was close to her mother, who was now cared for her only son and lived alone though she suffered from angina and diabetes. While she had turned to her extended family in Egypt to intervene in the past when Ehab abused her, migration distances and stigma now limited her appeals for their assistance. Both she and Ehab felt guilty that they could not send more financial help to their families in Egypt who imagined their Canadian life as prosperous and successful.

Ehab, was a handsome, thin, well-groomed man, who had been on a disability pension for his depression since coming to Canada. He came from a lower-middle class family and was raised in a rural village until he was 9 years old when his father died from myocardial infarct. Ehab was brought up by his nine elder siblings. He was well educated and had had a career as a business executive. He often traveled internationally for a large Middle Eastern consortium and had successful senior management career. However, tribal rivalries and family business politics appeared to have undermined his position in the company. It was unclear how he finally lost his job and made the decision to move his family to Vancouver. During his business travels, he had often visited Europe and North America, but preferred to move his family to Canada when his Middle East job fell apart. He was attracted to Canada as a peaceful, multi-cultural society. Ehab was struggling to complete a master's degree in computer science and had remained unemployed since moving to Canada. He felt his cultural background and age had been impediments to finding employment and increasingly he had a hopeless helpless attitude about building a successful future for his family in Canada.

Both parents had multiple somatic problems. Ehab suffered from chronic back pain, diabetes and hepatitis C. He anticipated a terrible death with hepatitis C and had sought expensive interferon treatment in Canada. Naz had chronic pain from fibromyalgia, fatigue and moderate obesity. As Ehab took his medications in a random and intermittent manner, his psychiatrist in Montreal now refused to treat him. Since the move to Montreal, he often threatened suicide to his family. He would remain in his bed for days at a time while intermittently screaming insults at his "noisy family who wouldn't let me sleep" and "wishing I was dead." His various combinations of medications had not improved his symptoms, and eventually we advised him to discontinue all psychotropic medications.

Naz had also been in various antidepressants, which her physicians thought might ease not only her depression but also her intermittent pain and "episodes". She had become progressively phobic in Vancouver, limiting her outings, as she was afraid she would swoon or lose consciousness during her djinn possessions, "they take over my body and I never know when it will happen," disclosed Naz.

She had grown increasingly dependent on her children, especially her eldest daughter Ayisha, as phobic companions. Abdul was often her daytime companion, as he was frequently suspended from school. She saw no connection between her own moods or djinn possession episodes, and his regressions. Her phobias and possessions had impaired her autonomy, consistent treatment, and visits to the mosque or parental functioning at home. Eventually I suggested she should begin a trial of fluoxetine, which she reported lessen her sedation, depression and panic episodes. Several of her healers and imams had counseled her to seek psychiatric care and take psychotropic medications, along with the parallel healing interventions of religious rituals, like sipping holy waters (prayed over with Qur'an hadiths or verses), using special herbs for fumigating or cleansing the body (b'Khour), using herbs that facilitating dreaming and relaxation, and doing her namaz (prayer) five times a day as prescribed in traditional Islam.

While Ehab was clear at our first family meeting that he had not wanted his two unplanned youngest sons, he did feel closeness with his eldest son Hamid who was named after his deceased father. In the past, he had demanded that Naz get abortions, which she refused. Their sexual relationship had then ceased about six years ago. They had continued to quarrel while Naz complained about Ehab's passive helplessness, and her overburdened role. Ehab had been upset about the acculuration of their children, and felt they were disrespectful and "too Canadian" in their clothing and attitudes. He also complained about the central role of the "black magic" in Naz's life.

Abdul

After moving from Vancouver (his birthplace) to Montreal in December 2003, Abdul at age eight had had a disastrous period in grade three in January to June 2004, before he came to us for a family consultation in July 2004. Abdul was a thin, delicately featured, almost effeminate boy who was active, engaging and lively. Despite one-to-one school support from a full time school aide, his aggressive, impulsive, oppositional-defiant, inattentive, and hyperactive behaviors escalated. He ran around the classroom, destroyed school property, could not make friends and was unable to learn. Despite normal intelligence with an absence of any specific learning disabilities according to his 2003 testing, he had academic delays in many areas. He had already had extensive treatment assessments and interventions in Vancouver from age 3, where he had shown similar behaviors progressing from early childhood. At age 3, he had been expelled from his daycare due to his unmanageable behavior. He had been diagnosed intermittently with conduct disorder, oppositional-defiant disorder, specific developmental learning disabilities (speech and language delays in expressive and receptive language), attachment disorder, attention deficit disorder and over anxious disorder. Trauma issues in the family system had never been elicited in his assessments.

At age 4 to 5, Abdul had been transferred to a specialized therapeutic day care in Vancouver for treatment of his aggression, swearing, biting, defiance, noncompliance, hyperactivity, delays in language and learning. In grade one, though he had had individual school aides and a reduced academic load (an individualized educational plan). He had not been able to manage in his classroom nor at home. His regressed behaviors and hyperactivity included crawling on the floor and making noises like an animal, attacking staff or peers unpredictably and frequently running out of the classroom until he was suspended (multiple times). He was sent home for significant periods furthering his academic delays. He was assessed for attention deficit disorder with positive results but a medication trial was not initiated in Vancouver.

Siblings

Yasin

Yasin was a healthy, lively, athletic boy who was doing well both socially and academically in grade one. He often advised his older brother Abdul on how to improve his behavior choices and control himself. He was far more subdued than Abdul and uncomfortable with the affective storms in the family often withdrawing into television watching or simply ignoring the eruptions. Yasin seemed to be more socially resilient and optimistic than his parents and brothers. In the midst of the family turmoil, he looked to his sisters for nurturing and closeness. He had good peer relations and thought Abdul's behaviors looked "crazy" and "silly" at school. While he was occasionally oppositional, he was generally calm and more compliant than Abdul.

Aisha

Twenty year old Aisha was the eldest sibling and a parental child. She was an attractive college student who dressed in jeans and T-shirts. Since migration to Vancouver at twelve, Naz had increasingly relied on Aisha instrumentally and she now helped the family with driving, cooking, cleaning and managing the home when her parents were not able to function effectively. She was often sullen, untrusting and withdrawn. She made it clear that she would never marry an Egyptian man nor tolerate repeating her mother's domestic abuse, thought she did admire modern Arab women like the former Egyptian President's wife, Jehan Sadat (1989).

Aisha had moved to Montreal to her father's apartment with Hamid, in September of 2003 to begin her first term at the university. She was angry with Abdul for causing so many problems at home including his noisy tantrums, which made studying difficult. She was "glad to leave him behind in Vancouver" and found his provocative behaviors and loss of control triggered her rage. She was often verbally abusive or tried to discipline Abdul as she felt her parents exerted "no control over him." She was determined to get an education and had refused to visit Egypt or the Middle East since her last visit for her maternal grandfather's funeral. During that visit with her mother, she had met a healer who had told her she was possessed with two djinns, but she refused to discuss this frightening encounter where she had dissociated and fell into an agitated state at the healer's shrine.

She consciously felt the roles and options of Egyptian women were "medieval" and found Canadian options more appealing. She had no interest in the marriage proposals that had already come to the family from Egypt. She suspected the motivations for marriage might be the new husband's access to a Canadian passport. Aisha feared domination of men in her culture and identified with her mother's predicament. She commented to me as an outsider to her cultural reality that "Arab men are abusive". She had many open fights with her father about the marriage offers and her clothing. During their affluent sojourn in the Middle East, Aisha said her father would rage that he didn't like his wife's cooking or felt she had shamed him by not entertained lashishly to promote his honor after the family had invited his business colleagues. She often attempted to intervene and mediate in these marital crisises when her father would beat her mother. Her father would sometimes listen to her and retreat into verbally abusing Naz. Since this pattern continued on reunification of the family in Montreal, Aisha was "fed up". She was torn between wanting to move out of the family apartment and worrying about her mother's ability to function. She was also negotiating the bicultural identity shifts bridging her experiences of a Muslim with both a Middle Eastern childhood and a Canadian adolescence.

Hamid

Hamid was the seventeen year old, eldest son and was beginning college in Montreal. As he had often skipped his classes, he was already failing in several courses. He was a good-looking adolescent who was passive and quiet in the sessions. He had spent the summer of 2003 in Egypt with his father, meeting his extended his family. This visit had in fact been a parental strategy to deal with his acting out and identity crisis in Vancouver, where he had begun to feel alienated and dislocated. He had moved from an elite Middle Eastern boy's school to a large public high school in Vancouver amongst mainly South Asian and Caribbean youth, who lived in lower income housing neighborhood. He had become close to some peers in a gang and was eventually involved in drug dealing and delinquent activities. When his mother went to Egypt for the terminal illness of her father, Hamid had been 15 years old. During his mother's absence, his gang had broken into his own family's home and stolen everything of value. This had been his first adolescent derailment and woke up his father to recognition of his emotional absence as a parent since their migration to Canada. Naz blamed Hamid's self-described desire to "become Jamaican," on Ehab's disengagement and her own self preoccupation, though she admitted that she had been "shocked" by Hamid's behaviour and lack of loyalty to the family. Both parents had suddenly realized Hamid's loneliness and his dislocation from Islamic values. They had not recognized his early signs of drug abuse nor understood that his late night outings were warning signals of his gang involvement.

In adult company he was a passive, insecure adolescent who was mourning a shift from a highly entitled past to an economically restricted welfare lifestyle where he shared a bedroom with his two younger brothers. He was insecure about his Islamic identity, avoided mosques, jettisoned his religious identity and was eager to "fit in" to Canadian life. Hamid joined his father and Aisha in the scapegoating of Abdul as the"family problem" and was not helpful to his mother.

Amina

Amina was an attractive, slightly built, shy 15-year-old girl who was having significant difficulty with school as she shifted from English schooling in Vancouver to French immersion in Montreal. She had had attentional problems, distress, insomnia and was becoming increasingly depressed. She nurtured Abdul at times but was often preoccupied with her own burdens. Her father had grown increasingly harsh toward her and Aisha, especially since Aisha often challenged his authority and told him "we would be better off if you leave the family . . . it was so much better when you were gone." Ehab often vented his rage on the more vulnerable Amina, particularly his anxiety that "her clothing was too revealing or sexually provocative compared to Egyptian women." This would cumulate in verbal abuse, with father calling her and Aisha 'whores'. Amina found this quite devastating and would weep, while Aisha grew more enraged. Naz felt powerless to set limits of Ehab's verbal abuse of her and the girls. The parent's frequent quarrels over these issues and her schooling upset Amina who would weep and withdraw. Our team tested Amina and established that she had a learning disability in reading. Her father refused to allow her to enter a special education stream, as he wanted her to go to university. He insisted that she should not stay late for extra tutoring offered by the school, as he was concerned that "she might start meeting Canadian boys." We found an empathic school counselor for Amina, who met her privately at the school. The counselor had previously consulted with us as he was following several South Asian and Middle Eastern adolescent girls in the high school who had stressful acculturation issues arising from pressure to accept arranged marriages or had other family conflicts arising from a dissonance of cultural values. Amina felt that this confidential relationship with the older male counselor was a source of solace and support in dealing with her father's rigidity, as well as her other home and school stressors. She did not have Aisha's assertive voice in the family and identified with Abdul's vulnerability.

Establishing Family Therapy as the Underpinning of Therapeutic Change

The family was initially engaged with a consultation that attempted to begin a narrative process (White & Epston, 1992), and engage in alliance building as well as realigning family boundaries (Bowen, 1978). Presented with a South Asian Canadian psychiatrist, there was immediate ambivalence as well as resonance, as the family felt Otherness was a common bridge of our immigrant identities. They had felt alienated as Muslims in a post 9/11 Noth American context and soon raised racism as a significant stressor in our initial discourse. They were curious about my third generation experience as a South Asian Canadian living in a francophone majority context. Though their children had been given eligibility for English language schooling as they moved from Vancouver, the parents wondered if they could cope with the larger cultural and language issues of francophone Quebec. Though they had spent most of their marital life in migrations, beginning with 12 years in a Middle Eastern Islamic country for father's successful business career, the transition to multicultural Vancouver and Montreal had coincided with a massive change in downward economic and social mobility. They also felt the stigma of their welfare dependent life and their current mental health problems could not be shared in their community.

At our first family consultation, Abdul flew about the room destroying play materials and disrupting my attempts to dialogue with his family. His decade long experience of the parent's serious marital tensions, his mother's djinn possession states, Aisha's open feud with her father and his own acting out at home, were the regular havoc of family experience. As a therapist I felt the first impact of disturbed mentation (Fonagy, & Target, 1996; Target & Fonagy, 1996) and the confusion in this noisy defense (Stirtzinger, & Mishna,1994), as I attempted to engage a child who appeared to be a 'whirling dervish', a mother who insisted she could contain him though he openly defied her, siblings who were largely silent or passive, and a father who nervously smiled and shrugged his shoulders as Abdul diverted attention away from any meaningful discourse. Our initial joining (Minuchin, 1974) in alliance, after our 9/11 and racism discussion, was the analogy of the "whirling dervish", and the family's Islamic values. Later on, I shared a story about the dilemmas of Anwar Sedat's wife Jehan, (Sadat, 1987) in order to engage with the eldest daughter Aisha, who held a strong affective position of sullen silence in the session. This was the story of a young woman trying to navigate a shift in values in a difficult time of Egyptian turmoil and this opened the family to speaking with me about some of their presenting distress.

For the initial weeks, the family felt reluctant to disclose to our treatment team, that they migrated with fourteen djinns that had inhabited Naz's body since her pregnancy with Abdul. His pregnancy had marked a transition in the couple's life journey as he was conceived in the Middle East where mother had been "poisoned" by a black magic potion, and was later born "in exile" in Vancouver, far from their cultural bedrock. In the beginning, we only spoke about issues of racism, Otherness, and Islam. Later, we started to discuss the essentials of their family conflicts, and the parents disclosed the secret of the djinns controlling their family life. Abdul then began to relate his traumatic anxiety about witnessing repetitive djinn possessions and his perception that his mother would die during one of these unpredictable episodes. The episodic crises of his mother's possession states had particularly terrified Abdul when he watched her fall to the floor with distressing somatic sensations of dissociative stupor, "burning head pain," breathlessness, chest pain and visions. While I had some familiarity with Islamic cultures and djinns, my co-therapists and I were both apprehensive and intrigued about co-constructing a meaning between cultural worlds and beliefs of this family and our psychiatric therapy strategies built on structural (Minuchin, 1974),

intergenerational (Bowen, 1978), narrative (White, & Epston, 1992), psychodynamic (Neill, & Kniskern, 1982), cross-cultural (McGoldrick, 1998), and strategic (Selvini-palazzoli, 1988; Papp, 1983) discourse.

The couple would comment later on the therapeutic alliance consolidated with
our team, as they reflected on their earlier therapeutic encounters in Vancouver,
where they faced an explicit suppression of any discussion of Islamic values,
dreams, djinns or any reference to their Middle Eastern heritage. They understood
the Vancouver therapists were making "well intentioned" efforts to accelerate the
family's "assimilation into Canadian society." Yet paradoxically this therapeutic
intervention in Vancouver suppressing any discourse on djinn possession or
cultural issues was a major impediment to their successful rebuilding and rework-
ing of family distress. Their previous psychiatric therapies had always focused
on Abdul's individual problems rather than seeking a systemic and cultural
formulation for his volatile behaviours. Abdul's relentless acting out of undis-
closed familial disturbances and his continuing testing of the failing family
coping strategies had escalated, eventually forcing a return to treatment. His
episodic regressions were helpful to our therapeutic team to identify recurrent the
emergence of posttraumatic triggers in his family system. Abandonment anxieties
and cycles of rage or shaming were recurrent themes for traumatic repetitions
experienced by both Abdul and his parents.

A Family Process of Progressions and Regressions

While in the initial interviews Abdul was clearly the identified patient and the
family scapegoat who caused distress with his "mad and bad behavior," the narrative of the couple and his siblings soon deflected this focus. The marital strain
and emotional divorce of the couple, the downward socio-economic mobility of
the family and the eruptions of djinn possession were hidden behind the family
stasis and the noise (Boszormenyi-Nagy & Framo, 1985; Stirtzinger, & Mishna,
1994) of Abdul's hyperactive acting out. Ehab's detachment from a paternal role,
his own longing for nurturing and his displacement of rage and blame onto his
wife for "ruining Abdul and the girls," were actively countered by mobilizing a
structural shift to empower him and mobilize his active rule in parental tasks.

In the second family session with family therapist Monisha (of South Asian
Christian Canadian origin), Abdul had run out of the clinic onto the street while
Ehab sat by passively. This gave the therapist an opportunity to establish a hierarchy of parental involvement as part of a structural reorganization of the family
system. The therapist asked the father as the head of the family to go to get Abdul,
who had now put himself in danger by acting out his role as a homeless waif.
When his father attempted to take charge of him, Abdul ran up and down the
parking lot and eventually locked himself in the family car. This initial family
therapy session was crucial to family engagement and coincided with Abdul's
admission to a four day per week day hospital. His father now became aware of
his role as indispensable to the therapeutic process and his mother shifted from

her position as a single parent with parental children. In her victim position, Naz had had a strong hold on the affective climate of the home, which had split the parents into a sadistic masochist couple, leaving the system with no leadership or effective instrumental parenting. The issues of the parental team now became the focus of family work while in the day hospital we addressed Abdul's anxieties, competence and social skills.

The couple was offered some sessions with me to understand their trauma, distress and conflict. Family therapy sessions continued to work on parenting, limit setting, problem solving and narrative. The undifferentiated ego mass (Bowen, 1978) of the initially passive family was now shifting to create spaces for the individual voices of the siblings and parents.

Day Hospital as Abdul's Sanctuary

When Abdul came to the day hospital, he had reported longstanding recurrent nightmares of monsters who were coming to eat him and his family. He thought he heard voices of the djinns and that they were coming to kill his mother. As the treatment progressed, his nightmares and auditory hallucinations paralleled anguished moments in his parents' tumultuous relationship, which was marked by periods of separation and reunion. At times Abdul reported that he could feel the monsters bite him in his sleep and he would show us bruises on his arm that were his evidence of "black magic". He repeatedly told us how he only felt safe in the day hospital.

Social skills interventions and art therapy were both approaches we used with Abdul in the day program milieu. Our focus as a team was Abdul's individual functioning, containing his mood lability, helping him with skills of emotional regulation, and supporting his school adaptation, as well as working with his family to understand and reduce his stress at home.

Neuropsychological testing indicated a mild learning disability in decoding and some attentional problems, which responded later in his treatment to a methylphenidate trial (5 mg bid). We were initially impressed by his anxiety (e.g. his fear that his mother would die while he was at school or his father would commit suicide) and emerging traumatic memories (e.g. marital violence and djinn possession states) co-morbid with his attention deficit disorder. He responded to the methylphenidate with both improved attention and reduced anxiety. His capacity for academic work improved.

For many months Abdul remained enormously burdened by his worry about his parents, sharing and seeking daily reassurance from our team, particularly his family therapist Monisha. He settled into more compliant and calm behavior on the unit once he felt his family concerns were being addressed by the therapists. He felt personally implicated in his mother's djinn possession, as these events had been long linked to his conception in the family narrative.

As the team worked on rearranging generational boundaries and strengthening parental teamwork on limit setting, his overburdened position shifted from parental caretaking and mirroring of his mother's moods to a more appropriate dependent child position. On admission, he had been overexcited, non-compliant or oppositional in his class or group activities and he was often unable to learn or manage even in a small class of seven students. However, he progressively settled at school and at home as family issues were exposed and deconstructed. He was comforted when his parents arrived at the day hospital unit for their couple sessions and he felt that we were "taking (his) problems seriously." He particularly attached himself to his family therapist Monisha, and Giovanni, the primary family management consultant, who a male child care worker and family therapist. Giovanni had also formed a strong relationship with Ehab supporting his role as father. He had worked with Ehab to build his parenting capacity and parental alliance with Naz. Giovanni and Monisha focused on family competence and allowed the parents time to slowly share their cultural beliefs and family dynamics.

Marital Turmoil and Djinn Possession

During Abdul's admission to day hospital, Naz began to make a conscious link between her domestic abuse and the arrival of the djinns as related elements of distress. In the course of family therapy, it was evident that Abdul was aware of his mother's depression, possession states, and house bound, phobic behaviors, which he related to the "black magic." The pattern of Naz's intermittent 'unpredictable' panic was not clear to us until Abdul related stories of the djinns, and Naz began to relate these experiences more explicitly both alone and with her husband in our sessions. However, the treatment process did not unfold without obstacles.

Resistances continued and the family often missed their meetings. We would receive calls from the family that Naz could not come as she had fallen into a coma or a djinn possession state. Instrumentally, Naz was overwhelmed and initially we learned that Abdul was physically abusing her just as his father had done. At that point, Giovanni made home visits whenever the family failed to arrive for sessions, linking Abdul's home and day hospital functioning as parts of alliance building. Since separations precipitated regressions in the system, he also asked the family to take care of our day hospital's pet birds as transitional objects during the Christmas holidays. Caring for the birds appeared to validate their functional and caring capacity as they took pride in returning the birds "in good spirits" after the break.

When the parents were initially confronted with their lack of consistency in response to Abdul's outbursts, Ehab would complain about fatigue and Naz insisted, as she was "possessed" by djinns or said, "The black magic was in charge." The family therapist would reframe their resistance as pessimism derived from traumatic repetition, previous failures and fatigue. She would also reframe their struggle to regain optimism, underlining their positive efforts as parents in limit setting. She also used as examples the consistency of Naz's religious devotion and Ehab's diligent efforts at university. Optimism and alliance was encouraged with validation of Abdul's positive behavior at school. Couple and individual therapy "held" their individual narratives and allowed them to reflect on their marital and individual traumas with their own long-standing dysfunction of blame, shame, despair and abuse.

Ehab had earlier emphasized his distance from a religious life, while Naz had found solace in Islam. He would mock her as superstitious, while he tried to connect with the therapist as a "modern and scientific woman." When the therapist took a validating interest in both Naz's Islamic values and the predicament of djinn possession, this ambivalent seduction shifted to Ehab's expressing his ambivalent adherence to his wife's belief system. Ehab then offered to get me a copy of the Qur'an in English and later, with my encouragement, he was willing to seek a suitable imam in Montreal to assist Naz. He met a young Moroccan woman in his classes who had also suffered from djinn possession and she directed him to a respected imam who ran groups for men and women separately.

Fluoxetine had helped to decrease, Naz's panic symptoms when she felt distressed by recurrent somatic symptoms or conflict but the underpinnings of her belief system about these symptoms were embedded in an explanatory motif of djinn possession. "Suspension of disbelief" (Witzum, Grisaru, & Dudowski, 1990), was a therapist position to neither deny nor accept the djinn possession as something we could solve but rather to accept the reality of this paradigm or belief system addressing its framework in a way that was acceptable to the patient. Cultural camouflage as described by Friedman (1982), was a helpful framework for the team to link the symptomatic elaboration of the family's traumatic distress and the complex cultural metaphors inherent to the djinn possession suffering. Both Naz and Ehab agreed their long history of marital dysfunction preceded the djinn possession states and needed to be addressed whether the djinns continue to inhabitate Naz forever or disappeared.

Abdul Leaves Day Hospital

Abdul had significantly improved between his admissions in Sept 2004 to March 2005 when he was discharged from our unit. Naz took a volunteer job in Abdul's school; she competently managed various family crisises, and returned to Egypt once for her mother's myocardial infarct in summer of 2005, leaving Ehab in charge of the family. This was a successful time for Ehab as a parent. He decided to take a job offer in the Middle East, after Naz returned refueled with hope from her trip. Abdul found his father's departure difficult and began to regress again at school. Despite many suspensions and an isolated molestation incident in the summer of 2005, he gradually improved as his mother continued to set firm limits and collaborated with both the school and the therapy team.

The older siblings had made use of the space in the family meetings to deal with their own issues. From early on in the treatment process, Aisha had used the family sessions to challenge her father's episodic rage. She had been her mother's champion when Ehab was physically and verbally abusive in Canada and in the

Middle East but now wanted to relinquish this role to the family therapists. Aisha's initial impenetrable silence shifted in the course of treatment when she later revealed both the secret of her own djinn possession and her experiences of intra-familial incest at the age of nine by a distant male cousin. Incest memories were triggered by Abdul's molestation incident. After leaving our day hospital, Abdul was sexually abused in a park by an older male peer. The perpetrator had attempted to penetrate Abdul. We had alerted Youth Protection to investigate this child abuse incident. Following this incident, Aisha had had a panic episode at her university. She was taken to a hospital emergency room with palpitations, shortness of breath, dizziness and chest pain, as she was afraid she would die. After this crisis, she was able to share her incest secret with her mother and sought individual therapy at her university health service. These events facilitated a new closeness with her mother. Aisha had harbored considerable resentment towards her mother as she felt unpro-tected at times of the incest. Earlier in family sessions, she had expressed her rage against her father's sexually intrusive remarks about the way Amina and she were dressing in Canada. His past infidelities and abusive behavior with her mother had appeared to be the triggers for her anger until the family incest incident revealed another level of identification between Aisha and mother as victims. Aisha was now seeking a more hybridized Canadian identity and was explicitly rejecting the religious beliefs of her mother.

As the family continued in treatment, the parents dealt with other family incidents. Hamid was scanning pornography sites with Abdul, he almost failed his college year and was lapsing into a depression. Once, while the father was away in the Middle East in 2005, he took the family car without telling his mother. This late night outing ended in an accident in a fashionable nightclub area in downtown Montreal. Though Hamid wanted to idealize his father and was exasperated with his mother's episodic crises and Abdul's demanding behaviour, he felt isolated in a family with no male confidants. His father was so preoccupied with other problems and depressed, that Hamid had felt psycho-logically abandoned and sought the excitement of adolescent encounters.

While earlier Hamid and Aisha had often refused to attend "Abdul's family therapy," they later individually sought out the team's support. Hamid felt the thera-pists could understand how he might be able to cope with his bicultural and familial distress. This shift in Hamid occurred only after both Abdul and his parents became more functional and the therapy reduced the high conflict level in the family system.

The incident of Abdul's molestation in the summer of 2005 had set some limits on Hamid's computer access, as his interest in pornography sites had continued. He sought private counseling in his college when he almost failed for the second time. He was still mourning his previous entitled life in the Middle East and it was hard for him to accept the constraints of welfare subsistence. Racism issues arose in his college life and he wanted to distance himself from his mother's Islamic practices. He was still constructing a meaningful identity within his Canadian peer group.

Naz began to feel empowered with the therapeutic team's encouragement to seek her extended family's support in order to lessen Ehab's abusive outbursts towards her. Ehab began to take on his own job seeking in the Middle East, with Naz's initial helping him through former friends. He was invited to come for a job interview in the Middle East in the winter of 2005, around the same time that he found for Naz the local imam who met "possessed women" in a group held in the mosque. The couple began to negotiate a separation that would allow them to create boundaries and reinstate Ehab's role as provider for the family.

Onset and Healing of Djinn Possession

As Abdul stabilized after discharge and the family made structural shifts, Naz's marital relationship transformed with her husband's re-migration to the Middle East. Ehab had become more solicitous as his role as a provider was secured and his paralysis of shame and failure had significantly diminished. Naz was then progressively able to discuss her djinn possession, and the turmoil of her Canadian migration experience. She was able to discuss her screaming uncontrollably at Ehab and the children in Vancouver and reflected that "the magic had made her a child abuser." At that time, her marriage had been mired in intense conflict when Ehab had proceeded to lose all their Middle East savings in a high-risk venture. She began to relate the chronology of events but she was unable to consciously relate the marital crisis to her disinhibited venting and "attacks." The magic or majnun (madness) nonetheless allowed her affects to be uncensored and the structural boundaries of the system were freely discarded. Since her personal mythology linked the black magic potion and entry of djinns to her Middle East traumas, I actively supported her exploration of past and current healing strategies.

Naz had achieved a spacious marriage, a sense of autonomy and additionally the support of her imam's women's group in Montreal. She had in fact gradually become the imam's co-therapist in the group. She commented that many women in the group had endured domestic violence, rape or trauma. Though djinn possession was their common discourse, from her descriptions, many of the women had secondary posttraumatic, depressive, phobic and anxiety symptoms debilitating their functioning.

She was able to discuss djinn possession individually in our sessions and she felt comfortable to recount her long quest for healers. She had sought out some eighteen imams and healers mainly in Egypt and a few in Canada. These experiences formed her knowledge base to assist the imam in the women's group as she disclosed, "I now had grown familiar with the questions they would ask and I could anticipate the things that were going to happen."

On the first of these healing quests, she visited a distant healing shrine in Egypt. Her mother and brother had reluctantly agreed to accompany her. En route by car, she had had an "attack" and the djinns had taken over her body. During this episode, she had felt extreme burning sensations at the top of her head, paralysis of her body on the left side, chest pressure, thirst and eventually fell into a "trance" (dissociative state) where she "could hear them calling her but could not answer them." Her brother and mother had been terrified that she might be having a stroke or dying. They had taken her to the imam who declared that she was possessed by a large number of djinns. The imam asked the family to prepare her for the healing by buying and preparing certain herbs, which were to induce dreams and cleanse her. He then had put his hand on her head and she had fallen into a trance where she could "see visions but could not move (my) body." The imam asked Naz questions, and told her that a group of djinns had entered her body through her head or mouth. He stated these djinns were refusing to leave her body and in any case, she would die if they were to leave. As a healing ritual, she was taught to use certain herbs, and instructed in certain Qur'an verses that she had to repeat. She was also told to use holy water (Qur'an verses were said over this water) when she fell into a "coma" or had somatic "attacks" by the djinns. She related that she had Ehab accompany her many years later to this shrine but he was found the place so "dirty and crushed with a great crowd of people", that he fled and refused to stay to meet this imam.

Naz had met many healers since her first encounter at that shrine. She related that while an imam would touch the top of her head, she would sometimes have a dream or a vision. She was asked to describe the vision and would offer her an interpretation of the origin of her suffering. Sometimes the djinns would speak in their own voices when the imam would ask them questions. First, the healer would ask where they resided in the body, and then from where they came or from which faith they originated from, what message they have brought with them and what was their mission. She said her "group of djinns included Muslim, Jewish and Christian members" who had spoken through her at various times.

Naz had been told at these healing encounters, that the djinns would kill her if they have to leave her body, that they will never leave her or that they might leave only after 14 years. The djinns had stated that they were terrorized by something or someone else and that they had left the mountain in Morocco and traveled for hundreds of miles to inhabit her body. She initially feared they could have caused Abdul's behaviour problems, but many imams had assured her that such a young child could not be possessed.

Naz also had dreams that were often related to the djinns attacking her. During healing visits with various imams and healers, she had had many experiences of dreams that foretold events or revealed frightening past events. Dream interpretation had been part of the familiar repertoire of both the vernacular television culture in Egypt as well as her healers in Egypt and later in Montreal (Al-Aharam, 2006; Marzaweh, 2006; Kakar, 1982; Dols, 1992). Naz felt that her dreams had confirmed that her life was cursed by the entry of the fourteen djinns and that this possession originated from her envious sister-in-law poisoning her during Abdul's pregnancy.

Naz was interested in dream interpretation as her healing interventions were focused on eliciting dreams or visions for interpretation (Dols, 1992). At several of her initial healing encounters, she had vivid dreams. One of these dreams was set in the home of her sister-in-law who was seen surreptitiously putting a black magic potion in her tea. The setting of this vision was her sister-in-law's living room and the vision-stimulated memories of a real event during her pregnancy with Abdul when she visited her sister-in-law in the same living room for tea. Another dream or vision involved the same woman pouring burning oil into the center of Naz's head while she screamed. At this recounting of her vision, the imam had sat down and wept, while he said that he could not cure her and that the presence of oil in such a vision was an ominous sign. In a third dream involving her sister-in-law, she pushed her hand into the earth and pulled out a snake, which she threw at Naz. Subsequently the snake wrapped itself so tightly around Naz's chest that she could not breathe. In each case, these visionary dreams were interpreted by the healers as confirmation of her possession and inferred that a death curse had been sent by her envious sister-in-law, though the healers would only say these were inferences from dreams.

Closure of the Therapeutic Process

On her last trip to Egypt in 2005, Naz sought out a senior imam in Cairo who was a renowned healer. He told that she should continue her psychiatric care in Canada and that she no longer had any djinns. She found his assessment hard to accept. He told her that the real source of her problems was her marriage to a very disturbed and suicidal man. He suggested that she had allowed his misery and distress to be absorbed into her psyche and that this had affected her body as well. He advised her not to live with Ehab anymore, and to maintain her boundaries from him as she would become mad if they would reunite. He told her that she must remain religious and observant rather than seeking the advice of healers or imams who could destabilize her. He also warned her that most healers were charlatans, gave her some herbs to calm her down, telling her that the fluoxetine was working well for her. She was laughing as she related to me, the curious parallels of the senior imam's understanding, which corresponded to insights from our individual and marital therapy sessions. Naz was not yet confident that her djinns had departed. However, she was relieved because she felt much better and her black magic states had ceased. She reflected that somehow she had now become a healer because of being possessed. She felt her djinns had tormented her for nine years but left her a better person and a more deeply religious Muslim.

Naz expressed her gratitude to the day hospital team for the family work that had helped her children. She felt therapy had given her tools to manage her family conflicts more effectively while making a distinction between madness and deep distress. She was pleased that Abdul was progressing in school after so many years of upheaval though she recognized his fragility. She felt that the earlier interventions in Vancouver forbidding her to explore the role of her beliefs and 'the magic' had been harmful, though she stated that she understood most psychiatrists were ignorant about "the magic" and "didn't want to know about this special knowledge.". She felt that our team indeed recognized that "the magic" could not be healed by them but that nonetheless it was a reality of her psychic life. She felt that integrating different and parallel healing approaches rather than judging her as "mad and bad" led to a securing and trusting alliance.

Naz wondered if she could teach me more as a healer by introducing me to her imam. She said, "You could learn from each other." She had taught me about "a shared world view" (Torrey, 1973; Sue & Sue, 2003) and hoped it would benefit others. Though she said most of the women in her group suffered similar distress, she felt that they were uneducated and terrified of psychiatry and that"they would never come to a place like this," because the stigma of mental illness in the community would harm their family relationships.

Naz talked about the visits with Aisha to a healer in Egypt at the time of her father's death and more recently with a healer once in Montreal. In Montreal Aisha had been very upset as she had fallen into a trance and begun to scream uncontrollably. She had had a similar response with the healer in Egypt. When both imams had suggested that Aisha had also been inhabited Aisha had been "terrified and silent." She was the only child who prepared the Qur'an holy water and had administered it to Naz when she fell into her comas or could not breathe. Aisha had refused to discuss this issue with the team and now had refused to continue this ritual with her mother. Ehab also had been diagnosed with djinn possessions in Egypt but had bluntly refused these formulation as he felt Naz's madness was basically superstitious beliefs. He felt his resolution was returned to a meaningful career in the Middle East.

Conclusion

The exploration of possession states and the culturally embedded meaning systems intrinsic to particular cultural spaces has been discussed in the context of many healing systems in Africa, the Middle East and India (Kakar, 1982; Obeyesekere, 1990; Greenberg, & Witztum, 2001; Witztum, Grisarul, & Dudowski 1990; Boddy, 1989; Csordas, 1987). The influence of deeply embedded historical legacies of majnun (Dols, 1992) or madness in medieval Islamic society is particularly relevant to Naz's location of illness meaning as presented in her elaboration of symptom meaning. Her systemic or relational universe and her intimate object relations were clearly implicated in her resolution of trauma and distress, which cascaded through the family system. The marital abuse she suffered was particularly harmful as she endured the loss of her idealized father, the stresses of downward migration, and isolation from her extended family supports. She felt the shame of her husband's infidelity and remained vulnerable financially and socially. Her symptoms and metaphors reversed her helplessness within the nuclear family by giving her a central affective role in the family just as Abdul had a similar role at school. Though Ehab exerted explicitly patriarchal authority, Naz implicitly ruled the affective life of her family until Abdul and her husband competed for the family role as the most disturbed member. Naz's fourteen djinns initially had adamantly refused to leave without killing her, but somehow exited with the orderly departure of her husband and her facilitation of maturation stages of the children. Her religious metaphors and beliefs systems were cemented to the symptom agenda.

As Sudhir Kakar (1982) has reminded us "the line of cleavage in the healing professions and amongst different healers is not simply between 'traditional' and 'modern' or between "Western," and "Asian," or between the healers belonging to different cultures. The real line of cleavage, cutting across cultures and historical eras, seems to be between those whose ideological orientation is more toward the biomedical paradigm of illness, who strictly insist on empirical and rational therapeutics and whose self-image is close to that of a technician, and others whose paradigm of illness is metaphysical, psychological or social, who accord a greater recognition to irrationality in their therapeutics, and who see themselves (and are seen by others) as nearer to the priest. Such a line of demarcation may indeed be an expression of an immemorial dialectic in the healing professions."

In addition to a fluidity of frameworks implied by Kakar (1982) and others, the role of the supernatural in the vernacular cultural of the patient must be accepted as a powerful belief system. In many developing countries mental disorders are often a source of fear and its causes are commonly thought to be supernatural which sometimes leads to a rejection of the mentally ill or a pessimistic attitude (Afana, 2006, personal communication). Greenberg and Witztum (2001) suggest that we work with patients from other cultures by readily acknowledging the relativity of our position (i.e. our belief systems) and be willing to accept that the patient lives, and will continue to live, within the code of his own culture. Every society or culture might have its own hierarchy, and a mental health worker must not imagine that its structure will be suspended to honor an illustrious expert.

Systemic interventions here were informed by family therapy (McGoldrick, 1998; Papp, 1983; White & Epston, 1992; Neil & Knishkern, 1982), though the role of healers and refueling with the country of origin were essential ingredients to the progress of the family's post migration adaptation. The therapeutic intent was to facilitate the family's capacity to find solutions by co-constructing meaning from the multiple dimensions of cultural, psychiatric and systemic agendas. The team validated elements of djinn possession, dream analysis (common in contemporary Egyptian milieus) and the role of black magic in the family's gestalt. At the same time, the therapists provided psychological holding (Winnicott, 1966) and worked at building parental capacity, competence, conflict resolution skills and facilitated transformations of identity. The collateral support of the healers and the dissonance resolved by the family visits to Egypt refueled their attachments and allowed them to process mourning and migration. Consulting traditional healers along with our team shifted the family towards a positive outcome.

The hybridization of meaning systems and the different points of view of the family ranged from identification, ambivalence or refusal. Their religiousness also varied and shifted in the course of therapy. Each family member had begun a third individuation process (Akhtar, 1994) to restructure and hybridize identity in the life long individuation of moving into an alternate cultural space.

This case illustrates how an individual diagnostic focus cannot have achieved a shift in the posttraumatic sequelae without the collateral work on family systems and acknowledging the meaning systems embedded in a family's cultural world. The identified patient initially may have appeared to have been Abdul, but the therapeutic process indicates that the symptom bearers shifted as we explored the underlying elements of affective distress.

References

Akhtar, S. (1994). A Third Individuation: Immigration, Identity and the Psychoanalytic Process. *Journal of American Psychiatry Association, 4*, 1051–1085.

Dream On. (2006, June 22 to 28). *Al-Aharam, Weekly Online.*, Issue no. 800.

American Psychiatric Association. (1994). *Diagnostic and Statistical Manual of mental disorders* (4th ed.). Washington DC: American Psychiatric Press.

Aslam, N. (2004). *Map for Lost Lovers* (p. 170). London: Faber and Faber.

Boddy, J. (1989). *Wombs and Alien Spirits: Women, Men and the Zar cult in Northern Sudan.* Madison: University of Wisconsin Press.

Boszormenyi-Nagy, I., & Framo, J. L. (1985). *Intensive family therapy: theoretical and practical aspects.* New York: Brunner-Routledge.

Bowen, M. (1978). *Family Therapy in Clinical Practice.* New York: Jacob Aronson.

Csordas, R. (1987). Health and the holy in African and Afro-American spirit possession. *Society Sciences & Medicine, 2*, 1–11.

Dols, M. W. (1992). *Majnun: the Madman in Medieval Islamic Society* (p. 294). Oxford: Clarendon Press.

El Khayat, G. (1994). *Une Psychiatrie Moderne pour la Magreb.* Paris: l'Harmahan.

Fonagy, P., & Target, M. (1996). Playing with Reality: I, Theory of Mind and the Normal Development of Psychic Reality. *International Journal of Psycho-Anal, 2*, 217–233

Friedman, E. H. (1982). The Myth of the Shiksa. In M. McGoldrick, J. Pearce & J. Giordino (Eds.), *Ethnicities and Family Therapies* (pp. 499–526). New York: Guilford Press.

Greenberg, D., & Witztum, E. (2001). *Sanity and Sanctity: Mental Health Work Among the Ultra-Orthodox in Jerusalem.* New Haven: Yale University.

Kakar, S. (1982). *Shamans, Mystics and Doctors.* Delhi: Oxford University Press.

Kleinman, A. (1991). *Rethinking Psychiatry: From Cultural Category to Personal Experience.* New York: Free Press.

Marzaweh, G. (2006, August). Une therapie pour le monde arabe? Freud rencontre l'islam (interview). *Courrier International, 822*, 50–51.

McGoldrick, M. (1998). *Re-visioning Family Therapy Race. Culture and Gender in Clinical Practice.* New York: Guilford Press.

Minuchin, S. (1974). *Families and family therapy.* Cambridge: Harvard University Press.

Neill, J. R., & Knishkern, D. P. (Eds.). (1982). *From the Psyche to the System: the evolving therapy of Carl Whittaker.* New York: Guilford Press.

Obeyesekere, G. (1990). *The Work of Culture: Symbolic Transformation in Psychoanalysis and Anthropology.* Chicago: University of Chicago Press.

Papp, P. (1983). *The Process of Change.* New York: Gulford Press.

Sadat, J. (1987). *A Woman of Egypt.* New York: Simon and Shuster.

Selvini-Palazzoli, M. (1988). *The Work of Mara Selvini Palazzoli.* London: Jason Aronson.

Stirtzinger, R., & Mishna, F. (1994). The Borderline Family in the Borderline Child, Understanding and Managing the Noise. *Canadian Journal of Psychiatry, 39*, 333–340.

Sue, D. W., & Sue, D. (2003). *Counseling and the culturally diverse: Theory and practice.* New York: John Wiley and Sons.

Target, M., & Fonagy, P. (1996). Playing with Reality II: The Development of Psychic Reality from a Theoretical Perspective. *International Journal of Psycho-Analysis, 3,* 259–279.

Torrey, E. F. (1973). *The Mind Game: Witchdoctors and psychotherapists.* New York: Bantam Books.

White, M., & Epston, D. (1992). *Narrative Means to Therapeutic Ends.* New York: WW Norton.

Winnicott, D. W. (1966). The Location of Cultural Experience. *International Journal of Psycho-Analysis, 48,* 368–372.

Witztum, E., Grisaru, N., & Dudowski, D. (1990). Mental illness and religious change. *British Journal of Medical Journal, 63,* 33–41.

6
Culturally Relevant Meanings and their Implications on Therapy for Traumatic Grief: Lessons Learned from a Chinese Female Client and Her Fortune-Teller

Catherine So-kum Tang

Human experiences, including traumatic encounters, are typically filtered through cultural lenses that help to define them and hence influence the pattern of coping and subsequent adjustment (Gielen, Fish, & Draguns, 2004; Hoshmand, 2006). Culture also impacts on worldviews of therapists and clients, their expectancies toward therapy, and the therapeutic relationship (Fischer, Jone, & Atkinson, 1998; Pedersen, 2003); which are salient factors influencing the effectiveness of psychotherapy and counseling (Frank & Frank, 1991; Torrey, 1996). As current theoretical models of trauma and their treatment implications have been generated from mostly middle-class English-speaking individuals, they may not be applicable to individuals from other socio-cultural background (Guilfus, 1999; Marsella, Friedman, Gerrity, & Scurfield, 1996). In this chapter, I will present a case example of a traumatically bereaved Chinese woman to illustrate how a lack of cultural sensitivity on the part of the therapist would impede her progress in therapy and led to a pre-mature termination. In subsequent sections, I will first summarize major theoretical and treatment models of traumatic deaths and traumatic grief. I will then discuss how principles from Taoism, Confucianism, and Buddhism influence Chinese cosmology and ontology. Finally, I will describe a case example with session by session summary and reflection.

Traumatic Death and Traumatic Grief

Many clients seek psychological services in order to cope with losses and deaths. Rando (1994) listed six factors that make a death circumstance traumatic. These factors include suddenness and lack of anticipation; violence, mutilation, and destruction; preventability and/or randomness; loss of a child; multiple deaths; or the survivor's personal encounter with death. Rando (1994) further argued that any one factor alone or in combination will generate post-traumatic stress disorder (PTSD) above and beyond that is found in uncomplicated grief. A traumatic death is also a high risk factor for developing complicated grief in survivors.

Traumatic grief, also known as pathological or complicated grief, refers to a syndrome of symptoms that are distinctive from those of bereavement-related depression and anxiety. According to Litchtenthal, Cruess, and Prigerson (2004), traumatic grief can be conceptualized as including symptoms of separation and traumatic distress. Separation distress typically includes preoccupation with thoughts of the deceased to the point of functional impairment, upsetting memories of the deceased, longing and searching for the deceased, and loneliness following the loss. Symptoms of traumatic distress refers to disbelief about the death; mistrust, anger, and detachment from others as a result of the death; feeling shock by the death; and manifesting somatic symptoms of the deceased. Traumatic grief is found to associate with enduring mental and physical health morbidity such as depression, anxiety, PTSD, and suicidality (Litchtenthal, et al., 2004). Thus, traumatically bereaved individuals will need therapists who understand PTSD, comprehend loss (physical, psychosocial, and secondary) and its consequent grief, and know how to intervene both areas separately and in conjunction.

Interventions for traumatic grief are often based on trauma recovery models (Figley, 1985; Foa, Keane, & Friedman, 2000; Keane, Fairbank, Caddell, & Zimering, 1989; van Etten & Taylor, 1998), and involve the application of cognitive behavioral therapy for PTSD management and grief facilitation. Important treatment components include; (1) providing psycho-education about traumatic death and traumatic grief as well as using medication to stabilize traumatically bereaved individuals and to establish their personal safety; (2) helping them construct a narrative account of the traumatic experience from physical, sensory, and visual memory fragments, (3) using primary relationships, natural healing environments, therapeutic support, and/or recovery groups to help them revise their assumptive worldviews and to create meaning of their traumatic experiences, and (4) forming a new identity, moving from seeing themselves as "victims" to "survivors" of traumatic grief, and reconstructing a positive sense of self and the world.

In recent years, concerns have been raised about basic assumptions of various psychosocial trauma models and their treatment implications which are based mainly on middle class White adults. Firstly, these models tend to assume a "benign universe" where traumatic events are infrequent and outside expectable life experiences (van der Kolk, McFarlene, & Weisaeth, 1996). The goal of therapy is to assist traumatized individuals to return to a pre-trauma level of functioning (Janoff-Bulman, 1992). Contrary to this assumption, multiple sources of stressors are often found in the physical, economic, social, political, and religious arenas for some individuals. For example, traumatic encounters such as natural disasters, interpersonal violence, political turmoil, and wars are prevalent among individuals residing in developing countries with few economic and political resources (Marsella, et al., 1996; World Health Organization, 2002). Thus, models with the "benign universe" assumption might be inappropriate for these individuals, with whom there is no definable "pre-trauma" to compare with "post-trauma".

Secondly, current trauma models assume that worldviews about self, others, and the world that are based on middle-class White adults are universal, and treat alternate assumptions as pathological (Gilfus, 1999). These models assume that traumatic events such as the death of love ones will shatter basic assumptions of survivors. Therapists then help these survivors rebuild shattered worldviews and develop a new positive identity by searching new meanings to traumatic experiences (Janoff-Bulman, 1992, van der Kolk, et al., 1996). Although these assumptions generally serve well, they are also at times over-generalized and over-applied. In fact, cultures differ regarding their dominant ideas about the ontology of self as well as relationship between self and others, between self and the universe, and between life and death (Hofstede, 1980; Hwang, 1999; Markus & Kitayama, 1991; Sampson, 2000; Triandis, Leung, Villareal, & Clack, 1985). Depending on one's culture, traumatic events may actually validate instead of violate one's assumptive worldviews (Neimeyer, 1998). Furthermore, current trauma models also tend to disparage the role of suffering in human development and use therapy as a means of ending suffering and restoring happiness. This is at odds with many non-Western cultural and religious beliefs that emphasize the inevitability of human suffering in order to achieve self and spiritual transcendence. For example, the Buddhist perspective views working through a problem as remaining present with one's suffering without trying to flee from it (Daya, 2005).

Thirdly, trauma interventions tend to over-emphasize the compensatory model of helping and coping (Brickman et al., 1982). Traumatized individuals are often seen as not being responsible for the occurrence of the trauma but are responsible for solutions and are believed to need power. The role of therapist is to alter traumatized individuals' maladaptive cognitive processes and to empower them through teaching them to set new standards, to develop new coping strategies, and to search for new meanings. However, these intervention strategies tend to create a high expectation of internal control and personal efficacy of survivors. These demands may then become additional sources of anxiety and depression for individuals who have few inner resources and/or live in constant disruption and violence. Alternate models of helping and coping as well as traditional and cultural healing practices may be more appropriate and in line with worldviews of individuals in some cultures (Gielen, et al., 2004; Moodley & West, 2005). For example, the enlightening model that views traumatized individuals as responsible for problems but unable to provide solutions (Brickman et al., 1982) may be more useful for cultures that endorse Buddhist worldviews. According to Buddhism, cravings for pleasure, material goods, and immortality are sources of human suffering, which can only be relieved through achieving Nirvana, a form of spiritual enlightenment about the true nature and causes of suffering (Daya, 2005).

In subsequent sections, I will describe my therapeutic encounter with a traumatically bereaved Chinese woman and the extent to which the above concerns were indeed valid. This case example also illustrates how a therapist's initial lack of sensitivity and understanding of his/her clients' cultural background and assumptive worldviews would impede the latter's progress in therapy. Before presenting the case summary and session reflections on the therapy process, I will briefly outline the three forces that shape Chinese cosmology and ontology.

Taoism, Confucianism, and Buddhism

Cultures differ in assumptions and definitions of self and its relationship with others (Hofstede, 1980; Hwang, 1999; Markus & Kitayama, 1991; Sampson, 2000; Triandis, et al., 1985). Western psychologists usually assume the self as an object of awareness. It enables one to examine one's differences with other objects in the world and to view oneself as a unique whole with a sense of personal identity. However, many Asian do not conceptualize themselves as independent entities in the world. On the contrary, they conceptualize themselves live in a network of interpersonal relationships. The self is situated at the center of the network, and is surrounded by dominant relationships with family members. In Chinese culture, the personal identity defined by the boundary of one's physical self is identified as the "small self", while the social identity defined by sanguineous ties with one's family members is called the "great self." The "small self" should defer to the "great self" in all matters at all times.

Taoism, along with Confucianism and Buddhism, are the three major forces in defining self and in shaping worldviews of Chinese (So, 2005; Yip, 2004). Taoism was founded in 604 B.C. in China by Lao-Tze, which means "old philosopher". It has a philosophical tradition and also a religious dimension with its own pantheon of gods. Its origins are obscure, but its roots probably developed within ancient shamanistic practices. It stresses the importance of devotional worship as a means of attaining a favorable afterlife. Taoists have always concerned with longevity and immortality. Taoists believe that people are good by nature and that one should be kind to others simply because such behaviors will be reciprocated in afterlife. Immortality can be attained by practices prescribed for longevity as well as by obtaining the mythical elixir of life. Chinese want to be important ancestors in Heaven after their death to help the living. Taoists seek answers to life's problems through inner meditation and outer observation.

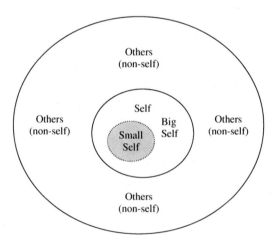

FIGURE 6.1. The Chinese conception of self and others

Taoism's focus on nature and the natural order complements the societal focus of Confucianism. Confucius, known as "master Kung", founded Confucianism in China around 500–400 B.C. Confucianism is a philosophy of life and a "code of conduct" to live. It has a tremendous impact on how Chinese live their lives and exerts great influences in Chinese government, education, and attitudes toward correct personal behavior and individual duties to society. Its "Golden Rule" is "what you do not want done to yourself do not do unto others". Every man should attempt to reach the ideal personhood by leading a virtuous life, by possessing a noble character, and by doing his duty unselfishly with sincerity and truthfulness. To be considered persons, Confucianism requires individuals to "control their desires and maintain Confucian norms" in daily social interactions. The major goal of Confucian self-cultivation is to socialize individuals to suppress personal identity in social interactions and to eliminate personal desires by following the Way of Humanity (Benevolence) proposed by the Law of Heaven.

Buddhism is a major global religion with a complex history and system of beliefs, spreading from Central Asia to China at about second century. The four Noble Truths comprise the essence of Buddha's teachings. Simply put, one's suffering exists because of one's craving for pleasure, material goods, and immortality as well as ignorance about the true nature of things. In order to achieve the transcendent state of Nirvana and free from sufferings, one has to behave with good moral conduct, practice meditation and mental development, and possess wisdom or insight. Buddhism denies the reality of a permanent self and views all things pertaining to the phenomenal world as undergoing constant transformation (Daya, 2005). The doctrine of reincarnation was adapted to Buddhism and Chinese Taoism around 3rd B.C. Reincarnation offers one of the most attractive explanations of human origin and destiny. It gives hope for continuing one's existence in further lives and is a source of comfort especially for those who lack resources. Karma plays out in the Buddhism cycle of rebirth, and refers to good or bad actions one takes during one's lifetime will bring about positive or negative consequences in the long run.

Filial Piety

Filial piety is a central concept in the Confucian ethical system and prescribes how one relates to their parents and ancestors. It is based on a simple fact of Chinese cosmology: Individuals' lives are the continuation of their parents' physical lives. One's body, including hair and skin, is derived from one's parents and exists solely because of them. Therefore, one should have complete obedience to one's parents during their lifetime and to take the best possible care of them when they grow old. Even after their death, one needs to perform ritual sacrifices at their grave site or in the ancestral temple. Filial duty to parents does not end when parents died; death merely alters the form the duty takes. Filial care is reciprocated by blessings from ancestors in the World of Heaven. One of the most important filial duties is to continue the family line, and dying without a son is a serious offence against the concept of filial piety. Because family members are conceived of as a whole body, members of a family residing under the same roof have an obligation to share resources with one another and to assist each other in difficult times.

Ancient stories about filial piety are documented in Chinese literal works, spread orally from generations to generations, and taught in schools. Even nowadays, Chinese children are knowledgeable about these stories and are thus subtly socialized to the concept of filial piety. Instead of emphasizing absolute parental authority, these stories typically described and glorified individuals who took great care of their parents, even if it required the former to put their own lives in danger. The following stories about exemplary filial conduct were among the twenty-four examples combined by Guo Jujing during the Yuan Dynasty in the fourteenth century while he was mourning the death of his father (Knapp, 2005).

Example 1: Fanning the Bed in Summer
The mother of a 9-year-old boy died before his father (167 B.C.). In hot weather, this young boy fanned his father's bed to make it cool before his father slept. And when the winter came, he first slept in his father's bed in order to make the bed warm.

Example 2: Fishing in Winter
Wang's (264 A.D.) step-mother liked fresh fish. In the winter time when there was no fresh fish in the market, he went to a nearby river everyday. He would then lie down naked on the ice of the river and prayed to Buddha. After several hours, the ice began to melt because of his body heat. He would then put his arm into the freezing water until he caught a fish for her step-mother. He would only catch one fish each time so that her step-mother would have a fresh fish every day.

Example 3: Calming the Dead Mother
Wang's (264 A.D.) biological mother had great fear of the sound of thunder. When she died and the voice of thunder happened again, he ran to her tomb and knelt down and called to his mother saying: "I am here, please do not fear!" He never forgot to do this throughout his life.

Example 4: Allowing Mosquitoes to feast on Own Blood
During the Chin Dynasty (4–5 A.D.), there was a poor family that could not afford a gauze net to keep away mosquitoes. The eight-year-old boy would sleep naked and let swarms of mosquitoes bit him without driving them away. In this way, the mosquitoes would not bite his parents.

Example 5: Getting Deer Milk
Yen Tzu's (1122 B.C.) parents were old and had eye troubles. The doctor recommended treating them with deer milk. Yen Tzu wore the fur of a fawn to pretend he was a child of a deer. In this way he would get fresh deer milk. Once he met a hunter who mistook him as a real fawn and was about to shoot him. He cried loudly and told the hunter the truth.

There are two types of filial piety. Reciprocal filial piety refers to physical, emotional, and financial care for one's aged parents out of gratitude for their efforts in having raising one. Authoritarian filial piety entails suppressing one's own wishes, complying with one's parents' wishes, and continuing the family lineage mainly because of role requirements. Yeh and Bedford (2003) argued that reciprocal filial piety may be related to beneficial outcomes such as better intergenerational relationships, lower levels of parent-child conflict, and greater financial, physical and emotional support for parents. In contrast, authoritarian filial piety may be associated with parental emphasis on obedience, impulse control, proper conduct, overprotection, harshness, and inhibition of children's self-expression, self-mastery, and all-round personal development. Ho (1996) also found that filial attitudes tend to moderately associate with over-controlling and harsh parental attitudes toward child training. People endorsing strict filial attitudes are also more inclined to endorse fatalistic, superstitious, and stereotyped beliefs.

Contemporary Chinese societies are undergoing rapid economic and social changes. Exposure to Western influences and expansion of capitalistic economies have no doubt led to increasing numbers of Chinese give up their traditional way of life and adopt Westernized ones. However, the extent to which these changes will also lead to new concepts of self and worldviews in Chinese remains unclear. Research seems to suggest that authoritarian filial piety may have declined, but the affective component of the reciprocal filial piety is still sustained or may even be strengthened (Yeh, 1997). Filial attitudes are more prevalent among people of low socio-economic status, and education has a significant negative relationship with filial attitudes. Women and older people tend to affirm stronger filial attitudes than do men and younger people (Ho, 1996).

Social, Cultural, and Contextual Background of the Case Example

An understanding of the social and cultural background of the therapist and client of the case example as well as contexts with which client's significant life events had taken place is vital in order to comprehend how two individuals sharing one cultural heritage might not share similar worldviews about self, life and death, sufferings, ways of coping, or conceptions of good and bad.

The client of the case example, Ah Ling, is a Chinese woman born in mainland China in the late 1960s. Her parents probably witnessed many historical events in the modern history of China, which was fused with civil wars as well as ecomomic, political, and cultural reforms. After almost 30 years of civil war, the Chinese Communist Party founded the People's Republic of China in 1949. But the construction of a new China was less than a smooth transgression into a new age. In 1958, the Great Leap Forward national plan was launched to stimulate agricultural and industrial productivity across the nation. This ended up being the greatest human-made famine in human history, with which 30 million Chinese were starved to death from 1958 to 1960. This directly led to the turmoil of the Cultural Revolution that was "officially" ended in 1969, during which China almost collapsed into anarchy. The politically charged atmosphere was maintained until 1976, when the new leadership began to address the need for reform and open policy in order to ameliorate life conditions of the Chinese population and to re-strengthen China's economy. During the early years after the establishment of the People's Republic of China, traditional Chinese culture was tolerated to some extent. When the Cultural Revolution began, all forms of traditional Chinese culture were suppressed. In the late 1970s, China urged for a revival of traditional Chinese culture as well as fostering economic and cultural exchange with other countries.

Ah Ling immigrated with her parents to Hong Kong in the late 1970s to "escape from the ruling of the Chinese Communist Party" when she was about 10 years old. Hong Kong, lying at the southern end of China, was a British colony as a result of a series of treaties between the British and Chinese governments in the 1880s. Hong Kong returned to the sovereignty of China in 1997 as a result of the Sino-British Joint Declaration of 1984, with which the Chinese government promised that the socialist economic system in mainland China would not be practised in Hong Kong under the "One Country, Two Systems" policy. Hong Kong's previous capitalist system and life-style would remain unchanged for at least 50 years, or until 2047. Hong Kong would enjoy a high degree of autonomy in all matters except diplomatic affairs and national defence. As a Crown Colony for almost one-and-a-half cen-turies, Hong Kong's educational, social, and political systems have been heavily influenced by the British model. Over the years, Hong Kong has become an afflu-ent metropolitan city with influences from both Western and neighboring Asian countries. People residing in Hong Kong also enjoys a high degree of religious freedom, nevertheless, the majority of her population practices ancestor worship due to strong Confucian influences. The official language of Hong Kong was English until 1997, when Chinese and English became the two official languages. However, Hong Kong Chinese speak with a local dialect called Cantonese and write in complicated Chinese fonts, whereas mainland Chinese speak Mandarin and write in simplified Chinese fonts.

I was the therapist of the case example. I am a Chinese woman born in Hong Kong. I lived in Hong Kong until the completion of high school. Like many of my peers, I spoke Cantonese and was taught to read and write in English since grade school. In high school, I took a popular curriculum – English literature was taught instead of Chinese literature and English history was taught instead of Chinese history. In the early 1980s, I went abroad to the United States to pursue my under-graduate, masters, and doctoral degrees. My graduate training program in Clinical Psychology at that time had an emphasis on the cognitive-behavioral orientation, although other theoretical and intervention approaches were also taught. The great majority of students and teachers in the Clinical Psychology program were Caucasians, but the program director was an African American. There was no special course on cultural psychology and little attention was given to cultural issues in psychotherapy. However, there were several lectures on race and IQ in the assessment course. My first encounter with cultural issues in therapy was during my internship year. I remembered that in one lunch seminar when a video-tape on time-limited psychotherapy was shown to clinical psychology interns, one African American intern commented angrily that "a White therapist will never know how a Black client feels when he/she is in despair." The rest of the seminar was then focused on whether the therapist and client should be of the same cultural background. Given my social and professional training background, I have few opportunity to take note of cultural assumptions and bias in various psychosocial theoretical and treatment models as well as to reflect on how my meagre understanding of Chinese culture would impact on my clinical work with Chinese clients.

Case Summary

Ah Ling was admitted to a psychiatric ward of a university teaching hospital about six years ago for close observation and drug treatment of depression following a suicide attempt. Upon her discharge from the hospital, she was referred to me for cognitive-behavioral therapy "to improve her mood and to correct her dysfunctional thinking." We met for a total of 12 sessions over a two-year time span, with many cancellations during the first year.

Ah Ling was born to a traditional Chinese family in Southern rural China in the late 1960s. Her family immigrated to Hong Kong when she was about ten years old in the late 1970s. Upon arrival in Hong Kong, she and her parents lived in a tiny room in an old apartment flat partitioned into many small rooms where several other immigrant families from mainland China also lived. She remembered that both parents were working all the time, and she was always left unattended and hungry. She did not go to school until one year later, as her parents were too busy to find a primary school that would admit new immigrants from China.

When Ah Ling was about twelve, her father came home one night saying that her mother had returned to China and would never see them again. Very soon, a woman living in the smallest room in the apartment flat, also a new immigrant from China, moved to live with her father. This woman gave birth to two girls during the following three years. When Ah Ling was about age 16, her father had an accident in the construction site where he worked and lost his right upper limb. He stopped working since then, while her step-mother had to take up two jobs to support the family. Ah Ling also needed to quit school and worked in a garment factory.

Ah Ling met a young man at work, and they got married after only a brief courtship because she was pregnant. Shortly after her marriage, she gave birth to a premature girl who lived for only a few days. She did not have much memory of her daughter as she was also hospitalized for childbirth complications. She only recalled that neither her father nor her parents-in-law visited her while she was in the hospital. After discharging from the hospital, relationship with her husband and in-laws became increasingly strained. The young couple often had strong verbal and physical fights even over trivial matters. Moreover, her mother-in-law also frequently complained about her inability to produce offspring because of childbirth complications. Two years later, when Ah Ling heard her step-mother deserted the family, she left her first husband and moved back to live with her father and her two younger step-sisters. She was only 21 years old then, and worked as a part-time waitress to support the family until her second marriage about 10 years later.

Ah Ling's second husband was a supervisor of a cleaning company. Shortly after her second marriage, her father had a severe stroke that left him paralyzed but with intact speech. He was in the hospital for about two months and was discharged to a rehabilitation home where he was extremely unhappy and dissatisfied. Ah Ling persuaded her husband to let her father live with them, who would then surrender his disability allowance to her husband. While her father's physical condition improved gradually, he became very irritable, demanding, and verbally abusive. He always complained that all women, especially his two wives and three daughters, had ill-treated him and tried to get back at him.

About three years later, Ah Ling's father was diagnosed to have terminal liver cancer and became increasingly jaundice with a "big tummy". He would at times become disoriented and thought he was still in China with his first wife. He had multiple home accidents and injuries despite Ah Ling's constant care. Her second husband eventually decided that he had enough of his troublesome and "foul-mouthed" father-in-law. He asked Ah Ling to send him to a rehabilitation home so that they could live a "normal life again." Before she made any arrangement, his second husband moved out of the apartment to live with another woman.

During the following two years, Ah Ling quitted her part-time waitress job to take care of her very sick father until one winter day when she found him lying unconscious and lifeless on the floor. Apparently, he had fallen down from his wheelchair while she was taking a shower. Since his father's death, Ah Ling would sit in his wheelchair all day and became almost catatonic. Her separated husband and two step-sisters took turns to visit her and brought her food to ensure she was all right. This lasted for about half a year, during which she lost almost 9 kg. When she learned that her separated husband's girl-friend gave birth to a baby boy, she asked him not to visit her and to spend more time with his new family. She then returned to work for about a month, but was advised by her employer to rest at home as she was very forgetful and made many mistakes when placing orders for customers.

Ah Ling then stayed home and slept most of the time, only to wake up with nightmares. She would then cry until she was exhausted. About nine months after his father's death, while her two step-sisters were at her apartment to pack all his belongings, Ah Ling suddenly became very upset. She rushed to the living room and attempted to jump out of the window (her flat was on the 25th floor of a tall public housing estate). Luckily her two step-sisters pulled her back to the apartment. The police was called to escort her to the hospital emergency room. She was then hospitalized and on drug treatment for depression.

Sessions 1 and 2: Intake Assessment and Initial Formulation

Ah Ling cancelled the first intake session four times, with reasons that she did not feel well. When she finally attended the first session, it was already three months after her discharge from the hospital. She repeatedly indicated that she had recovered and did not think it was necessary to see me. Her reluctance to enter psychotherapy and flight to health were common responses for most Chinese clients. This may be related to social stigma associated with mental illness and preference for coping within the family among Chinese (So, 2005).

My usual strategies to engage "unmotivated" and "reluctant" clients were to invite them to talk about their perceived major life problems and then to decide together the need for therapy when the initial assessment was completed. I did the same to Ah Ling and she seemed quite agreeable to my suggestion. We then spent two sessions on gathering information about her significant life events as summarized in previous sections. Despite her initial reluctance, Ah Ling was quite spontaneous in offering factual information, but needed prompting and relatively long time to describe her thoughts. She had no spontaneously mentioning of her feelings and emotions in relation to her life events. This again was not uncommon among Chinese clients with lower social-economic backgrounds, who tend to express mental distress through bodily symptoms than to verbalize them (So, 2005).

After integrating the factual information, I noted that Ah Ling had experienced repeated sudden losses and traumatic deaths in her life. The most recent one was the traumatic death of her father about 9 months prior to the intake session. His death, although somewhat expected as he had terminal liver cancer, was sudden as Ah Ling probably did not anticipate it would happen during her brief absence. After his death, she had manifested symptoms of traumatic grief, including separation distress (e.g., having repeated nightmares about his father's falling down from the wheelchair, being unable to care for herself, and making mistakes at work) and traumatic distress (failing to accept the death of his father, refusing to attend his funeral, remaining catatonic as if she was paralyzed, and avoiding social contact). Ah Ling also had an earlier traumatic death of her premature daughter when she was only 18, but she did not manifest symptoms of traumatic grief at that time. She also experienced multiple losses of love objects during her growing up – loss of her biological mother at age 10, loss of her first husband and step-mother at age 21, and loss of her second husband about 6 years ago. At the time of the intake session, she also reported clusters of symptoms that fulfilled the DSM-IV criteria for PTSD and Major Depression.

During Ah Ling's growing up, her parents were probably unable to provide nurturance, support, nor supervision. When the family first immigrated to Hong Kong, her parents were too busy at work. Her father probably had an extra-marital affair with this other woman who later became her step-mother. Their affair might have driven her biological mother away. Her step-mother was also probably too busy with her two young daughters to attend to Ah Ling's physical and emotional needs. Ah Ling's adolescent years were also in great turmoil with her father's disability, her step-mother's absence from home because of work demands, herself dropping out of school, as well as having to care for her father and two younger step-sisters. I speculated that these multiple sources of stress at home might have made her want to leave home. This was made possible by becoming pregnant and getting married at age 17. Given her circumstances, Ah Ling probably had difficulty in forming an integrated sense of self.

After I had some initial formulation of Ah Ling's problems and assessment of her inner resources, I decided to adopt the common protocol for working with PTSD and traumatically bereaved individuals. In achieving various sub-goals, I relied on trauma recovery models (Figley, 1985; Foa, et al., 2000; Keane, et al., 1989; van Etten & Taylor, 1998) to provide a skeletal structure of therapy and the cognitive-behavioral approach to program specific strategies (Fleming & Robinson, 2001; Foa, 2006; Scott & Stradling, 2004). My tentative therapy plan was as follows:

1. To assess safety – to assess risks of suicide attempts and other self-injuries behaviors, risks of re-traumatization, stressors in triggering new traumatic experiences, and the extent of support network;
2. To prioritize therapy goals – Following Rando (1993), intervention for PTSD should precede the management of traumatic grief and mourning, then follow by mood management if necessary;
3. To work on PTSD – especially coping with intrusive thoughts, nightmares;
4. To educate about traumatic deaths and traumatic grief;
5. To search for new meanings of various traumatic experiences; and
6. To integrate new meanings with shattered assumptions.

Sessions 3–6: Embarking the Intervention Program

Session 3: I discussed with Ah Ling about my initial formulation of her problems and the tentative therapy plan. In order to achieve various goals, I suggested bi-weekly meetings for about 8 sessions and longer if necessary. I then asked for her comments and feedback. She said she needed time to digest as I had given her plentiful information, but promised to let me know of her decision in the next session. She also indicated feeling very remorseful of her suicide attempt as she had no real intention to kill herself at that time. I told her that regardless of whether or not she continued therapy, we needed to assess her safety in terms of whether she would attempt to commit suicide again, whether she would encounter stressors that might trigger those "awful feelings and behaviors", and whether she had someone to help or to talk to should the previous two situations arise. She said she was very grateful that I cared so much about her. After assessment, I decided that she was quite "safe" in that she had no further suicidal ideations, there was no immediate stressor that could trigger a traumatic encounter, and her two step-sisters visited her quite frequently.

Toward the end of the session, I briefly explained to Ah Ling about the rationale of the homework assignment. I explained to her that by documenting the time and content of intrusive thoughts/memories and her reactions to them, she would be more able to channel the aroused physical state into more constructive way such as generating alternate coping strategies or seeking support from others. The homework assignment was a way to cope with various intrusive thoughts and memories (e.g., nightmares) of the traumatic death so that they would not overwhelm her and impair her functioning.

In general, I was quite satisfied with this session. I was able to engage Ah Ling, who seemed physically and emotionally in tune with me. I felt we had started to develop a therapeutic alliance.

Session 4: Ah Ling came two weeks later and brought along her completed homework assignment. Although written down in short phrases, her homework assignment provided much information about her intrusive thoughts, memories, and nightmares. She was particularly detailed in describing her nightmares, which usually occurred in early mornings. They were mostly about blood, deaths, and ghosts. She typically woke up with these nightmares, became very frightened, and cried until she was exhausted. Sometimes she would return to sleep, but a lot of times she would just lie awake in the bed for hours before getting up to prepare her breakfast. Intrusive thoughts and memories happened almost every afternoon. They were mainly about things she routinely did with her father before his death, such as feeding him, cleaning him, and helping him getting out of the bed to sit in the wheelchair. Sometimes, these intrusive memories included "bad things" that her father had said to her when he was in bad mood. She usually did nothing to dismiss these intrusive thoughts and waited for them to dissipate naturally, or she would just cry.

In order to manage her PTSD symptoms of intrusive thoughts and avoidant state, I first worked with her in generating alternate ways to cope with intrusive thoughts and memories. However, little progress was made. We also started to identify her avoidant behaviors and examined how they might impede her working through her traumatic death and grief. An avoidance hierarchy was then developed in collaboration with Ah Ling to facilitate her acceptance of her father's death. Visiting her father's grave was rated by her as the least anxiety-provoking and difficult, and discarding her father's belongings was the most anxiety-provoking and difficult. Overall, Ah Ling's progress with therapy was satisfactory. She was more responsive and receptive to concrete suggestions and assignment such as documenting the prevalence of intrusive thoughts and constructing the avoidance hierarchy. However, she was still unable to label or identify feelings associated with intrusive thoughts and memories. I also noted that the frequency of various trauma-related intrusions was quite steady over the last two weeks.

Session 5: Ah Ling arrived on the scheduled date and time. She said she had visited her father's grave twice. She gave detail accounts of how she had planned these visits. Contrary to her fears, she did not lose control of herself at her father's grave. She also planned to pack her father's belongings in her apartment in the next few days. The frequency of intrusive thoughts and memories were about the same, but she did not cry as much as before. I pointed out that she had made significant progress in therapy and praised her effort. I suggested that in the coming 2–3 sessions, she would proceed to search for meanings in her father's death, using a positive focus. Ah Ling did not directly respond to my last suggestion, but asked whether she would stop her homework assignments that required her documenting her intrusive thoughts and nightmares. I asked her to reflect upon purposes of these assignments, to take note of whether these purposes were achieved, and then to decide whether to continue working on these assignments.

She said she had less time to do these assignments because she needed to visit her father's grave more frequently, to tidy her apartment, and to go back to her part-time job. I pointed out that this might be indicative of her improvement with the PTSD symptoms, as she was not as overwhelmed by these intrusions as before. More importantly, she was taking more control of them and was able to make constructive plans of her daily life. Ah Ling did not respond to my last comments nor told me her decision about the homework assignments.

Sessions 6–8 Impasses

Session 6: Ah Ling cancelled three times before she finally came for her 6th session. I had expected her first cancellation, but was quite surprised by her subsequent two defaults. I rationalized that she might be showing resistance, as she was about to venture into more sensitive and anxiety-provoking topics. I also asked myself whether I might be moving too fast with her. She might need time to integrate new behaviors into her daily life. With my interactions with her in previous sessions, I anticipated that it would be more difficult for her to move from a concrete and behavioral level such as documenting intrusive thoughts and constructing avoidance hierarchy to an abstract and verbal level of searching for meanings and putting them into words. Psychologically, it would also be more anxiety-provoking and threatening to her as she would be confronted with her father's death and what it had meant to her. This would probably trigger her pent-up emotions toward her father and his death.

When Ah Ling finally came for her 6th sessions, she apologized for her three cancellations. She thanked me for taking time to see her, but did not think the therapy would help her. She said that after our last session, she asked her two step-sisters to help to pack her father's belongings. They had a big argument over things that needed to be discarded. Finally, the two step-sisters stormed out of the apartment, leaving Ah Ling alone with her father's belongings scattering everywhere. The two step-sisters returned a few hours later to help her tidy the apartment and stayed with her for the night. Since then, memories of her father lying dead on the floor as well as incidents of previous accidents and injuries that he had incurred at home kept flashing back. She also had nightmares almost every day. Her only relief was to visit her father's grave when she would "talk" to him. She said she would like to stop therapy, as she did not think it was an appropriate treatment for her. She said she liked talking to me and she knew I cared about her. She asked if it was possible to come for 30 minutes instead of 50 minutes, and just talked about events that had happened between sessions.

My initial reaction to her request was disappointment. I thought she had made significant progress in the last two sessions and was close to reconstruct her "shattered" assumptions about self, others, and the world; or might even be on her way to "post-traumatic growth". I thought we had implicit agreement or therapeutic alliance to move along this direction. My disappointment in her must have shown through my non-verbal cues, as she was apologetic throughout the session. I reminded myself that one of her "dysfunctional thoughts" would have been

"I am useless, I am a failure." With her life history, she probably would have developed these thoughts and found evidences to confirm them. Thus, I did not relate my disappointment to her. Instead, I repeated my observation about her progress in previous sessions, noted the returning of intrusive thoughts, thanked her for letting me know that therapy did not help her, and praised her for taking control of deciding what would be more appropriate for her. We agreed to continue bi-weekly 30-minute sessions to discuss things that she felt important.

Sessions 7–8: Instead of bi-weekly sessions, Ah Ling actually came every other month because she continued to make last minute cancellations. Both sessions went similarly, with her narrating factually about her nightmares, intrusions of past memories, visits to her father's grave, and fights with her two step-sisters. At the end of Session 8, Ah Ling asked if I would be angry if she stopped coming. My gut response then was to ask her why she thought I would be angry, but I expected that she would probably refer to her own dysfunctional thoughts again. I genuinely told her that I was not angry with her. I saw a lot of strength in her and knew she could handle her life without coming to see me, though with ups and downs. I would miss her and wanted to know how she coped with her life. She would contact me again if she decided to resume therapy. She then thanked me for my patience and understanding, but did not make appointment for the next session.

I asked myself lots of questions after she left.

1. Was I angry with her? Probably not, but I might be disappointed with her. Why would I be disappointed with her? Was I expecting too much from her? Did I impose my own standard of competency on her? Was I being too ambitious with her? Did I disappoint her, as she had continued to see me for about a year despite her initial reluctance? Was this a counter-transference on my part, did she trigger my own fear of disappointing others?
2. Was I angry with myself? Probably yes, I might be angry with myself for not being able to help her. Was this a failing case for me? Probably not, she had learned alternate ways of handling her intrusions and avoidance behaviors. Was this also a counter-transference on my part, did she trigger my fear of failure?
3. Was I correct in my initial conceptualization and treatment plan? Probably yes, I had adopted these models to work with other traumatized clients with satisfactory outcomes. Then, what had gone wrong that drove her away? Was it getting too close for comfort for her? Was this her defense to avoid getting in touch with her feelings about her father, his death, and other things in life? Where would she go from now? Was it a counter-transference on my part, did she trigger my sense of insecurity and doubts about my clinical competency?
4. More fundamentally, did we really have a therapeutic alliance? Did we share common expectancies toward therapy and its outcomes? Did Ah Ling really want to be empowered from a "victim" to become a "survivor"? She seemed more comfortable and energetic in describing her intrusions and nightmares than identifying her associated feelings. Would it be possible that she might be more comfortable with these intrusions and nightmares than without them?

Session 9: Turning Point

I received an unexpected telephone call from Ah Ling about four months after our last session. She asked if I would see her again. I was quite apprehensive about her coming back for therapy, anticipating that she might have another traumatic experience as she seemed vulnerable to sudden trauma. I probably had a sense of guilt for letting her terminate the therapy prematurely. When Ah Ling came, she seemed more relaxed than I saw her in previous sessions. She was again apologetic for not continuing therapy and thanked me several times for seeing her again. No special event had happened in the past few months. Intrusions and nightmares occurred regularly, though less frequently when compared with the last session prior to her premature termination. She now visited her father's grave almost every other day, except when it was raining. Her two step-sisters came to see her every now and then, and they still disputed about whether to discard her father's belongings.

I began to puzzle about underlying reasons that motivated Ah Ling to resume therapy, and I directly asked her about this. She then offered reasons along themes such as that she came because she knew I cared about her. I asked her to describe the most memorable events that had happened since our last session. She then carefully pulled out a small piece of red paper from her purse. She said that she had visited the Wong Tai Sin Temple during the Chinese New Year a month ago. She used to visit the Temple with her father before he was paralyzed. Using the fortune-stick method, she asked Wong Tai Sin for New Year blessings and guidance regarding what she should do with her life. As interpreted by the fortune-teller, Wong Tai Sin wanted Ah Ling to continue doing things that she had been doing with a wise woman. She said she seldom had positive experiences with women, and all women she knew could not be classified as "wise". The only "wise" woman that she had done things with was me. Thus, it was Wong Tai Sin's instruction that she should continue to see me.

Before I proceed with the session summary and reflection, I will present some background information about this popular fortune-telling practice in Hong Kong. The influence of Wong Tai Sin, an indigenous Chinese God, spread from the Guangdong Province in mainland China to Hong Kong in the early twentieth century (Lang & Ragvald, 1993). With his mercy and power, he is said to grant whatever is requested. It is also said that he punishes evils, heals the wounded, and rescues the dying. The Wong Tai Sin Temple was built in Hong Kong in 1915 by Taoist priests, and it is now known for its fortune-telling. Many people who visit the temple come to have their fortunes told, especially during the Chinese New Year. Generally, worshippers entreat the fate of the same year as well as ask for guidance to solve problems. They light worship sticks, kneel before the main altar, make a wish, and shake a bamboo cylinder containing fortune sticks until one falls out. The fortune stick is then exchanged for a piece of red paper bearing the same number of a fortune-poem from the set of numbered poems compiled for this purpose, which contains Wong Tai Sin's answer to worshippers' question. These poems typically refer to incidents from Chinese history and legends as well as teachings from Taoist and Confucian masters. However, they seldom provide any clear answer to worshippers' question, and hence it is necessary to resort to a "fortune-teller" (a professional interpreter of meanings of poems) to explain how these poems encode Wong Tai Sin's commands and guidance for worshippers. The fortune-teller can shift his/her diagnosis and advice in response to cues from clients. When worshippers' wishes eventually come true, they should return to the temple to express their gratitude. When worshippers get warnings of bad luck from Wong Tai Sin, the fortune-teller can also perform certain rituals to undo the bad luck on behalf of Wong Tai Sin.

I felt a little irritated and offended when I learned that Ah Ling resumed therapy because her fortune-teller told her to do so. She must have also detected my non-verbal cues, as she quickly apologized for not following my previous suggestion to continue therapy. I was at a lost as to how to proceed with Ah Ling. I then decided that if I could just let Ah Ling talk about her fortune-teller and temple worshipping, I might pick up some important information to guide my subsequent plan for therapy. I then reassured and encouraged her to talk more about Wong Tai Sin and her fortune-teller's stories. I first asked her what had led her to visit the Temple weeks ago after all these years. She related that as she was packing her father's belongings before the Chinese New year, she saw an old picture of a couple with a young girl holding the fortune-stick cylinder in front of the Wong Tai Sin Temple. She guessed it must be a family picture taken when they first arrived in Hong Kong in the early 80s. She then started to have strange nightmares of a pregnant rabbit being chased and hunted down by people. She would then wake up with cold sweats. She remembered she used to visit the Wong Tai Sin Temple with her father and had their fortune told during the Chinese New Year before he was paralyzed. The fortune-tellers always told stories about animals.

Ah Ling decided to visit the Temple to ask for blessings and to make sense of her nightmares. She brought the fortune stick to an elderly lady fortune-teller, who asked about Ah Ling's birth date and time. She then looked up a book to interpret the message from Wong Tai Sin. Basically, the message said she should be benevolent to all living things. She had done the "right" things in the past and should continue to do so. A wise woman would guide her all the way. Ah Ling said that this fortune-teller was also very wise. She would very quickly identify that either Ah Ling or someone in her family must have some misfortune. She also offered to read Ah Ling's palm without a fee to get more information about her future course of action. According to Ah Ling, this fortune-teller very quickly knew that she once lost a child and would no long bear children. Ah Ling went on to tell the fortune-teller's interpretation of her nightmares. According to the fortune-teller, Ah Ling's previous life was a baby rabbit inside the womb of a rabbit. The nightmares were about her previous life. Because of the bravery of saving her baby rabbit in her womb, the mother rabbit was reincarnated into the highest form of living, a human man. However, the baby rabbit was wounded and defective. So the mother rabbit begged the Heavenly Gods to also reincarnate the baby rabbit as his human offspring so that he would take care of it. Ah Ling went to great length in citing circumstances in her life that would support this fortune-teller's story. For example, her father did mention that he had to fight with several Red Guards to stop them from harassing his young pregnant wife during the Cultural Revolution. She also recalled that when she found her father lying dead on the floor, he did look like a pregnant rabbit – a curled up body with a protruding "big tummy" and one arm around his head as the rabbit's long ear.

As I was listening to Ah Ling and her fortune-teller's story, I was asking myself, "What is going on here?" Ah Ling was showing so much excitement and confidence about what she needed to do (basically to continue what she had done in the past). What was missing in my previous sessions that the fortune-teller was able to provide in order to energize her? I asked Ah Ling if she would need to visit her fortune-teller and the temple frequently. She said the fortune-teller told her there was no need to visit her again if she continued to behave in accordance with Wong Tai Sin's teachings. I asked her what she would like to accomplish if she were to continue therapy. What she told me next really surprised me, "I want to know more about teachings of Wong Tai Sin." I told her that I did not have much knowledge about this Chinese God, but I was aware that she was very excited in learning more about his teachings. Her visit to the Temple and fortune-teller had made an impact on her. I suggested that we both read about Wong Tai Sin and his teachings prior to our next session. Ah Ling agreed to the suggestion. We decided that we would meet monthly thereafter, as she was also planning to return to the part-time waitress job.

After the session with Ah Ling, I kept asking myself what was going on. How should I proceed from now? Should I continue with the original intervention plan – to search for new meanings of her traumatic experiences? Were we really going to discuss Wong Tai Sin and his teachings in subsequent sessions? As I reflected more about this case, I began to take note that the fortune-teller had used Buddhist concepts of reincarnation as well as ways of thinking and teachings of an indigenous Chinese God to communicate with Ah Ling and to explain events that she could not make sense of. On the other hand, I tried to accomplish similar outcomes using theoretical models and strategies that I learned from American clinical training programs. Given Ah Ling's upbringing in a traditional Chinese family that was relatively uninformed of Western influences, her worldviews would probably resemble traditional individuals in mainland China than that of the general public in Hong Kong. She probably related better to Chinese mythologies and stories, Chinese philosophers, and Eastern religious ethics than concepts like "empowerment", "victims", and "survivors".

I decided that it was necessary for me to learn more about traditional Chinese cultural thinking and Eastern religious beliefs in order to communicate with Ah Ling in a medium that she might be more familiar and thus more comfortable with. I then read books and articles in relation to Wong Tai Sin, Taoism, Confucianism, Buddhism, and Chinese traditional healings etc. I even located a website with a computer program that one could have one's fortune told by Wong Tai Sin. I tried several times with the fortune-stick method and found that many fortune poems also alluded to Confucius teachings and Taoist principles. I began to note that Chinese philosophy, religion, and folklores provide fairly comprehensive frameworks in explaining events and happenings, especially those that were not easily accountable by logical and rational thinking. Their teachings and advices often prescribe generic codes of ethics and behaviors that are easily applicable to a wide variety of circumstances. Many of their conceptions and teachings are not new to me, as I often heard from my parents and in grade schools during growing up. Some might even have their parallels in other cultures. However, I was seldom consciously aware of their relevance and made references to them during my clinical work, as my clinical training and experiences have mostly focused on the cognitive-behavioral and psychoanalytic traditions that were grounded in Western theoretical framework and models. Did my lack of cultural sensitivity and understanding lead to a long and winding road in my clinical work with Ah Ling?

Sessions 10–12: Searching for Culturally Relevant Meanings

Ah Ling attended the next three sessions as scheduled with significant improvement. Frequencies of her nightmares had decreased to once or twice between sessions, although intrusive memories of her father still occurred during the day. She now worked part-time and was planning to change to a full-time job. Her relationship with her two step-sisters also improved, and they had visited their father's grave together for the first time during the Ching Ming Festival. This festival is also known as the "Remembrance of Ancestors Day" or "Grave Sweeping Day", an important Chinese festival normally falling on the 4th or 5th of April every year when the whole family would visit ancestors to continue their filial duty of caring for their deceased parents and ancestors.

Throughout these sessions, I encouraged Ah Ling to talk about her thoughts about Wong Tai Sin and his teachings, as well as the extent to which she would relate them to her life circumstances. Despite the fact that she was only in her early 40s and had resided in a Westernized metropolitan city for about 20 years, she still maintained traditional Chinese cultural thinking and beliefs. Her worldviews had been heavily influenced by Taoism, Confucianism, and Buddhism; and she held very rigid views about filial duties. I was also increasingly impressed by her knowledge about Chinese history, culture, and religion. In fact, her father was a high school teacher in Chinese Literature in mainland China before the Cultural Revolution, and she had plenty of exposure to traditional Chinese cultural thinking and writings since an early age.

Ah Ling now eloquently explained that her nightmares and intrusive memories were to remind her that she and her father belonged to one body (a baby rabbit inside the womb of the mother rabbit), and she had dutifully fulfilled her filial obligations to care for her father throughout his sickness. She also saw her various losses and deaths as experiences (sufferings) that she had to go through in this world, either as reminders that she should not crave for worldly transient pleasure or as punishment for her wrong deeds in her previous lives. Most important of all, she now comprehended that the death of his father only meant he was changed into another form of being. All living things and events in the present world were not permanent but subject to change, her present life was a continuation of her previous lives, and good things that she did in this life would be rewarded in her next lives if not in her present life. She said she now realized that many of her life circumstances were tests of her understanding and adherence to teachings of not only Wong Tai Sin, but many Chinese great "masters' (which we usually refer to Chuang Tse, Lao Tse, and Confucius). She had tried her best to adhere to these teachings and filial duties even when facing great life difficulties. She was glad that Wong Tai Sin approved of what she had done and instructed her to continue to do so.

At the end of Session 12, Ah Ling initiated the termination of therapy as she planned to relocate back to China to live with her 70-year-old biological mother. She was remorseful about neglecting her mother in all these years, and was ready to make up for the lost days. We then spent some time in summarizing issues that we had discussed, changes that she had made, and ways to cope with PTSD and depression symptoms. Before saying goodbye, Ah Ling said, "I did not forget the instruction from Wong Tai Sin, I will continue to do things with a wise women. I have always wanted to take care of my mother, and she is a very wise woman."

When I reflected upon these three sessions, I found myself having better connection with Ah Ling as I became more sensitive to her cultural background and beliefs. It was also quite easy to engage her to work on her traumatic grief and related encounters. In line with the original intervention plan, she was taking an active role in confronting and contextualizing her traumatic encounters in these sessions. Instead of searching for "new meanings", she was looking for affirmation of "old meanings" in her traumatic experiences. When viewed with the Taoist, Confucian, and Buddhist perspectives, the death of her father and other traumatic events would indeed reflect the inevitability of human suffering, the constant transformation of the phenomenal world, and the action of karma and reincarnation. These perspectives, especially in Confucianism, also validated her suppression of self and worldly desires to fulfill filial obligations in order to lead a virtuous life. It was possible that her long-held cultural and religious beliefs were temporary laid dormant due to her hyper-arousal and avoidant state following the traumatic death of her father. Thus, she was unable to utilize these beliefs to make sense and to cope with the traumatic event and her daily life. The visit to the Temple, the fortune-teller's story, and teachings of Wong Tai Sin might serve to re-activate her assumptive worldviews. Furthermore, these three sessions also enabled her to focus on utilizing these culturally relevant frameworks to make sense of the past and to plan actions for the future. As she was better able to give meanings to her life experiences, her intrusive thoughts and accompanying disturbing emotions also improved.

Post-Therapy Information

Ah Ling contacted me about two years ago for an urgent appointment in relation to the death of her biological mother in China. She defaulted twice because she needed to be in mainland China to prepare her mother's funeral and related matters. She subsequently decided that there was no need to have this urgent appointment. I contacted her about six months ago to obtain her verbal consent to present her case for this book chapter. She now works as a full-time cashier in a restaurant in a southern city in mainland China.

Overall Reflection

As described in previous sections, there are essential incompatibilities between basic assumptions of Western trauma models and dominant Chinese cultural and religious beliefs in the conception of self and its positioning within the larger social contexts, inevitability of human suffering, life and death, and the "benign universe" etc. Despite these incompatibilities, Western psychosocial approaches to trauma management have been adopted for use in Chinese societies with little investigation into its cultural appropriateness and efficacy.

The case example illustrated that Western trauma models are useful in providing a general framework for structuring the course of intervention. However, certain assumptions of these Western models might not be applicable to some Chinese, especially among those who adhere rigidly to traditional and indigenous worldviews. In working with Chinese clients, unless the therapist is sensitive to areas of incompatibilities between Western and Chinese assumptive worldviews, the therapeutic process may be disrupted and the client may decide to terminate the intervention prematurely. The therapist's cultural understanding of concepts from Taoist, Confucian, and Buddhist perspectives can greatly enhance his/her ability to reach "empathic attunement" to Chinese clients' world schema and internal psychological states – an ability that has been argued as a requirement for effective post-traumatic psychotherapy (Wilson & Thomas, 2004).

Current trauma models tend to focus on the compensatory model of helping (Brickman et al., 1982). Given Chinese attitude toward healing is pluralistic and pragmatic with a propensity toward multiple treatment modalities (So, 2005), the therapist should also be open to alternate models of helping. It is not uncommon for Chinese patients to visit a Buddhist temple, consult a fortune-teller or feng shui master, or even engage in shamanic rituals to relieve their physical ailment and mental distress (Barnes, 1998). In the case example, visiting a temple to worship an indigenous Chinese God, seeking guidance with the fortune-stick method, and consultation with a fortune-teller had been therapeutic in terms of restoring the client's sense of meaning in her life circumstances, validating and affirming her past behaviors, and assisting her to plan her course of actions. As it remains unclear whether it is more effective to follow indigenous healing practices than to adopt Western psychotherapy for Chinese (Shek, 1999), the therapist thus may need to incorporate both traditional and indigenous healing practices into current psychosocial trauma inventions in working with Chinese clients.

To summarize, this case example reflects that scientist-practitioner understanding and practice of trauma work as well as narrative knowing through cultural meaning-making from myths and stories are both important in working with Chinese clients (Hoshmand, 2006). The therapist's cultural understanding will influence the therapeutic relationship and his/her sensitivity to aspects of incompatibility between assumptive worldviews of the client and Western trauma models, as well as patterns of traumatic responding and trajectory of recovery on the part of the client.

References

Barnes, L. L. (1998). The psychologizing of Chinese healing practices in the United States. *Culture, Medicine, & Psychiatry, 22*, 413–443.

Brickman, P., Rabinowitz, V., Karuza, J., Coates, D., Cohn, E., & Kidder L. (1982). Models of helping and coping. *American Psychologist, 37*, 368–384.

Daya, R. (2005). Buddhist moments in psychotherapy. In R. Moodley & W. West (Eds.), *Integrating traditional healing practices into counseling and psychotherapy* (pp. 182–193). Thousand Oaks, CA: Sage Publications, Inc.

Figley, C. (1985). *Trauma and its wake: The study and treatment of post-traumatic stress disorder.* New York: Brunner/Mazel.

Fischer, A., Jone, L., & Atkinson, D. (1998). Reconceptualizing multicultural counseling: Universal healing conditions in a culturally specific context. *The Counseling Psychologist, 26*, 525–588.

Fleming, S., & Robinson, P. (2001). Grief and cognitive-behavioral therapy: The reconstruction of meaning. In M. Stroebe, R. Hansson, W. Stroebe, & H. Schut (Eds.), *Handbook of bereavement research* (pp. 647–670). Washington, D.C: American Psychological Association.

Foa, E. B. (2006). Psychosocial therapy for posttraumatic stress disorder. *Journal of Clinical Psychiatry, 67*, 40–45.

Foa, E. B., Keane, T. M., & Friedman, M. J. (2000). *Effective treatment for PTSD: Practice guidelines from the International Society for Traumatic Stress Studies.* New York: Guilford.

Frank, J. D., & Frank, J. B. (1991). *Persuasion and healing: A comparative study of psychotherapy* (Rev. ed.). Baltimore: John Hopkins University Press.

Gielen, U., Fish, J., & Draguns, J. (2004). *Handbook of culture, therapy, and healing.* New Jersey: Lawrence Erlbaum Associates Publishers.

Gilfus, M. E. (1999). The price of ticket: A survivor-centered appraisal of trauma theory. *Violence Against Women, 5*, 1238–1257.

Ho, D. (1996). Filial piety and its psychological consequences. In M. H. Bond (Ed.), *The handbook of Chinese psychology* (pp.155–165). Hong Kong: Oxford University Press.

Hofstede, G. (1980). *Culture's consequences: International differences on work-related values.* Beverly Hills, CA: Sage.

Hoshmand, L. (2006). *Culture, psychotherapy, and counseling: Critical and integrative perspectives.* Thousand Oaks, CA: Sage.

Hwang, K. (1999). Filial piety and loyalty: Two types of social identification in Confucianism. *Asian Journal of Social Psychology, 2*, 163–183.

Janoff-Bulman, R. (1992). *Shattered assumptions.* New York: Free Press.

Keane, T. M., Fairbank, J. A., Caddell, J. M., & Zimering, R. T. (1989). Implosive (flooding) therapy reduces symptoms of PTSD in Vietnam combat veterans. *Behavior Therapy, 20*, 245–260.

Knapp, K. (2005). *Selfless offspring, filial children and social order in medieval China.* Honolulu: University of Hawaii Press.

Lang, G., & Ragvald, L. (1993). *The rise of a refugee god: Hong Kong's Wong Tai Sin*. Hong Kong: Oxford University Press.

Litchtenthal, W., Cruess, D., & Prigerson, H. (2004). A case for establishing complicated grief as a distinct mental disorder in DSM-V. *Clinical Psychology Review, 24*, 637–662.

Markus, H. R., & Kitayama, S. (1991). Culture and the self: Implications for cognition, emotion, and motivation. *Psychological Review, 98*, 224–253.

Marsella, A. J., Friedman, M. J., Gerrity, E. T., & Scurfield, R. M. (1996). *Ethnocultural aspects of posttraumatic stress disorder*. Washington, DC: American Psychological Association.

Moodley, R., & West, W. (2005). *Integrating traditional healing practices into counseling and psychotherapy*. Thousand Oaks, CA: Sage Publications, Inc.

Neimeyer, R. (1998). *Lessons of loss: A guide to coping*. New York: McGraw-Hill.

Pedersen, P. B. (2003). Culturally biased assumptions in counseling psychology. *The Counseling Psychologist, 31*, 396–403.

Rando, T. (1993). *Treatment of complicated mourning*. Champaign, IL: Research Press.

Rando, T. (1994). Complications in mourning traumatic death. In I. Corless, B. Germino, & M. Pittman (Eds.), *Death, dying, and bereavement: Theoretical perspectives and other ways of knowing* (pp. 253–271). Boston: Jones and Bartlett.

Sampson, E. E. (2000). Reinterpreting individualism and collectivism: Their religious roots and monologic versus dialogic person-other relationship. *American Psychologist, 55*, 1425–1432.

Scott, M. J., & Stradling, S. (2004). *Counselling for Post-traumatic Stress Disorder*. Thousand Oaks, CA: Sage Publications, Inc.

Shek, D. (1999). The development of counseling in four Asian communities: A critical review of the review papers. *Asian Journal of Counseling, 6*, 97–114.

So, J. (2005). Traditional and cultural healing among the Chinese. In R. Moodley, & W. West (Eds.), *Integrating traditional healing practices into counseling and psychotherapy* (pp. 100–111). Thousand Oaks, CA: Sage Publications, Inc.

Torrey, E. F. (1996). *Witchdoctors and psychiatrists: The common roots of psychotherapy and its future*. New York: Harper & Row.

Triandis, H. C., Leung, K., Villareal, M. J., & Clack, F. L. (1985). Allocentric vs idiocentric tendencies: Convergent and discriminant validation. *Journal of Research in Personality, 19*, 395–415.

Van der Kolk, B., McFarlane, A. C., & Weisaeth, L. (1996). *Traumatic stress: The effects of overwhelming experience on mind, body and society*. New York: Guilford.

Van Etten, M. L., & Taylor, S. (1998). Comparative efficacy of treatment for post-traumatic stress disorder: a meta-analysis. *Clinical Psychology and Psychotherapy, 5*, 126–144.

Wilson, J., & Thomas, R. (2004). *Empathy in the treatment of trauma and PTSD*. New York: Brunner-Routledge.

World Health Organization. (2002). *World report on violence and health*. Geneva: World Health Organization.

Yeh, K., & Bedford, O. (2003). A test of the dual filial piety model. *Asian Journal of Social Psychology, 6*, 215–228.

Yeh, K. H. (1997). Changes in the Taiwan people's concept of filial piety. In L. Y. Chang, Y. H. Lu, & F. C. Wang (Eds.), *Taiwanese society in 1990's* (pp. 171–214). Taipei: Academia Sinica.

Yip, K. S. (2004). Taoism and its impact on mental health of the Chinese communities. *International Journal of Social Psychiatry, 50*, 25–42.

7

The Story of Alex, an Armenian Man Who Encounters Evil Every Day

Boris Drožđek

First Impressions of Alex

Alex is a 40-year old Armenian man, born in Azerbaijan, where he had lived until 7 years ago, when he came to the Netherlands, escaping from political and war violence, in search of asylum and safety. He is married to 36-year old Anna and is father of David, a 10-year old boy. In Azerbaijan, after completing high school education, he helped his father in the family business. At present, he is a refugee with a temporary residence permit and no right to work. He is still uncertain about whether he will be repatriated.

Alex is a small man, very anxious, sweating, his body trembling constantly, his legs moving restlessly. The smell of his sweat penetrates the air as he sits in the chair at my office. He has big, brown, wide-open eyes that look out at the world fearfully. He looks as though something awful has happened to him just a second ago, as though he has just encountered evil or been confronted with death and annihilation. He has looked like this throughout the 6 years of our acquaintance – the period during which he has visited me for treatment at the outpatient department of our Trauma clinic.

We talk to each other without help of an interpreter in English, and occasionally in Russian or Dutch. At home back in Azerbaijan Alex spoke Armenian and, at school or in public, Russian. He speaks Azeri as well and he learned good English from his mother, who was an English teacher. In the Netherlands, he has picked up just some basic words in Dutch. When with his wife and son, he speaks Armenian.

English is not my mother tongue either. Originating from Croatia, I was of course brought up speaking Croatian. Since this is a Slavic language, and because, through the years, I have treated many Russian-speaking clients (with help of interpreters), I now manage to understand a lot when people speak to me in Russian, but I can only speak a few words of the language. Living and working in the Netherlands for the past 14 years, I speak Dutch well – as well as English, French, and Italian.

The History of Alex's Complaints

Alex cannot tell precisely when he started to feel bad. Actually, he says that before he was confronted with violence in Azerbaijan, 17 years ago, he felt much different from the way he feels now. He felt good and was healthy, but now he suffers from fears inflicted by the violence he has survived back at home. Talking to his wife, I heard that in the years following the outbreak of ethnic cleansing in Azerbaijan, Alex functioned pretty well, and that she did not think of him as being a sick person.

However, only a month after his arrival in the Netherlands, Alex was referred to the psychiatric services by the medical staff within the asylum seekers' reception centre (AZC), where he was living at the time. He was referred after a routine medical check-up because of evidence of high anxiety, sleeping problems, and social isolation. Alex himself did not ask for a referral, but did not resist it either.

The first medical records from the Crisis Department of the general psychiatric hospital of which our Trauma centre is a part, describe Alex as being very anxious, almost of psychotic intensity, paranoid and depressed. He was haunted by nightmares and could barely sleep. He isolated himself from others within the AZC and he was extremely alert. He expressed a wish to be dead, but still it was possible to make a non-suicide agreement with him.

Alex has never before been treated for psychological problems. As far as is known, there is no history of psychiatric illness or hereditary psychiatric problems in his family.

At that time he was given medication (Thioridazine, Levomepromazine and Citalopram), and he was seen a couple of times by a colleague of mine. Alex was diagnosed with complex posttraumatic stress disorder (PTSD) and depression. Soon he was referred to the more specialized setting of the Trauma Clinic for continuation of his treatment. Upon referral, I was appointed as his therapist. This is when and how Alex and I met for the first time.

Biography

Alex is the only child of married parents. He does not know why he has no brothers or sisters and has never asked the reason. In his country, it is usual for there to be more children in a family. When it was suggested that, as an only child, he might have had a lot of attention, his answer was that his parents had loved him very much.

According to Alex, in the town where they lived, his father was a famous man with a jewelry business. Alex finds it important to add that his father was also a clever man. He says that his mother was an English teacher and was also very intelligent. After he was born, she stopped giving lessons at school and stayed at home to look after Alex and the house. Both his parents are now dead.

When he was young, Alex had no close friends, although there were boys who said that they were his friends, he told – but when they came to his home and saw how well he and his family lived, they were jealous. In his parents' house, there was beautiful furniture, and an imported television and fridge, paintings, etc. Alex puts this jealousy down to the communist idea that everyone must be equal. Therefore, he stopped inviting them to his home. Another problem at least as big was that these friends also might hear what people said in Alex's house and could pass this on to the neighborhood police officer, who would be sniffing like a hungry dog in search of any sentiment not complimentary to the communist regime. In those days, said Alex, it was not unusual for children to spy on their parents and vice versa. He points to corruption in the communist era and says that his father often had to pay hush money to the local police officer. If he had not done that, the family would have had problems. From a very young age, Alex was taught by his father that if he saw anything that might bring problems, it was better not to get involved in order to avoid that possibility. He also taught him to be careful what he said in public, and that "the Azeris are jealous of the Armenians because Armenians are diligent people, successful in business and rich, whilst Azeris are poor and lazy, but still boss in their own country – Azerbaijan".

At home the family were members of the Armenian church (Christian orthodox), but that too was something that was not quite acceptable in the communist era even though there was a church to which they would go now and again. All the rituals and festivities connected with their culture and ethnicity had to be conducted secretly within the four walls of their home.

Alex cannot tell much about his sports, hobbies and free time activities. He says he does not have many memories about that. Every now and then, he went swimming and at home, his mother taught him English language and literature. That is why he can speak quite good English. He describes his English lessons, too, as an activity that had to be kept secret from the outside world. For holidays, the family would make short trips to Russia or would go to their summerhouse on the coast of the Caspian Sea. Alex said that they would often come home earlier than planned because his father would be afraid that their house would be robbed.

On enquiry, it appears that, as a child, Alex was usually frightened, but there were no specific anxiety-driven dreams. He cannot tell any more about this. "That was so long ago that I don't know, and it's also not important any more. What are important is how I feel now and what my life now is," he says repeatedly.

Alex progressed through school in his land at that time from the age of 7 to 17 without having to repeat any years. At school, he did not feel happy because the teachers did not like him and other children bullied him. Alex said that the reason for that was that, on the one hand, they had their own jeweler's business, his father was not a good communist, was not a Party member, and was in fact not at all interested in politics. On the other hand, his grandfather on his father's side fought with the Soviet army against the Germans in the Second World War. Then he was taken prisoner and interned in Germany. At the end of the War, the Americans freed him. When his grandfather came back to the – at that time – Soviet Union, he was questioned about what he had been doing all that time in Germany and he was accused of being a traitor. As a result, he spent a long time in the Gulag in Siberia – an event that has had consequences for the family.

The family got a bad "anti-revolutionary" stigma. Many years later, grandfather came home with a Russian woman whom he had met in the Gulag and divorced his wife. His grandfather died when Alex was still little and Alex can remember only the stories about him.

After getting his school certificate Alex did two years' military service. He served in northern Russia far from his home. His parents came to visit him sometimes but in that period, he himself did not go home. He was an ordinary soldier. The regime in the army was very strict and, besides that, the Russians regarded the people from Alex's region, the Caucasus, as inferiors and called them "the blacks". He felt that he was discriminated against; he kept his distance and had little contact with his fellow soldiers.

After his military service, Alex went to work in his father's business. He made jewelry. When asked whether this was his own wish, he answered that otherwise, he would have made his father unhappy, but he himself would have preferred something less dangerous. In order to be able to continue doing his business, his father sometimes had to smuggle gold or buy off officials. Alex was afraid of that. In spite of that, his father was an example to Alex and he adds that his father was an exceptional man. As an example, he quotes the fact that whenever his father went to the barber or the shoemaker he always paid more than he needed to. His father gave this extra money to those people (mostly Azeris) because they were poor. Moreover, these people, says Alex were in fact the first to turn against them when animosity began between the Armenians and the Azeris.

When he was 21, Alex married. His wife Anna is four years younger than he is and has the same education, plus a period at music school because she intended to go to a higher academy for music. Owing to the constraints imposed by war, nothing came of this. He knew his wife from their time at middle school. She lived in the same neighborhood. She is from a mixed ethnic background. Her father was Azeri and her mother Armenian. Her father abandoned the family when Anna was still very young and took no further part in caring for her. After that, her mother died and her Armenian grandmother brought her up in relative poverty. She grew up to be a nice, somewhat timid, physically fragile, caring person. Alex fell in love, but his parents (mostly his father) were at first against the relationship and the marriage, because she was from a mixed ethnic background and came from a broken home. Alex says that it was then that, for the first time in his life, he rebelled against his father in order to persuade him to agree to the marriage. He shut himself away for three days in his room and refused contact with his family. In the end, his father agreed to Alex's wedding plans. After the marriage, Anna came to live with Alex and his family. She helped in the household and had good, intimate contact with Alex's mother and a respectful but somewhat distant relationship with his father, who was and stayed the head of the family – a true *pater familias*. Later Alex and his wife had one son, who is now 10 years old. He was born after the beginning of the conflict in the country and during the time that Alex and his wife were living in hiding.

The History of the Conflict

The armed conflict between the Azeris and Armenians in Azerbaijan began in 1987 when Alex was 21. In 1987, Armenia attacked Azerbaijan and overran the Nagorno-Karabakh region, where most of the Armenian minority lived. The Russian army was also involved in the conflict since both republics were then still part of the Soviet Union. Azerbaijan later regained its independence in 1991 at the time of the collapse of the Soviet Union and became a republic. In 1994, Azerbaijan had to resolve its conflict with Armenia over Nagorno-Karabakh, and definitively lost the region. More than a million were killed and over 800,000 people became refugees. After that, the tensions between the Azeris and Armenians who lived in other parts of Azerbaijan increased and the Azeris began to show their dissatisfaction with the Armenians publicly. There followed a series of incidents in which Azeris attacked and killed Armenians, the aim being the ethnic cleansing of Armenian people from Azerbaijan. The Armenians were cast in the role of scapegoat, with all the dissatisfactions of the Azeri people being blamed on them. Armenians were openly painted as enemies and profiteers who had misused Azeri hospitality for centuries in order to further their own – particularly economic – interests (since Armenians were traditionally small businesspersons and tradesmen). This conflict also had a religious dimension because the Azeris are Muslims and the Armenians are Christians. Azerbaijan had to be cleansed of Armenians.

Alex's Immersion in Violence

The first actions against Armenians took place in 1998. The wave of violence quickly spread throughout the whole country and reached the town where Alex lived, too. Alex talks how he was afraid and says that he repeatedly asked his father's opinion about the possible danger to the family. The father kept repeating that they just had to carry on with their work and that in their town most probably nothing would happen. Nevertheless, sometimes father said that whatever was going to happen he was not planning to leave his business and his house. Once his father told him that if the Azeris raped the women of the house they should take their own lives. A woman who has been raped shames the family, said he.

Then the animosity in the town between the Azeris and Armenians began with the breaking of Armenians' shop windows, demonstrations by Azeris and the burning of the Armenian Orthodox cross. The Armenians then gathered in the streets to block the way to the Armenian church. The women and children went to the Armenian Church in search of safety and the men began to defend the building. Alex and his father were among the men. During that fight Alex and his father were taken prisoner by the Azeri police. One police officer known to Alex and his father took them aside. He suggested that he would let one of them go in exchange for money from his father. Otherwise, he would kill both of them there and then. Alex says that his father spat in the police officer's face and said that he would not give the money and that the police officer could kill him and let Alex go. The next moment, according to Alex, his father's head was severed with an axe in Alex's presence. Alex received a blow to the back of his head and fell unconscious. He thinks that another policeman hit him with the butt of a rifle.

When he regained consciousness, he found himself inside the Armenian church with his wife and mother. He learned that the Russian soldiers, who had intervened in the battle between the Armenians and Azeris, had found him unconscious and brought him to the church. In the meantime, the Russians had surrounded and protected the church against the Azeri mob. His mother and wife asked about his father, but Alex said nothing about his fate. He said that he knew nothing about it and at some point in the fighting had lost sight of his father.

There was panic in the church; women were praying loudly. No one knew what was going to happen next. People's fear of death was almost palpable. At a certain moment a number of people shouted at Alex and his wife, saying that they must leave the church because they didn't want an Azeri whore in their midst. Alex's mother went to a Russian soldier and asked for protection. She asked for her and her family to be taken to a village outside the town where a good friend of her husband lived. He would take in the family and protect them further. The Russian soldier agreed and drove Alex and the family away in a military jeep. The shop and their own house were left behind them and they took only some documents, jewelry and money with them. They have never gone back to their town.

Life in Hiding: Adik's House

Their father's friend was a Jewish man, Adik, who lived with his wife in a big house. Alex and his family had the basement and Adik lived above them. They stayed in Adik's house for ten years and, apart from going into the garden, they could not go out. Even in the house they had to talk very quietly. Adik regularly reminded them of the fact that all this time Azeris were looking for Armenians and that he was risking his life to protect Alex and his family. And that only because of his good friendship with Alex's father. Now and again Adik took Alex and his family to an old house that was out of the way in the country where they could spend a few hours outdoors, but that was it.

The money and jewelry that they still had were given to Adik, but Adik thought that they had more money because he believed that the father would have been clever enough to take care of that. That was not the case, but he kept putting pressure on them about it. The relationship with Adik's wife was good. She was ill and confined to bed. During their stay in the house, she died of cancer. At the beginning of their stay with him, Adik had promised to find a solution so that the family could go away, but that was not happening. He thought them ungrateful, threatened them with the police and humiliated them.

After a while, Adik began to demand more often that Alex's wife should come to his part of the house to help care for his sick wife. Alex's wife was forced into sexual contact with Adik. This was how she had to pay for the roof over their heads.

In the beginning, Alex did not realize this, but his mother told him indirectly and warned him to accompany his wife whenever Adik called for her. She did not say why. Alex did this but was repeatedly sent away by Adik. He did not dare confront him because, amongst other things, he was scared that Adik would murder him. Also, as a good friend of his father's, Alex respected him, did not want to be ungrateful and hurt him, and besides, was unsure whether to trust in his own suspicions about rape. He was afraid to be turned out of Adik's house onto the street where, as Adik said, th156e Azeris were still sniffing for Armenian blood. Alex was not certain whether his wife was indeed raped by Adik, but the story was told – and confirmed by the wife herself – during a session with both of them together.

After a few years, Alex's mother died, probably of heart disease, and Alex's son, David was born in the hiding place at Adik's house. The mother was buried in Adik's garden.

Finally, Adik organized an escape route for Alex, Anna and David out of the country, but thought it too dangerous for all three of them to go together. Alex had to go first and his wife and child would come afterwards. Alex did not like this in the beginning, but Adik pressured him ("if you love your wife, then you will do this") and finally he agreed.

Journey to the West

Alex was then hidden alone in a truck. He was told that he was going to the Netherlands. He remembers that the journey lasted a long time (about 8 days) and that he had to stay silent, but he no longer knows how the journey went or precisely how long it lasted. He was dropped off close to an asylum centre in the Netherlands where – according to the truck driver – he would have to report.

Adik had promised him that his wife and child would join him in a couple of months, and it was 4 months after his departure that the family was reunited in the Netherlands. Throughout that time, Alex had no idea how or where they were. He arrived in the Netherlands in 1999. He was then 33 years old.

One month after his arrival in the Netherlands Alex was referred to the Trauma Clinic for treatment.

Course of the Treatment

On our first appointment, Alex walked slowly into the room and immediately showed behavior that was marked by somewhat variable but always latently present tension, nervousness, suspicion and fear. His facial expression, especially at first, appeared cramped, sometimes almost a spastic grimace with tic-like movements. He frequently scratched himself with both hands on his upper body and head. He had shaking knees and in his eyes a fixed look of fear. He was very wary and looked around the whole time, checking for danger, and expressed his suspicions immediately. He asked which country I came from and added that

I certainly worked for the KGB (secret services) and am a Russian because my name is Boris. I gave him a short summary of my background and about our clinic that gives help to people who have undergone terrible things in war and because of that have had to leave home. This calmed him down and we could continue with the conversation, but when the door rattled slightly because of a draft, that immediately brought a reaction of freezing and panic in Alex.

In short, during our first meeting Alex showed an extreme preoccupation, almost an obsession, with seeing a deadly threat. We talked further about his problems and I tried to find out what he thought of himself, his health, and the reasons why he was sent to me.

Our first meetings were spent in developing feelings of trust and safety by giving broader explanations about our institution and answering Alex's questions. His complaints were also aired. He complained about tension and fear, and that he could not sleep. He said that in the asylum centre he felt threatened and unsafe, and that other asylum seekers were watching him. That is why he rarely leaves his room and keeps his curtains closed. He lives with his family and 300 other asylum seekers in an ex-army barracks divided into units with small bedrooms, and a common living room with television, common kitchen, bathroom and toilets per unit. He has a small room with a little window and three beds, one table and one wardrobe. He does not dare to go to the toilet or to have a shower because he is frightened of the other residents. He only does these things when necessary – and then preferably at night when most people are asleep. At the end of one of our sessions, I offered Alex medication (Mirtazapine, Thioridazine, Risperidon).

He accepted medication despite the fact that he did not consider himself to be ill, but rather broken by war, violence and flight. He wanted to stay alert to prevent danger. I explained that, thanks to medication, he would feel somewhat calmer and that would give him more strength to stay watchful. I think that he also accepted the medicines out of respect for my authority as a doctor. We agreed that we would see each other once a week in my office to talk about how I could help him with his problems, and that I would also come to visit him in the Asylum centre to see his living conditions. He agreed to that.

In the months that followed, Alex always came on time to his appointments, accompanied by his wife and son, both of whom mostly stayed in the waiting room, although sometimes they were present at the sessions. Conversations about his past and painful experiences alternated with necessary interventions and mediation with institutions and authorities in order to improve Alex's daily life. Thus, a bigger room was found for the family and letters about the state of his health were written to his asylum lawyer and the asylum authorities. I noticed that Alex, in spite of his lack of trust and fear, talked a lot and in great detail about what had happened to him in Azerbaijan. Sometimes I even had to slow down the pace of his painful recollections in order to prevent dissociation and even more inundation by fear.

Initial Transference

It was noticeable that after a few sessions Alex could no longer remember what he had told me before and was surprised when I reminded him of certain details of his life. It frightened him that I knew this, but he did not become suspicious towards me. He put it down to my expertise and this was for him the proof of my strength and special gift to empathize. He said regularly that, since he no longer has any parents or other family, I am his most important adviser and protector. I am not his doctor, but his family, told he. Alex also thought that we had a special attachment because I could understand him better than others did now that he is so far from home. He said that we both grew up in communist countries and knew how that system functioned and what dangers people had to watch out for. Moreover, this despite the fact that the societies of the former Soviet Union and ex-Yugoslavia had only peripheral similarities. In addition, I would be able to understand him well because we both belonged to a sort of "Slavic brotherhood". And this in spite of the facts that his national identity is not Slavic and our religious backgrounds are also different (Alex is Orthodox Christian and I am Catholic).

Alex did not feel comfortable growing up in the former Soviet Union, but it seems as though he is idealizing the "old times" before the disintegration of the country. These were the times of peace, relative safety and order. They were also the times of corruption, double lives, times when it was necessary to have a public and private self in order to survive, but people were not murdered. Alex told me that even in those times Armenians and Azeris did not like each other, but nobody dared to do anything about it or say anything publicly for fear of the KGB, which kept watch over the different peoples of the country. In the Soviet times Alex could behave as an Armenian mostly in private, almost in secret. After the break up of the country and the formation of the states of Armenia and Azerbaijan suddenly it was possible, and even important, to express publicly one's national identity. One could be more himself and show more of himself. Soon this ended in bloody national conflicts. Now in the Netherlands, Alex and other asylum seekers were told that they were free and could freely express themselves. The tradition of Western democracy made that possible. However, considering Alex's earlier experiences in life, how could he believe that? To him it seems safest to follow the only example of safety known to him from Soviet times by reacting to the new environment in a careful and suspicious manner. In his eyes, I was a powerful combination of a transitory object representing the safety of the Soviet times and a father figure who could be his guide in his "new life" in the Netherlands.

Alex Wants to Die

During that time, Alex twice tried to commit suicide. Both times, he intended to cut his wrists with a razor blade. It did not succeed because his hands began to shake. He said that he was a bad man who did not deserve to live. He had failed as a son and husband because he could not protect his father and his wife. He thought only of himself and how to save his own life. He is a coward. A successful suicide would be for him proof that he is not a coward. He did not manage to take his life and became even more convinced of his own worthlessness as a human being.

The suicide attempts brought us to the topic of guilt that burdened Alex. This topic will be present for a long time in therapy and regularly return in our talks. Alex especially reproached himself that in the few seconds before his father's murder he did not say to the police officer that he should kill him and let his father live. A grateful and good son who respects his elders would have to do that. In addition, in his culture, Alex said, respect for your elders is very important. Instead of that he said nothing because he was afraid to die.

Actually, from fear of death Alex froze up and years after that he still finds himself in this frozen state. The first attempts to reframe his thoughts about his feelings of guilt were successful and his suicidal behavior disappeared. It was suggested to him that he should not commit suicide precisely because of respect for his father who had given him the gift of life. The father wanted Alex to live, and to take his own life would be a sign of ungratefulness and cowardice. Alex was also given an explanation about the automatic reactions that people exhibit when confronted by extreme stress – such as the freezing up that happened to him and his father's fighting back by spitting at the police officer. Alex does not need to feel guilty about something that is biologically determined, I suggested.

Systemic Aspects: Alex's Life at "Home"

During my visits to his home, I got a better insight into how Alex functioned inside the family. At home, Alex mainly occupied himself with taking care of the family's safety, but in an extreme fashion. He checked that the doors were locked, took care that the windows were always shut and the curtains drawn and he listened to the noises from the corridor to be able to recognize possible danger in time. This behavior kept them safe back home in Azerbaijan when the conflict began. He spent little time with his son and wife and spoke of nothing but safety. He talked about how he was teaching his son, then six years old, to be prepared for all the evil in life and the inescapable threat of violent death. He wanted to pass onto him the strategies for survival. He also told his son that he must not live his life as the son of "bad" parents. The son did not understand him and ran repeatedly to his mother looking for protection. That angered Alex, who felt powerless because a child should listen to his father, as he himself had listened to his father's words. He felt that he was failing as a parent. He was also unclear about his role as a husband. He told me that inside the family Anna completely took over control of the household and did not listen to him any longer. And in his parents' house his father's word was law. Alex wanted Anna to ask his permission for everything and to leave the room as little as possible. The necessary contacts she had with the personnel of the asylum centre and their lawyer, he considered both unnecessary and dangerous. "Anna is a good woman, but she is stupid because she trusts people. She is also becoming dangerous inside the family because she is pulling all the power to herself," said Alex.

It appeared that Alex had an ambivalent relationship with Anna. This had to do with his suspicions that Adik had raped her. The father had once said that women who had been raped should take their own lives because otherwise they would bring shame to their own family. Anna did not do that. In the traditional segment of Armenian society, the picture that Alex's father sketched out did prevail, but there is also another way to avoid shame. The husband of the raped woman should kill either his wife or the rapist, and in that way cleanse the family's name. However, Alex cannot and does not want to kill anyone, neither Anna nor Adik. He still loves Anna, he has become dependent on her and, after all, she still looks after their son well. Is this one more sign of his weakness; is he failing again, as a man? Alex reminded himself of his grandfather, who was accused by the Soviets for collaborating with the Germans during the war whilst he was a prisoner of war in Germany. It was said that, for a Russian soldier, it would have been better to commit suicide than to fall into enemy hands; he was a traitor. The theme "it is better to be dead than to bring shame" seems to have deep roots in the history of Alex and his family. Besides feeling guilt for the death of his father, Alex was also burdened by a feeling of guilt for not protecting Anna, and for leaving her and their son behind when he left for the Netherlands.

Encounters Unfolding

I confronted Alex with another perspective concerning rape as part of the politics and violence of war. I told him of the systematic rape of women that is part of ethnic cleansing, for example in Bosnia, and that the culprits, when they let the raped women live, do it on purpose, taking into account the traditional way of thinking rooted in the victims' society. They know that these women will have no life left and will have no more children. I told him about the "blaming the victim" strategy and the paradox of the secondary victimization by their own culture. He said that I was trying to soften his feelings of guilt, whilst he "must" feel the guilt – and only God can forgive him.

The relationship between Alex and God was characterized by dependence and ambivalence. Alex believed in God and was brought up in a religious background, but now he asks himself if God is good, because He has allowed so much violence, pain and loss in Azerbaijan. For Alex God became a fearful symbol of punishment, someone who protects bad people. Alex became afraid of God and in that time he went regularly to church to pray. He was afraid that otherwise God would punish him even more. At the same time, he expected a sign from God one day soon that He would forgive him all his sins. Obviously, Alex was also ambivalent towards himself as well. He considered himself to be a bad person, but at the same time he didn't expect God's protection which, according to Alex, was given only to bad people.

As time went on Alex felt more and more under pressure, because of the cumulating of stress in his everyday life. It was decided that, as well as our individual consultations, two colleagues would, in addition, start both family consultations and individual consultations with Anna. The family agreed to it, but at that time Alex was getting steadily worse.

He was even more frightened and developed thoughts about having cancer in his bones. In his youth, he knew a boy who died of this form of cancer. In addition, Adik's wife had died while in a lot of pain with cancer. He taught that cancer was the punishment that he deserved for his shortcomings as a son, father and husband. His preoccupation with cancer was so strong that during our sessions Alex left hardly any space for topics other than cancer. I thought that he was psychotic and falling apart and I prescribed him ever larger doses of anti-psychotics. However, medication had little influence on Alex's thoughts. Consequently, I suggested admission to a psychiatric hospital, but he refused that. He could not desert his family and leave them unprotected as he had done with Adik in the past. In the end I went along with his argumentation and did not try to bring him to a different way of thinking any more; instead I tried to modulate his existing ideas. All right, he had cancer, but I as a doctor could see that it was a form of cancer that grows very slowly. With it he could certainly live for another ten to twenty years. At that, Alex became calmer and his fear decreased. He was again open to talking about other aspects of his life. In the following period now and again, his preoccupation with cancer would increase in parallel with the increase of stress in his everyday life. He could always be calmed down by reminding him of the slow development of his "illness". It was possible gradually to reduce his anti-psychotics down to a maintenance level but I did not dare to stop them altogether. The pills helped me probably to moderate my feelings of powerlessness in my dealings with Alex.

A few months later in family therapy the great family "secret" was disclosed. Anna told of her rape by Adik. Alex did not react with panic. He asked for advice about how to go on living with this knowledge and shared with me his misgivings. He was preoccupied with three dilemmas – the fact that Anna, as a woman, is not "clean" any more, his feelings of guilt because of having failed as a protector, and his ambivalence towards Adik who was at the same time his/their protector and the culprit. During this period, Alex began more often to ask himself questions about his relationship with his father. He allowed himself to have doubts about his father's moral integrity. He took it against his idealized father that sometime has cheated his customers, among them Azeris, and that he did not prevent the tragedy to the family by, for example, leaving the town on time, as had a number of their Armenian acquaintances. The father thought the money and his possessions more important than his family, said Alex, disappointed.

I interpreted the emergence of ambivalent feelings in Alex as progress and the beginning of the mourning process for his many losses. However, one could not look after all the wounds at the same time and Alex soon stopped sharing his thoughts about Anna's rape with me. It seemed that this topic did not preoccupy him any more and that he started to suppress it as he had done in the past.

In the following months, Alex's state was variable and there were many changes in his life. One of these was the fact that the authorities refused his asylum application and his lawyer started a new procedure based on medical grounds. It has to be said that Alex understood little of the asylum procedure and it was mainly Anna who was in touch with the lawyer. In addition, the family was transferred to another asylum centre because the previous one was going to be closed. The change in his circumstances was very stressful for Alex and his psychological state deteriorated. Once again, he was preoccupied by the fear of cancer and felt threatened by the people in the new asylum centre. He taught that these people want to get him in order to get to his father's money and maybe even Adik himself will come to the Netherlands to get the money. They do not believe that he does not have the money and because they will not find anything, they will murder him and his family. It was difficult to influence these thoughts of Alex and the dosage of anti-psychotics went up again. That numbed and calmed him down somewhat.

I asked myself whether Alex was psychotic or whether his cognitions were a logical consequence of the experiences he had gone through in his life. Alternatively, are his cognitions the result of the changes in his core beliefs with just an added psychotic "edge" whenever there is an increase in stress in the here and now? Would he ever get better? Should he be getting anti-psychotics at all? He found his fears and preoccupations with danger entirely logical. "Because I was alert in Azerbaijan, I managed to survive. I cannot afford to let that control go now. Moreover, what you say about the Netherlands not being Azerbaijan and that there is no war here, that is no argument. In Azerbaijan, everything began very suddenly and people who used to be your friends became your murderers. So control and alertness are essential for survival, Alex told me repeatedly. In addition, because the anti-psychotics were not having the desired effect, I gave in to Alex's reasoning and the anti-psychotics were again reduced.

Transference Developing

At the same time, I was becoming aware of my fears that I would never be able to help Alex get better. I also developed several fantasies about how to save Alex. In the event that Alex and his family did not get asylum in the Netherlands, I would get in touch with acquaintances who worked in television to make a program that would attract public attention to his case. In order to protect Alex I would write protest letters to government ministers and to the association of medical specialists. I asked myself as well whether I could continue my work as a trauma therapist after such a disappointment. However, at the same time I was afraid to attack the authorities. My own upbringing and growing up in ex-Yugoslavia played a role in that. I had learned that the government always has power and the citizen has only limited freedom to express his own opinion. And in the end the government always wins. I asked myself if I, a person of foreign origin, would dare to risk confronting the Dutch authorities. During my team's intervision session I became aware of the parallel processes in my relationship with Alex. We were both suspicious of the power structures and I was trying to compensate for his failures as a protector. And maybe, as a therapist, I was already doing everything that I could for him in the given circumstances – by having created a safe haven for him where he could share his fears, learn again to trust his fellow men and get stronger in order to be able to pick up his life again. Finally, even if rejected for asylum in the Netherlands, it doesn't mean that he has to go back to his own country to be killed there, or that he will commit suicide. He could still disappear into illegality or get enough money together to emigrate illegally to another country. Our contacts continued.

One of the focuses in our sessions was to list the remaining strengths in Alex's self with the intention of improving his daily ability to function (empowerment). Partly at his suggestion, his relationships with Anna and his son were examined, and we searched for points that could be improved on. It was noticeable that Alex adopted a regressive position. He had no knowledge of what a healthy adult relationship should look like. He could not remember what his relationship with Anna was like before the war, or what his parents' relationship was like. He asked me to give him concrete advice about how a grown up man should behave in the family, and what were his responsibilities. I had to tell him literally, how he could show his affection to Anna, how he would have to express his love and care, how he would have to play and talk with his son. It seemed that Alex understood my advice but he always asked for a delay in putting it into practice.

Alex did hardly anything with this advice in his domestic situation. His only – and the most important role – at home was that of a protector and he did not see any other aspects of his role as a father and husband.

A Better Future?

When, after four and a half years in the Netherlands, Alex was the only one in the family to receive a temporary residence permit based on his bad psychological state, and he could exchange his one room in the asylum centre for a family house in a small neighboring town, his behavior and habits hardly changed. At first, yet another change in his life gave him great difficulties. "All the changes up until now have led to problems; why should this one lead to improvements?" he asked me. After some time, he was happy with the improved safety. In his house, he could have a shower and go to the toilet without being disturbed. He even went alone for a walk more often, but he restricted himself to doing this only when it was raining. Then there were fewer people in the streets and he felt himself less threatened. At home, he spent most of his time behind the large window in his living room, keeping an eye on the street from behind the blinds. Often he told me with pride about how good he had become at taking care of his family's safety. It seemed as though he had finally found a territory in which he could assume an identity and show competency. He was "the protector". At a certain moment, he was even ready to share with me the responsibility of safety. "The world is too big and I can't deal with all of it. You take care that you get a good insight into the dangers that exist in the world and I shall limit myself to the safety in my immediate surroundings," suggested Alex in one of the sessions. After that, this became the agreement between us. Alex became more relaxed and our relationship seemed to resemble a more balanced partnership between two adult men.

Gradually relinquishing the need for control in his life became the new target of Alex's therapy. We analyzed the difference between how to guarantee safety in time of war and in times of peace. Are his vigilance and the control that he used in times of war to stay alive the most appropriate survival strategies in his present life? Does he dare to trust me, after his disappointing experiences with protectors in his earlier life, and can he share areas of control with me? Would he ever feel safe enough to go through life without an external protector and could he internalize his feeling of safety? The terms "war mode" and "peace mode" within which he could function were introduced. How could he switch on time between the two modes, for example on the first day of an imaginary future war? Can he behave in peacetime as though it is peacetime, and in war as though it is wartime?

Alex told me about the first signs of unrest in Azerbaijan. Public transport ground to a halt, Armenians' passports were taken away, the symbols of his nation were destroyed, crosses were burned, Armenians' shops were smashed, there were riots in the streets. Only after that did the Azeris begin to kill. Therefore, there was time to escape and avoid the danger. Alex, as the experienced "danger specialist", has time to switch from "peace mode" into "war mode" if he is aware of these signals. He does not need to interpret everything as a threat and to generalize danger. Along with that, he can rely on my estimate of danger in the arena of world politics and take into account the fact that I will warn him in time. I also used the metaphor of "the commander and the soldiers on guard duty". The commander orders the soldiers when to be on guard and when not to be. He tells them when to relieve one another. Alex is always on guard duty, he takes no rest and because of that, he gets tired, exhausted and no longer capable of doing his guard duty well. Then he is not able to function well as a father and a husband. Although in the beginning Alex had difficulty in accepting these new ideas, in small steps over the course of time I could see changes in his way of thinking and his behavior.

He also realized that his suspicion might have something to do with other things as well and not only with his war experiences. Suspicion is something he had inherited from his father and is a historical legacy: on one hand, from the life lived by Armenians in Azerbaijan and, equally on the other, from life in the ex Soviet Union where people lived in great fear of the secret service (KGB). In addition, he began to see the relativity of circumstances to the expression of evil in people. Only during war do people change en masse into beasts whilst, when not at war, they can hate each other but are rarely destructive on a large scale.

In one of the sessions we looked back to Alex's own explanatory model for his problems. He does not consider himself a psychiatric patient, although he knows that I am a psychiatrist and helping him. He comes to me because he has problems with the governments of Azerbaijan and the Netherlands, is too weak himself, and not influential enough to solve them. I am a doctor, but above all, for him I am a warm human being on whom he can rely and who will always be there for him. I also live in a town and he in a village. In the event of riots (that mostly take place in towns, he says) I can give him and his family a timely warning to flee. Then we shall flee together, says Alex. In terms of illness, Alex suffers from cancer but I cannot help him with that. The biggest secret kept from his family is his fear of failing them as a protector. By looking after them well, he wants to reduce his feelings of guilt and shame in connection with his previous failures as the protector. I tried to suggest to him other actions (rituals) that could rid him of guilt and would have no connection with his family. What could he do for the world, with his experience whom else could he help? Whom else could he care for? However, Alex was not open to that. At this moment he wants to focus on what more he can do for his family and he wants to think more about that. The world and the people outside his family and his therapist hardly interest him at all.

Only recently, interesting changes occurred in Alex's treatment. David started asking Anna for help with his math homework. Since Anna could not be of help, she referred him to Alex. Alex was at school always good in math, but did not understand David's assignment written in Dutch. This frustrated him so much, that he asked me for advice. He wanted to help his son and learn the language, but was afraid of loosing control over the "safety issues" while concentrating on studying. At that point, we have made an arrangement with Anna. While Alex is learning, Anna has to focus on the "safety issues". Alex is going to learn in blocks of 45 minutes, interrupted by 15 minutes breaks wherein he can take care of the "safety issues" by himself. This arrangement worked out well and Alex became the appointed person in the family when it comes to David's math homework assignments. He started to learn Dutch almost every day for a couple of hours, and he expanded his spectrum of activities at home beyond the role of the protector. He is now vacuuming the house and playing chess with David, who recently got interested in this game, while Anna is sitting on his place behind the large window in their living room, keeping an eye on the street from behind the blinds, and relaxing.

Some Concluding Remarks and How to Proceed

This is the point that Alex and I have reached after having talked for five years. Following his rapid attachment to me in a superficial manner and his telling me the story of his life in detail at the beginning of our contacts, it took many years to build the foundations for a relationship of trust. Alex was brought up in a protected way and in an atmosphere where it was even necessary to maintain a strict division between his private and public self. In addition, his soul was torn apart because of the violence to which he was nakedly exposed, and someone in whom he had trusted deceived him. This is why he needed a long time before he dared take risks and once again form an attachment with someone. He also needed a long time because he was forced to leave his country and found himself lonely in another – for him – unknown country, confronted with a different culture, language, society and political system. In the person of the therapist, he found a number of symbolic "lost certainties". These are the understanding of the Russian language and knowledge of Slav peoples and cultures. Also, there were in his view equivalents between him and the therapist in terms of growing up in a socialist/communist society and being a migrant.

Alex strongly idealized me because I formed a protective layer around his tumultuous self, a cocoon to contain his chaotic feelings. With the passage of time, our relationship became more balanced and a partnership was formed concerning the guarding of safety in life. Later Alex developed ambivalent feelings concerning his father and Adik, the two important protecting figures in his past, so that, in my view, the way is now open for mourning the disappointments and losses he has suffered.

After five years of therapy, in small steps Alex begins to investigate the world around him and to rediscover himself in this world. He dares to share with me the responsibility for control over his life, which will hopefully leave more room to take up again his roles as husband and father. In family therapy, on which I haven't focused in this chapter, the rape of his wife Anna was revealed and discussed, but apart from reducing tension in the relationship, this brought no significant changes in the way the couple were functioning with respect to each other. The secret was spoken about, but remained laden with shame and guilt. Alex remains the dysfunctionally functioning protector of the family, Anna the driving force who makes survival in the Netherlands possible. She cares for her husband as a patient and looks after their son David, who is a somewhat lonely boy trying to build the foundations for his life in the Netherlands by getting good marks at school and forming a few friendships with Dutch children of his own age.

Besides the consultations that are going to be continued, Alex is still treated with medication (Setraline, Topiramate, Clopixol in low maintenance doses). These drugs will hopefully protect him from the "psychotic edges" that currently manifest themselves at moments of great stress. They are a sort of "glue" that holds Alex's broken soul together as he wrestles with the demons from his past and carefully examines the vacuum of the present, trying to find a road to the future for himself and his family.

Comments on the Cultural Formulation of Diagnosis

Alex's Cultural Identity

Alex is Armenian and belongs to the minority in Azerbaijan, the land of his birth. The history of the Armenian people and their presence in what we now know as Azerbaijan goes back approximately 3,000 years. "Historic" Armenia (the area traditionally inhabited and, for very brief periods of time, ruled by Armenians) encompasses the eastern-most part of Turkey, southern Georgia, Armenia, most of Azerbaijan and north-western Iran. It is uncertain whether the Armenian people were the original inhabitants of this area or were migrants from Europe and Mesopotamia. The Armenian language has developed from a very early form of Indo-European and the alphabet was developed around 400 A.D. largely out of fear of losing their Armenian identity after being partitioned by the Byzantine and Persian empires. The uniqueness of the alphabet and language along with the Armenian religion have allowed the Armenian culture to survive for 3,000 years in the face of nearly constant occupation and foreign rule.

In the third century A.D., the Armenian dynasty adopted Christianity in order to limit the influence of the Iranian resurgence of the Zoroastrian religion. This resulted in an invasion of Armenia and the destruction of their capital. Rome intervened on behalf of the Armenians leading to the eventual division and sub-jugation of Armenia to Rome (Byzantium) and Iran. The adoption and strong adherence to the Armenian Church has distinguished the Armenian people and has contributed both to their history of genocide at the hands of the Turks and to their close historical ties with Russia.

The more recent history of Armenians in Azerbaijan includes the Nagorno-Karabakh conflict, which like so many territorial disputes in the Caucasus, has its roots in the "divide and rule" ethnic policies of Stalin and the Soviets. In 1918, Armenia experienced a brief period of independence, but this ended in 1920 when the entire region was invaded by the Bolsheviks and incorporated into the Soviet Union. Soviets divided Armenian territory between Azerbaijan, Georgia, Turkey, and the area which eventually became the Armenian Soviet Republic and was based on the administrative district of Yerevan, a backward and impoverished area. Since most Armenian wealth was located in the cities of Tbilisi (Georgia) and Baku (Azerbaijan), Armenia became one of the smallest and one of the least influential of the Soviet republics. Through Soviet rule, the Armenian economy was transformed from agriculture to industry and the Soviet authorities under Stalin made every attempt to break Armenian culture and heritage. Despite this, Armenian culture survived and prospered, 99% of ethnic Armenians listed Armenian as their primary language. Additionally, Armenia as a whole pros-pered, their per capita income was higher than that for the Soviet Union as a whole and 70% of Armenians were urban. Because of their prosperity, despite the early hardships suffered under Stalin, Armenians continued to be very pro-Russian. In the case of Alex, the Soviet Union symbolizes the peaceful times of his past, when life still seemed to be controllable.

Alex cannot identify himself with Dutch society, above all because he is afraid of everything that is unknown to him. He feels unsafe and that feeling does not seem to depend on the situation in which he finds himself. In that sense, he shows no interest in the context of his life in the Netherlands and he remains preoccu-pied with safety and the protection of his family. Despite the fact that the only connections he has are with his family, his therapist and the system therapist attached to the family, Alex does not feel alone in the Netherlands. For him, more contact means less clarity and the greater the risk, and that is why he avoids it. For these reasons, Alex has not been able to take on the identity of a migrant in the Netherlands. His identity is that of a victim of violence and of a failing protector, pierced by feelings of fear and guilt.

Alex does not understand the asylum procedure in the Netherlands and does not feel involved in it. For example, he does not know the difference between the status based on political grounds and the status based on medical-humanitarian grounds, or what falls under the Dutch government's policy concerning trauma. Alex has not seen his lawyer for about two years. He does not find the asylum procedure important. The procedure is a peacetime phenomenon that has to do with the future, whilst in terms of his feelings Alex is still in the war and is solely focussed for the moment on survival.

Alex's native language is Armenian. He also learned Russian and Azeri at home and at school, and English from his mother. Because of fears, attention and concentration disorders on the one hand, and the unavailability of language courses for asylum seekers on the other, he has not started to learn Dutch. He has only learned a few words from the television or from his wife and son. Only recently, he started to learn the language by himself at home in order to restore his paternal role.

Alex has no contacts with his compatriots or with the Dutch because of mistrust that can be seen as a damaged core belief or basic assumption (Janoff-Bulman, 1983) within the framework of his complex and chronic post-traumatic damage.

Cultural Explanations for Alex's Complaints

The terms that Alex uses most often to describe his complaints are tension, fear and sleeplessness. He does not consider himself to be ill or a patient. He is broken by the war, violence and enforced flight. He does not see his excessive vigilance and suspicion as ego-dystonic, but as a logical consequence of the experiences in his life and an important part of his survival strategy. He feels that he is a bad man who, according to the norms and values of his culture and upbringing, has failed as son, husband and a man. The somatic complaints in the form of pain and itching that Alex often presents, have a partly organic basis (eczema), but he puts them forward as symptoms of cancer. Cancer is the punishment for his failure in life.

The fact that Alex does not consider himself a psychiatric patient and does not see his therapist as a psychiatrist but as an advisor, might also have to do with the standing of psychiatry in the former Soviet Union. Alex is afraid of psychiatry because it was an instrument of oppression. Enemies of the state and dissidents were declared psychiatric patients and were locked up in psychiatric hospitals and tortured.

The culture from which Alex derived his identity is a culture in transition form a collectivist "We" culture to an individualistic "I" culture. In the communist Soviet Union and the traditional cultures of the Caucasian nations collective norms and values were seen as the most important and most valued, and as such were the basis for the creation of the public self of the individual. The group and the society expect of all its members that they will share the same morality and accept and respect the same norms and values. Those who do not hold to that get personally punished, but their misdeeds can also have consequences for their descendents. The stigma can be attached to the descendents by the political system (the "anti-revolutionary" family), religion (God's punishment) and by the culture (the family's name must be purified). At the same time, Alex also had a more individualised identity, a private self that he could only use "underground" and within his family life. He was aware that he was "different" from his environment because he belonged to the ethnic minority and to a family that cherished anti-revolutionary and intellectual values.

Whilst in an individualised "I" culture the individual is himself held responsible for his behaviour and its consequences, in the "We" culture the responsibility is also assigned to the family and the group. In the "We" culture illness is a social, not just an individual, problem. In Alex's case, both explanations are valid. Alex could not protect his father and wife against, respectively, the death of the former and rape of the latter, and for that, he has to pay. Because his faults are irreparable, his punishment is an incurable illness – cancer. Alex had internalised the feelings of guilt that are prevalent in his culture, and this formed the basis for his depression and hypochondriac ideas. At the same time, Alex tries to correct his faults and relieve his feelings of guilt by being obsessive about the protection of his family in the Netherlands. The improvement of his own ability to function is Alex's reason to accept professional help.

The fact that Alex has psychological complaints and is being treated for them has influenced his asylum procedure and has led to an – at the moment – temporary residence permit. Nevertheless, the influence of his illness in other areas, has not until now been reflected in the way his therapy is unfolding. Above all Alex is focused on looking for solutions for his psychological, relational and physical problems and not on obtaining a residence permit. At the same time, the therapist is clear about his role in terms of formulating of his competencies and defining his professional boundaries. However, he is also prepared to support Alex's asylum procedure by sending the medical findings to the relevant agencies – that is to say the lawyers and the Medical Advice Bureau of the Ministry of Justice.

Cultural Factors in the Psychosocial Environment and Functioning

Alex misses his parents and especially his father, in the past his most important advisor. He does not miss the broader social context of his people and his country because he grew up with suspicion towards the outside world. That is now getting in the way of his integration into the new society in which he has arrived as an asylumseeker.

In Azerbaijan Alex was the breadwinner. Because of his enforced migration, illness and the seven-year period in the Netherlands during which he has been dependent on the support of the authorities, he has lost his social role as the breadwinner. In addition, his roles within the family have changed, because of the facts that he cannot be a good partner for his wife or a good father to his son. Alex is only "the protector" of his family and that comprises his total identity. That gives him a certain satisfaction, although from time to time he seems to be aware of his incompetence in fulfilling the other roles that a grown up man with a family should have. He asks for practical advice in that area, which makes me think that he has never possessed these competencies. He was never separated from his parents and became stuck fast in a dependent position during his development towards adulthood. In practice, Alex does almost nothing with my advice in connection with his relationship to his family. Psychological damage and strong anxiety are standing in the way. It seems that his wife and son have gradually abandoned their expectations towards him, and do not press him to behave in a different way.

Cultural Elements in the Relationship Between Alex and the Therapist

In the trauma clinic, Alex has individual therapy, but the therapist discusses the progress of the therapy with his team. The trauma clinic's team has a western education, but has a lot of experience with intercultural therapy and is used to thinking and working in a culturally sensitive contextual way. This makes it possible for them to recognize and interpret culturally dependent phenomena in Alex. Cultural sensitivity confers an attitude whereby the therapist structures, conducts the therapy, and at the same time is open to information from the patient related to cultural problems. Alex is the therapist's guide in all culturally dependent matters. The therapist's personal background is therefore not of great importance, but in Alex's case it facilitated bonding between client and therapist.

Alex considers the therapist to be an authority and idealizes him. This attitude stems from his need to be protected because of his post-traumatic psychological regression, but it can also be partly culturally determined. In Alex's culture the doctor is an authority figure who has to be respected – more so, for example, than is the case in western society.

It is clear that communication becomes more difficult the greater the cultural differences between therapist and client. However, if the therapist is prepared to be open and to develop sensitivity towards cultural differences between him and the patient, communication improves. He must combine his western professional knowledge with the norms, values and expectations that the patient brings with him to the therapy. The therapist should as a matter of course dare to take into account the experiences of the patient and from those analyze the signals and symptoms step by step.

General Conclusions about the Role
of Culture in Diagnosis and Treatment

Alex is a barely independent individual who, because of various traumatic experiences, has developed a spectrum of complex and chronic post-traumatic damages in combination with aggravated depression. These damages exceed the diagnostic criteria for post-traumatic stress disorder, as defined by the DSM classification (APA, 1994). For Alex, the exposure to trauma resulted in his ego being drowned by anxiety, and a regressive psychological state. The question is whether or not, Alex is suffering from a psychotic decompensation triggered by the traumatic experiences and stressful life events later on in life. In the case of psychosis, drug therapy with antipsychotics should be adopted, reinforced by a supporting, structured psychotherapeutic approach. Interventions focused on the trauma should be set aside or only be gradually employed during the course of therapy (gradual exposure).

In my opinion, Alex is not suffering from psychosis, but at the most, he develops phenomena at the edge of psychosis at moments when his fears are increased by actual stress. One could consider these phenomena as one of the many different "faces" of PTSD, and on a continuum of the same disorder. His conviction about having cancer can be interpreted in that way, although this conviction itself has, above all, to do with feelings of guilt and the conviction that he deserves punishment. The feeling of guilt by survivors is the well-known universal phenomenon in victims of trauma, and it is culturally determined. According to the norms of his culture, Alex had failed as a son and husband. He had not shown enough respect for his father when he "let" him die and he had not protected his wife against repeated rapes. In addition, he had not done anything to purify the name of his family following the rape of his wife.

Alex's suspicions are also not of a psychotic nature, but can be ascribed to his upbringing and to his socio-cultural background. The suspicion is also a consequence of the porttraumatic damage done to his core beliefs. At the moment when a person is confronted with the evil in his fellow beings, he/she begins to generalize this experience and to position him/herself, whatever the cost, in such a way in life as to minimize the risks of any future confrontation with evil.

In spite of all this, Alex has always been treated with antipsychotic drugs. Their function can be to "glue" together the broken parts of Alex's ego and to prevent a threatening psychotic fragmentation. He is also given other medicines to counteract symptoms like flashbacks, re-experiencing and nightmares, and alleviate dark moods.

During his treatment, Alex often could not remember that he had already shared with the therapist some of the most emotionally loaded moments from his past. Although this could point to the presence of dissociative phenomena, with Alex it is more probably a case of isolation and suppression as defense mechanisms against nasty, painful memories. Dissociative states are not something that Alex is known for, and his wife confirms this. Alex is also projecting and shifting, in order to make bearable the inescapable self-reproach about what has happened to him over the past years. There are some narcissistic characteristics noticeable in Alex's personality structure. It seems that there is a suggestion of narcissistic compensation for his powerlessness. In addition, it is evident that he is strongly preoccupied with himself, often to the point where he makes himself completely reliant on the support of his wife, omitting to reciprocate with efforts of his own to get himself out of a given situation. The way in which he gets himself tied up in his problems shows the characteristics of masochistic self-torment.

Alex's treatment will continue for a long period. The outcome will depend on the support given by his wife and on the presence of various disruptive factors such as the stresses of everyday life and the progress of the asylum procedure. Moreover, even in the best case the question that remains is whether Alex's soul is irreparably broken.

References

American Psychiatric Association. (1994). *Diagnostic and Statistical Manual of mental disorders* (4th ed.). Washington DC: American Psychiatric Press.

Janoff-Bulman, R. (1983). The aftermath of trauma: Rebuilding shattered assumptions. In C. R. Figley (Ed.), *Trauma and its wake. Vol. 1* (p. 15–35). New York: Brunner/Mazel.

8

Loss, Reconnection and Reconstruction: A Former Child Soldier's Return to Cambodia

Edvard Hauff

Clinical History

Introduction

This chapter will describe the narrative of a young Cambodian man, Mony, who sought therapy when he probably was 30–31 years old (he had no papers regarding his real birth date). He was at that time working as a technical expert in Phnom Penh. The patient sought therapy because he suffered from pathological gambling. During a course of brief therapy he unfolded a life history characterized by periods of danger and tragedy, separations and losses – but also of new opportunities, fulfillment and satisfaction. He may be described as a traumatized war child, a refugee, an adoptee, an immigrant and as a returned expert to his native country.

As a child he had been incarcerated in a Khmer Rouge labor camp for children where he was recruited as a child soldier. Subsequently he was exposed to war incidents during the Vietnamese invasion in Cambodia in 1979, and then managed to flee across the border to Thailand where he stayed for 2 years in an orphanage. Then he was received as a refugee in the US and was adopted by an American family. After having completed his college education he returned temporarily to his native country to contribute to its reconstruction. Thus Mony had experienced a complex set of life events related both to extreme trauma, uprooting, forced migration and resettlement – and in this respect his story may be helpful in illustrating several of the challenges forced migrants are faced with, and which are expressed in therapies with these patients. He could have sought therapy in the US, or in Europe for that matter. But would his story and the way he told it be the same? How were his narrative and the clinical encounter, in which it was told, characterized by the context, by the fact that he was back in his native country in a completely different position than when he left it?

I will try to retell parts of his story, and I do this with a certain measure of humility, not the least because my contact with the patient was of a short duration. It can be difficult enough to giving proper justice when retelling the stories of patients with whom we have had long term therapies – even if we feel we share most of the socio-cultural context with them. In our case we were intertwined in a discourse of a marked degree of cultural complexity.

History of Present Illness

Mony, an athletic and healthy looking young man, was probably 31 years old at the time of our initial contact, although he thought he might be 1–2 years younger, and he had no official information about his birth date. He was working as a technical expert in his native country Cambodia, having returned temporarily from the United States. He was accompanied to the therapist by a friend, a North-American lawyer, who had insisted that Mony needed treatment when the patient had confided in him about his gambling practices and debt. I was at the time practicing as a Senior Psychiatrist for the Cambodian Mental Health Training Program in Phnom Penh (Hauff, 1996; Hauff, 1999) and the examination took place there.

The patient agreed that he was ill and that this heavy gambling which had lasted for about a year, had to stop. He had been introduced to gambling two years ago, but initially no large sums were involved. Now he had lost all his savings, however, about USD 25 000, and had run debts. He was also worried about potential threats from loan sharks in the future. He described how his hands started to shake of excitement when he entered the gambling halls. "I feel I want the power (of winning). It is like sex, like the feeling that I just got to have that girl". He was preoccupied with gambling, needed to gamble with increasing amounts of money to achieve the desired excitement, became restless and irritable when he tried to cut down on the gambling, was "chasing his losses" (returned another day to get even), lied to conceal the extent of his gambling, jeopardized significant relationships, because of the gambling, and relied on others to provide money to relieve the desperate financial situations he got into. However, he did not report that gambling was a way to escape from particular problems or to relieve dysphoric mood. He also denied to have committed illegal acts to obtain money for gambling. During the initial interview his mood did not appear markedly lowered, but he stated that he felt depressed at times. However, he reported considerable insomnia, poor appetite, he felt low in energy and felt everything was an effort, worried a lot, felt trapped and blamed himself for his present problems.

He denied any substance use, however, and stated that he was particularly careful not to drink because his father had been drinking too much at times. He also denied using any illegal substances and he did use tobacco. He suffered quite a bit from headaches, but had only mild symptoms of anxiety, feeling a little shaky and nervous at times.

Psychiatric History and Previous Illness

Mony first felt depressed for a period during his high-school years in the United States, but did not consider it serious. In college, however, he started feeling very depressed. He had a Vietnamese girlfriend for 2 years, but eventually her parents demanded that she should marry a Roman-Catholic man and she wanted to terminate the relationship with the patient. He was arguing a lot with his girlfriend about this, and one day he lost control, went to the library where she was studying and started slashing her books with a knife. Subsequently he was admitted to a private psychiatric institution for two weeks. He remembered little from this admission, but apparently he did not receive any course of anti-depressant medication. He did not have any further psychiatric treatment after this.

Social and Developmental History

The patient was born in Phnom Penh and also spent part of his childhood in Pailin, a provincial town close to the Thai border. He felt very close to his father, who gradually became a wealthy businessman, also having businesses in Thailand. He has one brother, approximately 4 years younger. He had fond memories of his mother, who died from tuberculosis in 1973. His father married again after that, and had two sons with his new wife. When he described his early childhood, he compared himself to the "rich kids" in Phnom Penh at the time of the therapy. "I did not know how the real world was out there, how poor people lived and how poor they could get, until the communists took over in 1975". Then the Khmer Rouge regime forced the family to leave the city, like the rest of the population there, and he was separated from his parents. He was placed in a group with 300–400 children. He managed fairly well at first. "For the first year, I don't think I was sick a single day". He was proud when in 1976 he was picked out to be a "volunteer" as a leader in the group and was subsequently offered to join the army, which he accepted. He felt powerful being treated as a leader. "They made you want to see that you are part of them. They wanted to give you ambitions to become like one of them". He liked his black uniform and was given a gun. "The gun was taller than me!", he disclosed. Then he was sent to become a guard in the mountains at the border between Thailand and Cambodia. Fortunately, he did not have to kill anybody since his unit did not capture any people who tried to get across to Thailand. But in other places he heard that they caught them every day, and when they caught them they killed them instantly. He was exposed to sleep deprivation with only two hours of sleep each night, and after two years in the mountains he became seriously ill. He could not urinate and became very skinny. "They only need you when you are healthy, and I could hardly walk. When I was very sick, I always asked for my mum and dad. And then that was not acceptable. The commander instead threatened to burn down the area where his parents lived. When his leader finally took him home, he first expected to be killed. "At that age it did not matter to me any more, because I'had seen so much. I mean, not so much, but I knew what it was like. So he took me with him. He had these knives, long knives – they were very sharp, and he could cut my head off with them because that's how they used to kill people. They did not want to use their bullets". However, the leader did not kill him, but brought him back to his parents.

He thought everybody expected him to die, and that he had tuberculosis at that time. He was hospitalized, but there was no medication. Mony then confirmed that life did not mean anything at that time for most people, and he did not really care if he would live or die. Surprisingly he regained his health and energy, and he was sent back to the youth group. They put him in a group that had to work especially hard, and they had to attend political meetings at 4 in the morning. "The young adults, 18–20 years old, they barely survived. They looked like the Jewish people with very skinny and old faces".

After a year he was permitted to visit his parents. When he approached their house he heard somebody say that the guards took some people away the same afternoon. They mentioned names familiar to him, and he suddenly knew that his fathers name was on that list. "They took my father away and I never saw him again". As the eldest child, he expected to be killed as well.

He then escaped with his best friend Socheata, a girl of the same age, whose father had been taken away at the same time. They were pretending to be brother and sister from another area whose parents had died from starvation. This was a highly dangerous journey. He was extremely scared and suspicious at the time. However, the people they met in the other area bought their story, and they survived. Eventually they met an old farmer who took them into his house pretending they were his grandchildren. This man apparently had a little freer relationship with the Khmer Rouge who barter traded with him. Mony got attached to his daughter, whom he started to call "mom". The old man was tougher, however, and demanded that he carried out a lot of missions for him into the jungle. "Sometimes this old man hit me, but they hit Anne Frank as well. My story is just like hers". He did not explain where and when he had heard of Anne Frank, but it is unlikely that he had heard of her in his early childhood in Cambodia. I expect that his comparison with her was part of his attempts to understand and come to terms with his own suffering in retrospect, during his adolescent years in the United States.

He remembered how he felt in command when he was riding the ox in the forest, looking for food. Then the Vietnamese army eventually invaded the area in 1979 and he saw a lot of corpses on his way. This scared him, especially when he once slept close to a corpse, since he was afraid of spirits and ghosts. These ghosts were dangerous and they could kill him or possess him. The presence of spirits and ghosts is part of the world view of many or most Cambodians today, as it was at that time. During my time in Cambodia I have heard numerous stories about how ghosts can interfere in the lives of the living, and I can easily understand that he was extremely frightened.

When he returned home one day, he saw that the house where Socheata was staying was hit by artillery fire, and she had died instantly. This was a terrible shock to him. "This was the saddest day of my life. I felt they took my soul from me". He felt that every time he got close to someone, they disappeared.

After the invasion of the Vietnamese army, he was brought to the Thai border by a family who visited the old man. That family looked after him for a while, until he subsequently was taken under the care of leaders in the border camp who later became senior politicians in Cambodia. He also connected with peers, who he now called foster brothers, and with whom he had resumed contact. He stayed in an orphanage in the border camps for approximately two years, before he was resettled in the US. He had high expectations of how life would be there, and dreamt about getting rich parents. However, he ran away from the first foster home, and was placed in another family instead. At the time of our encounter he asked himself what kind of power and influence he might have had if he had returned to Cambodia instead of going to the US. Obviously he felt that the "American dream" did not come through.

Mony seemed in a way to continue his fight for survival in the United States, but this time more in the sense of dealing with the feelings and memories of the past, as he at the same time struggled to "make it" and be successful academically. He struggled with the English language, only knowing Khmer, his mother tongue. He could not speak any English when he started school in the 7th grade, but still his results gradually improved. He had mostly Southeast-Asian friends in school. He found college especially difficult, and several times he almost gave up completing his education, but he graduated with a degree in a technical field.

He had several girlfriends in the US, stating that he felt it safer to have two girl-friends at the time, so he would not feel so bad when one of them left him, since he expected them to do that. He felt that the important persons in his life had always left him– by death or otherwise. He fathered a son with a Cambodian girl-friend in the US, with whom he had had several conflicts, and he did not cohab-itate with her at the time when he left the US for Cambodia. The son was almost 5 years at the time the patient was in therapy. He loved him deeply and he also visited the patient in Cambodia on one occasion.

When he returned to Cambodia for the first time to work there he met his younger brother by chance, and since then they kept in touch. He assisted both him and his family financially, as well as one of the half-brothers. He knew that his step-mother was alive and living in the country. He postponed to contact her, however, because he was afraid that her expectations of him were too high, and that he would not be able to support her completely. He did not clearly state if this was primarily financially, or also emotionally, but my understanding was that his worries were related to both of these types of support. He expressed a deep anger towards the regime that killed his father, but he did not explore his fantasies about his father's death during this brief therapy. He seemed to be more inclined to hold on to a somewhat idealized image of his father, instead of exploring the image of his father as a victim. Mony was ambivalent towards working in Cambodia. On the one side he wanted to serve his people. On the other side, however, he stated that "sometimes I do not know what I am doing here, because I hate this country! But I have to try to forgive – otherwise I could not live here".

Course and Outcome

The patient underwent a short term therapy which totally consisted of 18 sessions (including the assessment sessions), mostly once in a week. The therapist attempted to explore the connections between Mony's presenting complaint, his problems in the past and his current interpersonal relationships. During the first part of the ther-apy we worked with simple behavior modification interventions, combined with a focus on emotional aspects of his coping attempts. Subsequently, he opened up to tell his childhood history, and then we also explored the possible relationship between this and his gambling behavior, as well as with his interpersonal difficulties and depressive symptoms. He soon stated that he did not feel the urge to gamble anymore. He spent more time at work, and reported some increased work satisfaction. His interpersonal relationships improved in quality, and he felt more stable emotionally and socially. Gradually he also slept well and had a good appetite. He still felt depressed, but was able to cope with it. This may seem to be a fast recovery. Although I had no reason to doubt that his level of functioning was improved, I also felt that the improvement to some extent was related to a wish to show me that he could deliver and achieve the objectives of the therapy. I felt he was eager to keep an image of me as a good helper, probably related to his idealization of his father. We both realized that he had not completely processed the painful memories related to the dramatic events in his life. He still felt bored without the gambling, but he partially coped with this by working harder in his job. Towards the end of the therapy he reported that he had been back to the casino once, losing USD 5000. He felt sad about it, and at the same time his sleep became more disturbed and he lost his appetite again. He also reported that he had problems with his girlfriend in Phnom Penh at that time, with whom he had had a relationship over the last two and a half years. Just after the last regular session, his girlfriend broke up with him, and initially he felt that history was repeating itself and that his life was falling apart. But after two additional crisis sessions he realized that he could cope with the loss. Aware of his vulnerability to losses and broken attachments, he was surprised about the emotional strength he experienced. He did not receive any antidepressant medication during this therapy.

Sixteen months later we had a follow-up session by telephone, when I was back in my native country. He had gambled again and had run a debt of USD 50 000. But during the last 5 months he had not been gambling, and reported that he did not feel any urge to go back now. He sounded otherwise content and had continued the relationship with his girlfriend in the US (the mother of his son). His son would soon be 6 years old and was going to school and doing well. My impression was that his return to his girlfriend to a large extent was related to provide a better family life for his son.

Social Psychological Dimensions

The Context of the Trauma

In his early childhood the patient was living in a more traditional Khmer context, characterized by Theravada Buddhism, a predominantly agrarian society, a strict social hierarchy, collective rituals and respect for the elders (Chandler, 1999). But soon the Vietnam War and the civil war in Cambodia led to an increasing fragmentation, corruption and uprooting (Bit, 1991). During the war the American planes dropped several hundred thousand tons of bombs over the country, contributing to the disaster, suffering of the population and disruption of the country's social and cultural fabric.

The major subsequent disaster set in immediately after the Vietnam war ended in 1975 when the Khmer Rouge took power over the whole country. The forced uprooting of the urban population, to which the patient was exposed, was implemented almost immediately.

An estimated 1.7–2 million people died during this regime, due to executions, hunger, exhaustion and treatable illnesses. The uprooted population was forced into camps with a strict regime of hard labor and very limited access to food. There were separate camps for children who were kept away from their parents. An outline of the modern Cambodian history including the period before and -during the Khmer Rouge reign can for example be found in Chandler's book on the tragedy of the Cambodian people (Chandler, 1991).

Although the Khmer Rouge regime imposed an extreme harshness and terror, the country did not have a uniform policy and there was a variation in the type and level of terror, depending upon the attitudes and practices of the local leaders in the different areas (Chanda, 1986). The peasants living in the more remote provinces were regarded as the Old People and were less exposed to the systematic terror. Population groups that were especially persecuted were the Cham (Muslim) population, Buddhist monks and the Vietnamese minority population. Eventually the Vietnamese army invaded the country and Khmer Rouge had to withdraw from most of the territory. This war created a rather chaotic situation in the border areas to Thailand where the patient was situated. There was a mass refugee exodus to the Thai refugee camps on the other side of the border. A large number of the refugees wanted to be resettled in a third country, but only a smaller number achieved this. Thus the patient was achieving a perceived benefit that was not available to everyone. The remaining refugees in these camps were later repatriated, like the surviving members of his family. During the years when Cambodia was dominated by the Vietnamese army and government, the country was quite isolated internationally, except in relation to the Soviet Union and other communist regimes. When the Vietnamese troops had been withdrawn and the Cambodian government appealed for assistance in the reconstruction from the international community, the United Nations played a major role through the UNTAC operation. This was the first time that the patient had the chance to return to his native country and reconnect with his brother. But the war was not over. There continued to be civil war incidents for a number of years in some of the Western provinces of the country, where the Khmer Rouge still had troops. There was a new democratic constitution, but the political climate continued to be full of conflicts and intrigues, and at one time led to battles between the two major political parties (1997). Thus at the time of the therapy the political future of the country was full of uncertainties. Although the opening towards the international community and the introduction of new market oriented economical policies took place, the country continued to be one of the poorest in the world.

When the patient contemplated his fate in case that he had returned to Cambodia instead of going to the US, he probably could have become a poor farmer just as well as a budding affluent businessman and politician in the new ruling class in Phnom Penh.

Societal Dimension

What were the patient's native and host cultures? Or perhaps better, which cultural spaces and contexts has he familiarized himself with, and moved in and out of? This question reminds us about the complexity of comparisons of cultural backgrounds. The patient's original cultural context was rooted in a Buddhist society with hierarchical social structures and with a strong adherence to tradition. Loyalty to and respect for parents, teachers and other authority figures were strongly emphasized, as well as strict adherence to social norms in public, with avoidance of public expression of aggression. The extended family unit was the main collective base, and inter-dependence in the family system, where the eldest son had comprehensive responsibilities, was emphasized. The belief in Karma was widespread in this Buddhist society.

From this traditional cultural space the patient and his family were thrown into a context of upheaval and tragedy, where the rulers intentionally tried to break down the traditional cultural patterns and create a New Man from the year Zero. The experiment failed, but not before the Cambodian population was reduced by two million people and the survivors were more or less emotionally and bodily scarred. The patient described his encounters with the Khmer Rouge predominantly as a space of power abuse and suspiciousness. As a child, Mony seems even to have been seduced by this power play, when they appealed to his strength and leadership qualities, and made him join the army, without knowing the implications.

In the border camps he encountered the context of a refugee camp, consisting of a mélange of Khmer survivors, international aid workers and Thai officials. This was a space where hopes for the future started to grow eventually, and where the patient nurtured his dreams of America.

In the US he appears to have encountered the traditions of the Mid-West including Baptist Christianity. But at the same time he appears to have had access to milieus consisting of a mixture of other young South-East Asians, probably partially creating their own original cultural spaces.

Finally he found himself in a socio-cultural context of his native country, but where the cultural fabrics were only partially repaired and modified and new patterns appeared. For example, processes of modernization were emerging with emphasis on internationalization, efficiency and industrial productivity. New media channels were formed and the internet was introduced. A new urban middle and upper class emerged, and in this new urban context gender roles started to change in a slightly more egalitarian direction. The international aid community with its human rights rhetoric was also clearly visible. At the same time there were intertwined processes of such rapid culture change but also of socio-cultural disintegration, such as increased corruption and crime, broken homes, and weak leadership (Leighton, 1998; Bit, 1991).

Mony experienced all these patterns and was part of these processes. Such a context-changing journey could easily have been confusing and leading to a sense of anomie. However, my impression of the patient was that he showed his survivor skills by handling these changes fairly well. It appeared more difficult and painful to come to terms with and mourn all the losses in his life, while also trying to make sense of his experiences during the Khmer Rouge regime.

Cultural Identity of the Patient

Regarding his basic outlook in life, he described himself as a Buddhist and a Christian, and underlined that his foster-father had been a Baptist Minister, but he did not give the impression that religion played any important role in his life. However, in psychotherapeutic encounters, references to religion may be down-played if the patient expects that the therapist does not have any particular interest in religion. This may have been the case in our encounter, in spite of my general interest in the psychological aspects of religion. But the fact that he described himself both as a Christian and as a Buddhist may indicate that he neither saw himself as a doctrinaire Christian nor as a traditional Buddhist.

He explicitly tried to combine and integrate some of the values that he met through his odyssey. When he worked in Phnom Penh he stated that he tried to work hard and systematic as an American, while at the same time he tried to honor some of the values of his childhood, like generosity and loyalty to the family. In this respect I think it must have been a painful dilemma for him not having visited his step-mother yet. He spoke English and Khmer fluently, but his verbal English had components of young American slang language.

Mony was to some extent preoccupied with his self-image and self-esteem, related to his many attempts to re-establish himself in different environments during and after the extreme traumatic incidents that he had experienced. He also had several compensatory fantasies of becoming a film star or obtaining other powerful positions. Thus he seemed to be struggling with issues of self-esteem regulation. This is a phenomenon I often meet as a clinician in my work with refugees and other immigrants.

Throughout his migration process he was several times faced with the challenge to adjust his self-image and cope with potential blows to his self-esteem. His relationship with women may have been another source of self-esteem as he seemed to find new girl-friends easily. However, this was not a very stable source considering he expected that they would leave him, in accordance with his previous experiences. There seems to have been a related streak of sensation-seeking throughout his life, starting as a child when he was enjoying the freedom and excitement while roaming the forest to find food. He was easily bored, and the tendency to sensation-seeking behavior may have been a decisive vulnerability factor regarding his pathological gambling. According to my observations, however, he was not likely to be in any major conflict with ethnic norms to the extent that he could be perceived as a "womanizer" and an adventurous gambling young man.

During the time of the therapy he appeared well established in his role as a technical expert in Cambodia. He mostly enjoyed his job, and this was a source of self-esteem for him. To some extent he participated in the expatriate milieu in Phnom Penh and had foreign friends like the lawyer who brought him to the therapist. As a Khmer-American he seemed to experience more social independence than his peers who had stayed in Cambodia. It might have been more complicated for many of them to spend a lot of time in a high-class casino. He actually reported that he became closer to his foster-brothers (from the camp) when he stopped going to the casino. He also kept an identity as a Khmer young man and related socially to his brothers and his Khmer friends. He probably identified more with the emerging middle and upper classes, which he originally belonged to, than with the poorer segments of the population, although this is not clear from the material. However, his ethnic identification as Khmer appears to be complicated in line with his ambivalent feelings towards the Cambodian society as described above. He gave an impression of striving towards social and cultural integration in Cambodia as well as in the United States, but that he oscillated between feeling as an insider and as an outsider in both contexts.

Cultural Formulation of Diagnosis

Cultural Explanations of the Illness

There is a wide variety of traditionally based emic concepts for suffering and health problems in Khmer and Khmer-American culture (Daley, 2005), and there are also a variety of traditional healers (Kru Khmer) and monks addressing emotional suffering, and a wide variety of culturally based healing practices. One example of a well known cultural idiom with its related healing practices is "wind overload", which Hinton and Hinton (2002) associate with panic attacks. Such explanatory models are also found among the most educated segments in the society (Hauff, 2001). However, the patient never referred to such traditional concepts, and to my knowledge did not consult traditional healers of monks neither for his gambling problem nor for his depressive symptoms.

Gambling is a prevalent activity globally, and it is described in different ethnic groups as well as among immigrants and refugees (Petry, Armentano, Kuoch, Norinth, & Smith, 2003; Raylu & Oei, 2004). Anecdotal evidence indicates that it also may be prevalent in Southeast Asian countries. Considering the problems presented by the patients in psychiatric outpatient clinics in Cambodia, pathological gambling is a cause of great distress for a large number of families in the country. Usually the problem is presented by the spouse and not by the gambler. Pathological gambling appears to be seen more as a moral problem than as an illness. The problem might also be perceived as a result of "bad Karma", a consequence of wrongdoings in a former life. There is a need, however, for more research on the explanatory models and related help seeking behavior for gambling in different cultural contexts.

Currently, depression may be perceived as a physiological disturbance, a spiritual problem or a psychological disturbance. The author had ample opportunity to observe the variations in symptom presentation and explanatory models during his work at a psychiatric out-patient department in Phnom Penh (Hauff, 1996; Hauff, 1999).

Cultural Factors Related to Psychosocial Environment and Levels of Functioning

Social Stressors

The difficult relationship with his present girlfriend and the subsequent break up was a pronounced stressful element during the last phase of the therapy. His economical problem, as a consequence of the gambling, was another stressful element in his life. The unresolved relationship to his stepmother was an issue that he did not elaborate on as a stressor, but it appeared to me that he might experience this as more problematic the longer he postponed contacting her.

Social Supports

Mony received sustained support from his closest friends in his attempts to end the pathological gambling behavior. He seemed to perceive himself mostly as supportive for his brother and half-brothers, at least financially, but it is likely that the social and emotional support was mutual to some extent. He had also bonded again with his foster brothers from the refugee camp and they seemed to represent his connection with the past, as well as s supportive network in his present life situation in Cambodia. The love for his son in the United States probably represented his deepest inter-personal commitment and thus also a strong support for his attempts to avoid bankruptcy and self-destruction.

Levels of Functioning and Disability

Mony was able to fulfill his work obligations throughout the therapy period, in spite of the gambling, the pain and the sadness he encountered when he told me his life story and upon the break of relationship with his girlfriend. He had at one stage an aggressive outburst at work, but otherwise he reported enjoying what he was doing and seemed to find it gratifying.

Cultural Elements of the Clinician-Patient Relationship

The clinical encounter can be seen as a polyphony of narratives, where the patient's and the therapist's multiple verbalized and non-verbalized stories are activated and often entangled into each other. During the therapy I sometimes felt overwhelmed by the drama and losses that Mony shared with me. I sometimes felt I could not quite follow the sequence of events and felt confused. A few times I also noticed that I started to doubt if the events really could have taken place in the manner

Mony described them. This mostly happened when I was overwhelmed by the material and felt that the patient was not emotionally involved in his story. When we listen to stories of extreme abuse, violence and loss we sometimes need to protect ourselves by creating a distance to the story and the story-teller, and I probably defended myself in this way at such times–even if I was already well informed about the atrocities of the Khmer Rouge regime. But there are no particular reasons to believe that Mony exaggerated his story. When I presented it to a Cambodian colleague, who also had survived the killing fields, his comment was that many survivors had experienced even more dramatic childhoods. In spite of the taped sessions I probably also have misunderstood part of his story, and I apologize to the patient and the readers for this. But most of the time I felt I was able to hold on to an empathic and listening position.

During the time the patient was in treatment, I was teaching and supervising Cambodia's first batch of psychiatric residents (Hauff, 1996). I was slightly frustrated not having my own patients in treatment, and was pleased when the opportunity arose to offer Mony a therapy which could be conducted in English. I think my willingness and motivation might have contributed to the patient's decision to embark on this venture. In spite of having been in psychiatric treatment briefly before during his brief admission to a psychiatric ward at the time of his crisis in college when his girlfriend left him, he did not seemed familiar with this type of self-revelation. In my eyes he was more Khmer than American in this respect. Thus the patient was ambivalent towards exploring his past and in the beginning often gave rather sketchy or vague accounts of events during his childhood and adolescence. However, gradually the material became more detailed, accompanied by a more emotional narration. It seemed that he allowed himself doing this by establishing an apparently altruistic reasoning. He wanted to tell his story so that he could give a voice to children like himself who had suffered in the killing fields of Cambodia. In a similar vein, other young Cambodians have made the painful effort to tell their childhood stories from the killing fields, too (DePaul, 1997).

As a therapist I was more familiar with the socio-cultural context of Mony's present life in Cambodia than with the context of his life in the US. I had visited Cambodia many times during the preceding four years, and had lived there for almost a year when we started the therapy. I was working closely with my Khmer students every day, and I also had Khmer friends who had returned from abroad to serve their country in a similar way as the patient did. Furthermore, I had visited the casino where he gambled away his money and was to some extent familiar with the urban young adult milieu that the patient was a part of. There were obviously cultural elements present continuously in our discourse, but these were not explicitly focused upon in the therapy to any great extent. Thus most of the time during the therapy I did not feel a great cultural distance between me and the patient. We had both sufficient cross-cultural experiences that we were able to maintain a feeling – or may be an illusion – of understanding each other sufficiently most of the time, for a meaningful dialogue to take place. However, in spite of having a considerable clinical experience treating traumatized refugees in Norway, as well as having lived and worked in several countries, I sometimes felt a vast experiential distance, as described above.

Overall Cultural Assessment

The patient sought therapy for a specified problem, i.e. his gambling behavior. The main diagnosis according to DSM-IV R was pathological gambling behavior (APA, 2000). Mony received a positive score on 8 out of 10 DSM IV criteria for this diagnosis. I did not find that he satisfied the criteria for any personality disorder (DSM-IV axis II). Physically he was very healthy (axis III). Summing up his psychosocial problems, he had childhood exposure to war and genocide, subsequently being a refugee, presently returned to the country where he was traumatized (axis IV).

Mony also had some depressive symptoms, and a screening for anxiety and depression respectively with Hopkins' Symptom Check List-25 (Mouantounoua & Brown, 1995) indicated that he might have a depressive disorder, but it did not indicate that he had any anxiety disorder. Clinically assessed, the condition was most in line with the criteria for Adjustment Disorder with Depressed Mood. He showed an improvement in his psychological, social and occupational functioning during the time of the therapy from moderate to mild symptoms and problems of functioning (DSM-IV axis V). Mony did not fulfill the full criteria set for posttraumatic stress disorder, although this disorder is highly prevalent in Cambodia (de Jong et al., 2001; Dubois et al., 2004). He did not complain about the classical symptoms of re-experiencing the trauma, nightmares etc. Neither did he show the main features of personality change after catastrophic experiences, including social and emotional withdrawal. His condition reminds us of the many faces of reaction to extreme trauma. Pathological gambling has to my knowledge not been described as a consequence of childhood traumatization. Obviously it is not clear that he would not have developed this condition if he had not been exposed to multiple traumatic events and situations in his childhood. He might e.g. have developed this condition anyway based on a genetic disposition towards sensation seeking. On the other hand, certain dynamic elements emerged, indicating that the condition could be, at least partially, a consequence of the trauma. Mony appeared to use gambling, to some extent, as an active defense against depression. There also seemed to be elements of re-enactment of his childhood drama in the casino. He compared the feeling of freedom and excitement he felt on the back of the buffalo roaming the forest for food and other commodities with the feeling he had in the gambling hall when he taught he was going to win, and when he won. He then felt a strong sense of mastery. However, in this way he might also have re-enacted his traumatic losses. The multiple traumatic losses in his life appeared to be the most painful memories he dealt with in the therapy. Death was a constant companion during a decisive period of his life. In accordance with his upbringing and cultural traditions, he also feared the spirits of the persons who had met a violent death and that he has met on his way.

Final Comments

When I read thorough the transcripts of the tape again, I was struck with a feeling of meeting a rather fragmented story. I remembered how I was struggling to get a sense of continuity and my attempts to help the patient to connect the fragments together. I wonder to which extent I understood how much the patient probably was struggling with this himself.

In the first sessions of this short term therapy the patient felt that it was a mystery to him why he gambled. Gradually he came to the conclusion that it was related to the sadness and losses he experienced as a child. However, it seemed that he regarded this more like a hypothesis rather than that it represented an insight on a deeper level. When he summed up his experiences in the therapy, he could see how he initially tried to avoid talking about the past to avoid the pain. But he eventually felt that the sessions also had helped him to mature a bit, as well as to process his feelings, especially in connection with the loss of his father and with his war experiences.

The patient had at least one relapse of gambling after the therapy ended. He was obviously not cured for his pathological gambling disorder. To achieve this, he might have needed a more systematic follow-up with a focus on further behavior modification. To process his childhood trauma and tragic losses on a deeper level he might have benefited from a longer term systematic psychotherapy. If the situation had been different and I could have offered him this, I probably would have done so, and I do not see this treatment as the optimal one for the patient. Was it harmful? I have not found indication that is was. Something happened in the therapy. There was a therapeutic connection and a sincere attempt of reconstructing a life history. The patient experienced this as meaningful, and he also discovered his emotional strength and coping capacity at the end of the therapy. At time of the termination of the treatment process, he was confronted with a new loss of a girlfriend, but this time he dealt with it in a different and less painful way than he used to deal with losses earlier in life.

I would like to express my gratitude to "Mony" for allowing his life history to be used in this chapter.

References

American Psychiatric Association (APA). (2000). *Diagnostic and statistical manual of mental disorders* (4th ed., text revision). Washington DC: American Psychiatric Association.

Bit, S (1991). *The Warrior Heritage. A psychological perspective of Cambodian Trauma.* El Cerrito, California: Seanglim Bit

Chanda, N. (1986). *Brother Enemy. The war after the war. A history of Indochina since the fall of Saigon.* New York: Collier Books.

Chandler, D. P. (1999). *A history of Cambodia.* Boulder, Colorado: Westview Press

Chandler, D. P. (1991). *The tragedy of Cambodian history. Politics, war, and revolution since 1945.* New Haven: Yale University Press.

Daley, T. C. (2005). Beliefs about treatment of mental health problems among Cambodian American children and parents. *Social Science and Medicine, 61,* 2384–2395.

De Jong, J. T. V. M., Komproe I. H., Van Ommeren, M., El Masri, M., Araya, M., Khaled, N., et al. (2001). Lifetime Events and Posttraumatic Stress Disorder In 4 postconflict settings. *JAMA, 286*, 555–562.

DePaul, K (Ed.). (1997). *Children of Cambodia's killing fields. Memoirs by survivors.* New Haven: Yale University Press

Dubois, V., Tonglet, R., Hoyois, P., Sunbaunat, K., Roussaux, J. P., & Hauff, E. (2004). Household survey of psychiatric morbidity in Cambodia. *International Journal of Social Psychiatry, 50*, 174–185.

Hauff, E. (1996). The Cambodian mental health training programme. *Australasian Psychiatry, 4*, 187–188.

Hauff, E (1999). Transcultural Perspectives of the Management of Mental Health Care: Challenges in Europe and in Low-income Countries. In J. Guimon & N. Sartorius (Eds.), *Manage or Perish* (pp. 95–100). New York: Kluwer Academic/Plenum Publishers.

Hauff, E. (2001). Kyol goeu in Cambodia. *Transcultural Psychiatry, 38*, 468–473.

Hinton, D., & Hinton, S. (2002). Panic disorder, somatization, and the new cross-cultural psychiatry: The seven bodies of a medical anthropology of panic. *Culture, Medicine and Psychiatry, 26*, 155–178.

Leighton, A. H. (1998). Recollections of culture and personality. In S. Okpaku (Ed.), *Clinical methods in transcultural psychiatry* (pp. 18–41). Washington DC: American Psychiatric Press.

Mouantounoua, V. L., & Brown, L. G. (1995). Hopkins Symptom Checklist-25, Hmong version: a screening instrument for psychological distress. *Journal of Personality Assessment, 64*, 376–383.

Petry, N. M., Armentano, C., Kuoch, T., Norinth, T., & Smith, L. (2003). Gambling participation and problems among South East Asian refugees to the United States. *Psychiatric Services, 54*, 1142–1148.

Raylu, N., & Oei, T. P. (2004). Role of culture in gambling and problem gambling. *Clinical Psychology Review, 23*, 1087–1114.

9
Silence as a Coping Strategy: The Case of Refugee Women in the Netherlands from South-Sudan who Experienced Sexual Violence in the Context of War

Marian Tankink & Annemiek Richters

Introduction

Sexual violence during war and other conflict situations is increasingly recognized as a severely traumatic event with serious consequences for the physical and psychological health of the person affected by it. A growing amount of research has been done on the functions and meanings of sexual violence in war and on how women experience this violence. Most of those studies have been carried out in conflict areas, however, and not among refugee women who fled to Western countries for their safety. This lack of research is understandable because, although many refugee women have experienced sexual violence during the conflict in their country of origin, during their flight or in an asylum seekers center, only a few will reveal their experiences to others and try to seek specific treatment. It is well known that sexuality and sexual violence are taboo subjects among many people, in some cultures more than others. They are connected with feelings of fear, shame, guilt and loss of respect. Most women who are traumatized by the experience of sexual violence do not trust other people, and are afraid that their secret will be passed on, resulting in accusation or rejection. Sometimes, while these women are still in a violent and traumatizing situation, such as war, they seem to be more willing to tell people outside their community what happened, presuming that testifying may lead to some help in ending the violence. However, the moment the women arrive in a peaceful environment in which they try to rebuild their life, the expected negative impact on their daily lives and their future of revealing sexual violence becomes an extra reason to keep silent. In other words, from the little we know, the coping strategies women adopt are not only culture-bound but also context-bound.

There is a lack of knowledge about the way in which experiences of sexual violence affect the personal lives of refugees, the relations they have with others, and their health and well-being. There is also little known about the kind of health strategies women develop in an attempt to overcome their health problems or live with them. In order to address these gaps in knowledge the first author did medical anthropological research among refugee women in the Netherlands from

Afghanistan, Bosnia, and South-Sudan who experienced sexual violence as part of the conflict in their countries of origin or during their flight.

This chapter deals with some of the results of this research by focusing on refugee women from South-Sudan.[1] The main question to be addressed is: How do these women cope with their experiences of sexual violence. Sub questions are: Why and to what extent do they hide or disclose their experiences of sexual violence in their contacts with others? How do those others react to the disclosure? What are the effects of their reactions on the women concerned? And how do the latter respond to these effects? On the basis of the life history of one South-Sudanese woman we will discuss these questions. The concepts of *cultural master narrative* (the story a particular social group has about itself) and *silence* will guide the analysis. First we will give some historical background of the conflict in South-Sudan.

Women and War in South-Sudan

After becoming independent from the United Kingdom in 1956, Sudan has been divided by protracted civil war. Only the period 1972–1982 was relatively peaceful. Since 1983 more than two million people have died because of war and famine and over four million people have been displaced. Many Southern-Sudanese fled to refugee camps in neighboring countries.

From 1983 up to 2005 the Arabic Muslims in the North and the non-Muslim (mainly Christian) Africans in the South have been fighting. The government in Khartoum considered Southerners to be anti-government rebels. The Southerners faced aggression not only from soldiers from the North but also from Southern military groups, due to a split along ethnic lines of the Dinka and the Nuer (the main ethnic groups in the South).

In January 2005 the Naivasha peace treaty granted the Southern rebels autonomy for six years, after which a referendum for independence is to be held. A separate conflict that broke out in the Western region of Darfur in Sudan in 2003 is a threat to the fragile peace in the South.

The position of women in South-Sudan during the war was problematic. Many households were headed by women, because men were fighting, had fled or died. Some women were involved in the war, not as soldiers but as suppliers of food and providers of moral support. The majority of women suffered from extreme

---

[1] Concerning refugees from South-Sudan, the first author has had several in-depth interviews with fourteen women and one man and seven focus group discussions with four groups of women, one group of men, and two groups consisting of men and women. Three out of four participants had residence permits; the others were still waiting for a permit or were illegal. Every Sudanese woman she has interviewed told her about cases of rape. All of them had family members, neighbors or acquaintances who suffered sexual violence at the hands of soldiers from the North, rebel groups, or various other categories of men while in jail. Most of the women she talked with are Dinka. Seven women told her they were raped during the war and/or their flight. From two women she knows that they were raped but they denied it during the interviews.

poverty, chronic famine, being uprooted, loss of many family members, lack of the most elementary health care, and a variety of other large-scale human rights violations. Villages were bombed and burned and residents chased away. Women were raped and young children and women were taken as slaves to the North.

Tensions experienced between soldiers and civilians were re-enacted in domestic violence. Women were not only raped by soldiers as a theft of male and family honor, but also by their husbands and other male family members after those men had been humiliated and sent away from their land and had lost their possessions. The men could not protect their women and they lost their dignity. The combination of frustrations with alcohol and/or drugs increased the incidence of domestic violence (Pol, 1998).

Since Muslim fundamentalists seized power in Khartoum, hundreds of thousands Sudanese people have fled the country. About 7.500 were granted refugee status in the Netherlands. There are probably thousands more Sudanese people in the Netherlands on an illegal basis. Of the Sudanese people with residence permits in the Netherlands, 34 per cent are women (Heelsum, 2005). Most refugees are Dinka, Nuer or people from the Nuba Mountains, although there are also people from other ethnic groups in the South.

Introduction of Ajak, a Dinka Refugee Woman from South-Sudan

Ajak is one of the few refugee women who were willing to talk about the sexual violence they experienced and its effects on and consequences for their daily life. Her story is an example of the use of silence as a coping strategy in the various contexts – in particular the group, marital, and intrapersonal context – in which the life of Sudanese refugee women unfolds.

The first author had contact with Ajak as a medical anthropological researcher. Accordingly, the interviews with her were not therapeutic, but were intended to gather information for anthropological knowledge production about her predicament, the meaning she gave to this predicament and the coping strategies she used to survive. Tankink interviewed her four times, for an hour and a half each time, and had several informal conversations with her in the year after the interviews. Because there is no official female Dinka interpreter in the Netherlands, a female relative of Ajak's translated on the first two occasions. Later, her relative left the country. Ajak did not want an interpreter from the Sudanese refugee group. Therefore she started to speak with Tankink in Dutch, even though her Dutch was very poor.

War Experiences

Ajak is 36 years old and her history is filled with horrific experiences. Her father, a policeman, was killed by soldiers from the North when her mother was pregnant with her. Her mother gave her a name that expresses the bitterness of that period, a common practice in South-Sudan.

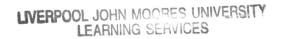

Ajak is the only child in the family who did not attend school. Her mother wanted her to work on the family's land. Ajak regrets this very much and it still makes her angry. From her second to her twelfth year there was no war in South-Sudan and her life passed with no remarkable events. When she was fifteen she was kidnapped by a man who wanted to marry her. Ajak refused the proposed marriage. She went back to her family. When it turned out that she was pregnant, her family decided that she had to marry the man, so she did. The marriage was not good and her husband never paid the bride-price of cows to her family, something that was very painful for both Ajak and her family. Her husband fled Sudan five years before Ajak; she (the first wife) and his four other wives had no contact with him after that.

During the war four brothers and two sisters of Ajak's were killed. Ajak witnessed the killings of four of them. Two of her brothers were tortured to death by being tied to the back of a car. The family could not bury them because they had to flee. Ajak cried when she spoke of this. "We suffered from a lack of food and water and had no shelter. It was very dangerous; we were often beaten by soldiers and there was no medical care at all. We had to flee but the soldiers got us and I got pregnant with a child whose father I don't know". This was her way of saying that she was raped and tortured by seven soldiers. Those soldiers killed other people and shot her two-year-old son in the leg. In Egypt Ajak gave birth to a daughter and asked members of her church if they would take care of this daughter. The Catholic church refused to adopt the child, but offered Ajak assistance to flee. She wanted to go to the Netherlands because during her childhood she had heard stories from her uncle about the Netherlands where everything was so green and where milk comes out of the tap.

The Asylum Seekers' Centre and Ajak's Psychological Condition

"In the asylum seekers' centre in the Netherlands I couldn't sleep and had terrible nightmares about the brutal murders of my brothers and sisters, and about the rape. I had too much pain in my heart and too many problems. I wanted to kill myself but couldn't do it because of my children. I had to take care of my children, although I could cry the whole day. The nurse at the centre suggested I should go a psychiatrist, but I wasn't mad; I was only very sad and worried, so I didn't go because if I did, other people would say I was mad".

Talking with other Sudanese people about her grief for her lost brothers and sisters gave some relief. People related her feelings of depression and aggression to these losses; no one had any idea that she was also carrying the secret about her other suffering, which she revealed in the interviews.

In an attempt to get more insight into her emotions the researcher tried to talk about her feelings, but this turned out to be very difficult. Even long explanations by the interpreter did not make it clear to Ajak what was meant by emotions and feelings. The interpreter explained that the Dinka do not have a word for most emotions. One of the exceptions is feeling ashamed, which is prevalent in Dinka culture.

"Rape is very bad; it is big shame, and so it's impossible to tell others about it. If I do that, they will say that it is my own fault. It will affect my relatives. They will lose respect too. I didn't dare see the doctor about gynecological problems because the doctor would write it down. I prayed to God to cure me". However, during the interviews Ajak explained that she was not guilty. "It was war, and our norms had been destroyed. Nobody respected the rules and norms of our community any more. I am a victim of war, just like many other women who also suffered from rape and other kinds of violence. In war you get victims. Me as a woman, I can't help it . . . it was something outside me. Those soldiers and rebels did it. I am not guilty, but I somehow feel guilty that I have not buried my brothers. But it was impossible. Their bodies were eaten by birds. I hope God will forgive me".

Ajak also feels guilty that she keeps her rape secret, because the Bible says it is a sin to lie. She feels the urge to tell other people what had happened ("So that the world knows, and my rape and the rape of others will not be forgotten"), but she does not dare reveal her secret. She is ashamed and afraid of being accused.

Ajak feels an intense bond with her relatives. She has a large family (her father had 7 wives and 46 children), some of whom are in the Netherlands and other European countries. When she talks about the consequences of sexual violence, she always explains that one may share one's secrets with particular relatives. "I have told two family members about my problems. One cousin started to talk with me about her own rape experiences because she trusted me. Another cousin I have told a few things too, I know she will keep silent". These relatives of Ajak's advised her not to tell anybody about her experiences and to forget them. They are afraid of gossip and also that they too might lose respect in the Sudanese community, because if a relative "does something wrong", all family members are held responsible for it.

When Tankink asked Ajak why she thinks she had to suffer from all those appalling experiences she said, "It is God; it's God's plan. God gives children and takes them away. God created the situation where war could arise and where we have to live with those Arabic people, and God will bring us peace". To the question of why God had let her suffer so severely she answered, "I have no explanation, but it didn't only happen to me, many people suffered. It is all God's work. He brought me in the Netherlands. He could have left me in Sudan. A better life will come. He helps me". When her memories or problems become too much, she starts praying. Every Sunday she goes to the Catholic Church. "Without my religion I wouldn't be able to continue my life. God has made me strong. I am a very healthy and strong woman. I am never ill. God gives me power. God helps me to forget". None of the church members know her secret.

Ajak tries to forget all the terrible experiences. "Talking means remembering and pain. Forgetting is the best I can do, but it is difficult". Often events in her life trigger her memories, although with the passing of years the painful memories have become less. "I can now look at the picture of my brothers without getting all the horrific memories back and without getting headaches. I think that's because it was some time ago and because I feel safe here. I try to forget my experiences by being active and trying to avoid being alone at home".

Ajak never went to a health care worker or a doctor with her problems. She has no idea what they could do for her. Besides, going to seek mental health care is difficult for her; it would undermine her strength and power, because in her vision only "people who are separated from their head", as Ajak calls them, need mental health care, and she managed not to go mad. Only recently she informed her general practitioner that she had been raped, but she turned down his suggestion that she go for psychological treatment.

The Reunion with Her Husband

After some months in the asylum seekers' centre Ajak came to know that her husband was also in the Netherlands, and she moved in with him.

"I had to tell him the truth about being raped, because we Dinka believe that if a married woman has sexual intercourse with another man she has to inform her husband, otherwise he will die after having intercourse with her. I told my husband and we asked an old man to perform a ritual. He boiled water in a calabash on glowing coals and he put two little sticks that were tied together into the water. When the water had boiled, the man sprinkled us with it. My husband told me he believes I wasn't responsible for the rape, but he didn't want to have my youngest child in the house. I took her to an uncle. She is living with him. I wanted her with me, but what could I do? I had to obey".

She tried to avoid having sexual intercourse with her husband, but as his wife she was not allowed to refuse. He started to have sex with her in a violent way and started to beat her. "I don't know if he was so violent because other men slept with me. He also experienced terrible things in the war. Besides, we had become strangers to each other after living apart for five years". Living apart from her husband, Ajak had developed survival strategies to cope with her situation. She did not want to adjust to traditional gender roles and responsibilities any more. "It was difficult for me to obey my husband. I often disagree with him, which led to a lot of tension. My husband wanted to continue with the old roles but I didn't want to be sent back to the kitchen. Maybe he was beating me because of that".

The domestic violence worsened. Ajak was beaten with chairs and belts and her husband constantly called her names. "But it was even more difficult that he didn't let me go out. He locked the door. He had no job and he did the shopping. It was terrible; sometimes we had only beans and lentils to eat for weeks. I had no shoes and the children had hardly any clothes to wear. My relative, who is married to his uncle, tried to talk with him but it was useless. I couldn't even visit my son when he was in hospital for three weeks because he had still serious problems with blood vessels in his leg where he was shot. When my son was released from hospital he was very angry with me. I told him that his father did not allow me to visit him. My husband argued that I did not know the language and the rules of the society and that he did not want me to become too Dutch. But he could not speak the language either". He also forbade Ajak to take Dutch lessons.

The battering continued to worsen and one evening when her husband had beaten Ajak very severely, her son called the police. After this incident the family members in Europe came together and decided that Ajak could divorce, and so she did. Her husband continued to harass her, however, and caused serious personal and financial problems for her. He spread rumors that her relative had pushed her to divorce him. Some people believed him, which was very painful for Ajak and her relative. "People came and told me that I was not a good wife and that I was putting my family to shame. One relative even told me that he could kill me because of that. So I tried to stay as quiet as possible. I thought I would go mad. I needed to talk, but I didn't dare say anything, because I was afraid other people would accuse me of not being a good wife. Sometimes I ask myself if my husband's behavior was because of me, but I don't think so, because he beats his new wife too".

Ajak and the Southern-Sudanese Community

As a form of protection Ajak did not give her daughter a special name that gives information of the situation in which she was born, as Ajak's mother did with her. However, "if other Dinka people knew that my daughter was born out of rape, they would give her a nickname that refers to the rape. Everybody would immediately know the situation my daughter was born in. If my daughter did anything dubious, other people would start saying that it's in her family. They would argue that I, her mother, was raped because there was something wrong with me, and therefore with my daughter too. Even my grandchildren would run the risk of being judged that way. I need to protect my daughter from these terrible judgments and so I remain silent".

"I need to keep my experience secret because people would definitely look at me differently and they wouldn't take me seriously any more. People would talk and gossip and they might even laugh at me. I am afraid people wouldn't believe me if I told the truth, and they would say I had made it up to cover up a secret sexual affair. I myself would like to tell my story; people need to know what has happened in South-Sudan. But my relatives have forbidden me to talk; they are ashamed. I only talk about pleasant things with other Sudanese people". At the same time Ajak wants the world to know what happened to her. That is one reason why she was happy with the interviews, which she considered safe.

When she attended a meeting of South-Sudanese in the Netherlands, she witnessed that another woman who spoke about her struggle with integrating into Dutch society was reproved during the meeting by a male family member. He was angry that she was telling a story that was not in line with cultural ideas of how a mother has to behave. This incident confirmed Ajak's opinion that it is better to keep silent.

"All Sudanese women gossip; it fills a substantial part of their life. I don't like gossip; you never know if the other person will keep your secret. For me gossiping is dangerous. It can ruin my respect and the honor of my family".

Living as a Refugee in the Netherlands

"After my divorce I immediately went to Dutch language lessons and although I never went to school, I can now read, write and speak Dutch on a low level".

Ajak always watches Dutch television and also has some Dutch friends (former neighbors and people from the church). She wants to spend the rest of her life in the Netherlands.

Unfortunately serious problems arose. The husband left her with the rent in arrears, and since he had never allowed her to learn Dutch and integrate in Dutch society, she did not know where to buy cheap food and clothes. More seriously, she did not know how to pay the rent or how electricity and gas payments are organized. She had never had electricity, running water or heating in Sudan. As she had already been in the Netherlands for more than four years, she received no more assistance from the organizations that support new refugees.

Ajak was not able to pay all her debts, resulting in increasing rent arrears. This situation has caused many problems. She cannot sleep because she does not know how to tackle her financial problems. Because of her current problems, the painful memories of her horrific experiences return more often. She is very tense and is in a cheerless state of mind.

Silence as a Strategy for Survival

The case of Ajak shows that she has many reasons to keep silent. The cultural master narrative of the South-Sudanese plays a determining role in how silence is played out in various contexts. Before we focus on what precisely happens in terms of silencing in a range of contexts, the concept of cultural master narrative and the related concept of silence as cultural censorship will be introduced.

The Role of Cultural Master Narratives in Fostering Silence

Every cultural group creates its own cultural discourse which is built up from cultural assumptions, the tracks of its collective past, cultural notions of femininity, sexuality, gender identity and roles, discursive and symbolic formations and practices, and ideas of how to deal with order and chaos. Equally important are ideas of the values of personal responsibility, of how to control the environment, of how daily life should be arranged, and of an orientation toward the future (Becker, 1999). Those narrative constructions, often called cultural master narratives, inform a person about what gives life meaning and what is inspiring, and also what is dangerous, risky or worth taking a risk for (Mattingly & Garro, 2000). Such a cultural discourse has the function of a "cultural script, a kind of social character" (Mattingly, 2000, p. 186), directing individual narratives, behavior and the making of meaning. Violence against women and reactions to it (by the women themselves and others) can only be understood by analyzing this cultural script, paying particular attention to what it prescribes in terms of gender relations.

It is important to realize that a cultural master narrative is not a fixed, static entity but the result of creative activity in which ideas and notions are developed and shared. Its production takes place in a continuous process of dialogue between individuals and the group they belong to; it is linked with specific contexts, and it is always culturally based. In the case of refugees, the dominant ideology or cultural master narrative is usually the one they bring with them from their country of origin. In general, as long as refugees are in a kind of transitional phase they tend to connect their self identity more with who they were than who they have become (Daniel & Knudsen, 1995). Since Sudanese refugees in the Netherlands consider themselves to be in a liminal space, as almost everybody believes that they will go back after peace is settled, they try to keep their Sudanese way of living as their 'lifestyle'. In addition, adhering to the ideology of the country of origin can also be a means for surviving the new situation they are in. However, this cultural ideology can be problematic for people who have to deal with experiences for which their culture has no constructive answer.

In public space (that is the part of life in which one is interacting with people other than close relatives) and with society at large, the South-Sudanese refugee group acts as if it is continuing to subscribe to the cultural master narrative of the homeland. By doing this, people can avoid having to recognize underlying tensions within their refugee group. In private, people may express a counter-narrative that does not match the public discourse and is therefore kept secret or only expressed to a select group of listeners, either close family members or non-Sudanese people, because they do not expect rejection, exclusion or further humiliation from such people. An example is the incident mentioned in the case presentation, where a woman was publicly reprimanded by a male relative during a group discussion. Afterwards, all the women the first author spoke to individually told her that they supported the point of view of the woman, but did not feel able to express this support in public or even to the woman herself.

This silence aspect of social relationships is very closely connected with the social ethics and values of a society. Rules and patterns of silence operate on different communicational levels (Saville-Troike, 1995). On the level of society as a whole, the pattern is connected with its social organization and with dominant attitudes in society, but also with social control and ritual interactions that are important for group identities. The individual use of silence in social groups depends on a person's position in that society. Aspects of that position which are relevant are role, age, gender, ethnicity and class. In Sudanese society young women, for instance, are considered to be people without power and are very vulnerable to public disapproval. They have to conform to various 'societal forms of silence', which are forms of silence dictated by institutions such as governments and religious denominations or by the members of certain groups (cf. Tankink, 2004).

Sheriff (2000, p. 114) introduces the concept of silence as cultural censorship. He argues that although " . . . there may be meaningful, even profound, psychological motivations underlying this silence, it is socially shared; the rules for its observance are culturally codified". The individual and communal forms of silence surrounding sexual violence can be considered to be cultural censorship. Unlike state-sponsored censorship, cultural censorship is practiced without explicit coercion or enforcement. With reference to Bourdieu, Sherriff (2000) argues that if people share the same cultural master narrative in which the speech is judged, then direct control of the speech of subordinate groups is rarely necessary. The silence needs to be considered as an acceptance of the dominant ideology. The use of language (and thus also of silence) has become a "lifestyle"; it has become "embodied" (Bourdieu & Wacquant, 1992, p. 149). Women who have been raped seem to be particularly aware of those processes.

Silence as Practiced in the Refugee Group

The group is very important for refugee women who lack emotional support and protection from of their own relatives in the country of asylum. They are dependent on the refugee group for their support and social contacts. Although the refugee group has taken over some functions normally performed by relatives – such as weddings, celebrations and funerals – the group members will not, in contrast to relatives, keep silent when women do not behave according to the prevailing cultural ideas, because they do not run the risk that aspects of honor and shame will cast a shadow on them too. It seems that asking for support from group members is only possible in the case of non-sensitive issues. The moment a woman expresses herself in a way that is different from that expected of her, she runs the risk of being criticized in public. This way of silencing women is very effective.

Although Ajak, like most women who have experienced sexual violence, disagrees in private with how they as women are positioned in the narrative construction of the group regarding sexual violence, at the same time she and the other women reproduce the group ideas over and over again in public. These women as a group have not constructed a counter-narrative, and as a consequence they cannot support each other. The only two strategies Ajak and other women think they have are to isolate themselves from the group or to just keep quiet about their own experiences.

The cultural form of silence at issue here is thus socially codified; but there are also psychological motivations underlying this silence, as we will discuss below.

Keeping Silent in Order to Avoid Gossip in the Refugee Community

Many South-Sudanese women, like Ajak, live in constant anxiety about the possibility that gossip will accuse them of having broken with cultural notions of maintaining their sexual integrity and their identity and respect as women. They are not only anxious about being the subject of gossip but about the consequences of gossip as well. The risk of public shaming and the subsequent risk of desertion or expulsion is high and is compelling if there are no alternative social relationships (De Vries, 1990; Merry, 1984). South-Sudanese women fear 'social death' within the refugee ethnic group they belong to. This 'death' does not always mean physical exclusion by the group, but can also mean loss of respect, strong disapproval and, above all, not being taken seriously, directly or indirectly. For some women the fear of gossip causes them to leave the group on their own initiative rather than running the risk of being abandoned by the group. This gives them the feeling of maintaining their dignity and control rather than being hurt again.

In individual encounters, women express themselves about their experiences differently in group meetings. The fear of gossip and actual gossip itself control individual behavior and morality, including sexuality, because as Manderson and Allotey (2003, p. 16) point out, "the stories of which it consists operate as moral tales for both the teller and the listeners: either might be the next subject of rumor". This can cast a slur upon the person's identity, respect and dignity, and it creates distance between people as well.

Although Dutch immigration policy and practice is a serious obstacle to a refugee's becoming a full member of the Dutch society, and the problems of unemployment, social deprivation, marginalization and discrimination are profound, Ajak feels equally restricted in her freedom of action by the social control of her own ethnic group.

The Need for Gossip and its Boundaries

Although most women experience gossip as a hindrance, gossip is an important element of communication, particularly for women, and serves a significant social function. "Gossip provides an important dynamic through which judgments and values of community life are transmuted and refined" (Tebbutt, 1995, cited in Manderson & Allotey, 2003, p. 4), and this has positive effects.

According to most women, the gossiping in the refugee group is worse than it was in South-Sudan. Gossiping helps to keep their personal problems at a distance because, when they gossip, they are concentrating on another person. This is regarded as positive and helpful for them. Another positive side is that gossiping helps them to get to know each other. Most refugees have no history together other than that they are refugees from the same country. They do not know and trust each other. It is often unclear what the political position of the other was in their country of origin. Gossiping is a way of getting more information about the historical background of other people, which is needed to create a sense of belonging to a group. Gossiping creates proximity. However, as we have seen above, this proximity also has a dangerous side, which silencing can keep at bay.

Silence and Disclosure as Practiced in the Marital Context

Sexual violence often destroys the sexual relationship between husband and wife; women are ashamed by the violence and afraid of negative judgment. They often suffer from a lack of self-esteem. Men might feel guilty that they were not able to protect their wives. Sometimes a woman is angry at her husband if she has been raped because of his political activities. The sexual relationship becomes often very problematic. Women frequently try to avoid a sexual relationship with their husbands, especially if they have not told them that they have experienced sexual violence out of fear of being misunderstood and rejected.

All of the men Tankink has spoken with stated that if their wives were raped by soldiers or rebels, the women could not be blamed for that and they would try to support their wives. Women are skeptical on this point, as they all know examples of women who were sent away by their husbands. However, the women who had told their husbands that they were raped indicated that men too make a distinction between public and private narratives and will also keep the experiences of sexual violence secret. Moreover, as Walter and Bala (2004) describe, it is not only the shame, fear and feelings of worthlessness of the woman that are at stake. Husbands can also have fantasies about the 'putative facts', which are often even more difficult to discuss than the women's real experiences. In short, paying attention to the feelings and meaning of the husband in a culturally sensitive way is essential. Because Ajak's ex-husband no longer lives in the Netherlands, it was not possible to ask for his opinion.

Ajak also did not dare to tell her husband that she was raped, out of fear that her husband would divorce her or become violent. But at the same time she had no choice but to tell him, fearing that something would happen to him if they did not perform the necessary ritual together.

Gender and Domestic Violence

Refugee couples have often lived separately for some time. During that time they may have experienced intrusive events that they cannot share. Furthermore, they may have developed new skills, and this can be problematic for their partners when they are reunited.

Though domestic violence is a problem not only for women who experienced sexual violence but for many refugee women, we want to pay attention to this particular form of violence. Women who 'become too Dutch' are kept on a tight rein by their husbands who use the cultural discourse about how women should behave in order to justify their actions. Sudanese men joke that the moment peace has come and they go back to South-Sudan, they will leave their wives at the airport and look for another woman. According to an informant, Acholi women, from a different ethnic group from South-Sudan, stated that "if their husbands do not beat them, then they don't actually love them". One woman said that such domestic violence "becomes a romantic way of expressing love". Such jokes and expressions make it difficult for individual women to be freed from this violence.

Notions of gender and sexuality play a dominant role in cultural ideology. Forced migration, unemployment and the newly available civil rights in the Netherlands put traditional gender roles under pressure. All of the women from South-Sudan referred to marital tensions, and most of those tensions are connected with their socio-economic position in the Netherlands.

Most men, educated or not, do not have jobs and feel that their social position and respect has dropped dramatically. They feel useless now that they have failed to take care of their families.

Awareness of women's rights on the part of women and the weakening of the position of men have had a negative effect on men's self-image regarding their masculinity. According to the women, men are anxious about losing their position and with it their control over their wives; this can result in men subjugating their wives, starting to beat them or forbidding them to find a job. Women feel restricted in their opportunities in the Netherlands. Domestic violence against women increases not only as a result of social and economic problems, but also as a result of trauma and stress.

Women are expected to do all the domestic work and the upbringing of the children and are not supposed to disagree with their husbands, because the husband paid bride wealth when they married. Many Sudanese men have difficulty with a wife who works outside the home. Their wives, even if they have jobs, are also fully responsible for all the domestic work and the upbringing of their children.

Making domestic violence public also puts women in a vulnerable position, because the woman herself is usually considered to be to blame: "if she had been a better wife he wouldn't have needed to abuse her". For the same reason, getting divorced is hardly possible. In public, many women denounce those women who have divorced, and many also consider a divorced woman to be a threat to their marriage. Therefore, women stay quiet in cases of domestic violence. Couples who have changed their gender roles a little – for example, where the man helps the woman at home with domestic tasks – keep their role changes private. Some, mainly young, Southern-Sudanese women said that their husbands help them with cleaning, cooking and raising the children, but the moment they have visitors their husbands will not lift a finger. Women accept this because otherwise their husbands will lose respect, and they themselves will lose respect along with them. There is a huge distinction between the private context and the public context. In public, women act in accordance with the way they think the group wants them to act, and by doing so they reinforce the 'old' cultural notions about gender roles instead of transforming them according to their own wishes or needs. Women tend to accept this and remain silent.

Silence as Practiced in an Intrapersonal Context

Ajak is very much aware of the existence of the group discourse of the group she feels part of. Although in private she reveals that she does not endorse the group's cultural master narrative, she will not express a private counter-narrative in public. She is therefore in continuous personal conflict between, on the one hand, her personal need to disclose her secret and her religion that forbids her to lie and, on the other hand, her acceptance that in her culture she cannot discuss issues of sexual violence and the pressure of her relatives to keep silent. This conflict causes tensions within her. The group narrative, which prescribes the silencing of rape issues in the group, means that speaking is not an option. Therefore, Ajak is unable to integrate her personal traumatic experiences of sexual violence into the public history and memories of the war. She is locked within her own psychological circumstances, which makes it very difficult for her to experience the appalling events as meaningful and therefore 'sufferable'.

Emotions

Ajak's history is full of traumatic experiences, which have affected her life up to the present. She can express her pain and grief over the death of her brothers and sisters. Dinka people do not, however, talk easily about emotions. The relative who interpreted on two occasions, a Dinka who has lived in the Netherlands for a long time and who speaks English and Dutch, explained that Dinka do not have words for many emotions. They say 'always crying' or 'looking sad' for somebody expressing sadness. Words such as 'feeling down', 'feeling sad', 'feeling tense' or 'depressed' do not exist in the Dinka language. In Dinka culture people also make little distinction between grades of emotions. Feelings are often expressed in relational terms; for instance, Dinka will not say "I am angry" but "he made me angry". Expressions for how they feel are often connected with their heart. Ajak feels pain in her heart because she has many problems. Emotions tend to be connected with very concrete experiences with another person or with things that cannot be said, and thus with silence.

According to Saunders (1995, p. 175), who analyzed silence among Italian families, " . . . silence may be an indication of conflicting or problematic emotions, emotions which must be monitored, controlled, or inhibited in expression because of their political consequences". Thus, in order to understand emotions, the whole context of the person must be taken into account (Richters, 1991). If we consider emotions as expressions of Ajak's relationships with her environment, and thus also of the problems in these relationships, then most emotions are related to the structure of society.

Shame and Guilt

Although Ajak feels that the rape is very shameful, as everything that is connected with sexuality is taboo, she does not feel guilty; and her sense of dignity and integrity seems not to have been irretrievably damaged. She feels it is shameful that she was not able to bury her brothers, because she has violated the cultural norm of giving the dead a proper burial. This hurts her a lot, but this shame is not connected with a taboo, she can talk about it and she will be heard with compassion by other Sudanese people who do not consider her responsible for it, knowing that she had no opportunity to bury them and had to save her own life and the lives of her children.

That shame is an important moving force in social interaction among the Dinka is expressed in the following anecdote told by Ajak.

"At a nice party with many people, nice food and dancing, a man farted. Everybody started to ask who did it and finally pointed at one man as the one who produced the fart. The man was so ashamed that he decided to leave the community. Three years later the man came back and the first person he met was a deaf man who was at the party and had seen everything but heard nothing. The deaf man said: "Oh, I haven't seen you for years, weren't you the one who let out a fart?" The man was shocked that the deaf man still knew. He was sure that other community members would still remember that incident and would probably talk about it. Therefore he decided to go away for good."

Shame can be a response to a violation of cultural or social values, while feelings of guilt arise from violations of internal values. This might explain why most Sudanese women who have experienced sexual violence do not feel guilty (it was outside their control) but do feel shame because of the cultural values they embody. Keeping experiences private protects women from shame. Shame can create a sense of a splitting of the self, resulting in a tendency to conform to the norms of the group or society out of fear of exclusion and public humiliation (Mahoney, 1996).

Self-Experience: The Family Self

The Western concept of the self is regarded as an organizing principle and as a concept of how a woman experiences herself and her self in relation to others. The Southern-Sudanese women in my research do not experience themselves so much as an individual in the Western sense of the term, but more as having a 'family self'. This concept is based on the "relational model which envisions intense emotional relationships within the family" (Roland in: Ramanujam, 1992, pp. 126–127). In contrast to the Western sense of self, it is a 'we-self' based on a strong identification with the values of one's family and social/ethnic group. Because the emphasis is on " 'we' rather than 'I', the experiences are considered more on the intersubjective rather than intrapsychic level" (Jackson, 2004, p. 53) Therefore, for Ajak, talking about her experiences would also affect her relatives. The private, individual self holds a less prominent place than the family self. In traditional Dinka culture the self is also represented as passively experiencing the impositions of external (mystical) agents and suffering is "objectified, and projected in something in the world outside the self" (Lienhardt, 1961, p. 149).

Making Meaning

As in many African societies religion plays an important role in the production of meaning for Dinka people (Tankink, 2007). Religion allows people to convey an internal feeling to something outside them, to God, which can help to reduce their pain. Religion offers "the formulation, by means of symbols, of an image of such a genuine order of the world which will account for, and even celebrate, the perceived ambiguities, puzzles, and paradoxes in human experiences. The effort is not to deny the undeniable – that there are unexplained events, that life hurts, or that rain falls upon the just – but to deny that there are inexplicable events, that life is unendurable, and that justice is a mirage" (Geertz, 1993, p. 108).

For Ajak, religion serves as a guide for how to suffer and "how to make physical pain, personal loss, worldly defeat, or the helpless contemplation of other's agony something bearable, supportable – something, as we say, sufferable" (Geertz, 1993, p. 108). Geertz (1993) talks about "models *of* reality" and "models *for* reality". He shows that religion has a dual function: it gives meaning to the social and psychological reality within a religious framework, and it adapts itself to the social and psychological reality. By explaining that everything is God's plan, Ajak gives a personalistic explanation for what happens to her; all suffering and misfortune, and also prosperity, is considered to be the work of God. This externalization (that is seeing it as something God has a purpose with) can help women to find a meaning for what happened. This meaning is not, however, strong enough to overcome the fear of social judgment.

Remembering and Forgetting

Ajak thinks that forgetting is the best thing she can do and that keeping silent is a way of trying to forget. For the traumatic memories about the killings of her brothers and sisters Ajak has an audience, because that kind of trauma is shared by the whole community, or in other words is acknowledged by the listeners. Thus there is a potential space for retelling. If a community agrees about the existence of traumatic events and makes it part of its history, then there will be a collective memory in which the individual memory can have a place or can be transformed. But if the listeners, the community or the family agree that the trauma did not happen, or if they have other ideas about what must really have happened, then the memory of the event will be separated from the collective memory, and this severely hampers the individual in his or her own recollection (Kirmayer, 1996). Memory is socially and culturally mediated. Therefore, it is always important to be aware of what is endorsed and what is denied. Remembering and forgetting are determined by those claims.

Sharing (as well as not sharing) experiences with other people shapes memories. As memory is deployed in order to heal, to blame and to legitimate, it is subjective, and recollection is not only an individual, internal psychological activity, as we often think, but also a social operation (Antze & Lambek, 1996). Talking can incite feelings of anger, sadness and embarrassment, and therefore people may try not to remember. Silence, in this case, is often considered a way of forgetting.

Social memory, as part of the dominant discourse, is a source of knowledge and provides categories in which, unconsciously, a group experiences its life and reflects on it (Fentress & Wickham, 1992). In other words, social memory influences both the expression and the concealment of individual memories.

Conclusion

The central questions we discussed in this chapter are: why do women hide or disclose their experiences of sexual violence in contact with others? How do others react to disclosure? And what are the consequences of that reaction? To find an answer to these questions the concepts of cultural master narrative and silence as cultural censorship proved to be an appropriate analytic tool. The cultural master narrative, the story a social group has about itself, has the potential capacity to help in coping with experiences of abnormality and disruption, by using narratives to reconstruct a sense of self and to find a place in the social group (Becker, 1999).

Silence as the dominant theme in the group's master narrative functions as cultural censorship. It is important to note that socially shared silence does not preclude agency. The daily reality in which the cultural notions of South-Sudan operate influence the women's risk perception and, consequently, their coping strategies. Everybody knows of unpleasant incidents that strengthen their opinion that they should keep quiet in order to protect themselves, their relatives and the future life of their children against more grief and pain. Silence can also be "a form of resistance to the dominant discourse" (Mahoney, 1996, p. 604).

A process of developing a new group narrative for rape victims when circumstances change, as Atlani and Rousseau (2000) describe for Vietnamese refugees, has not taken place among the South-Sudanese refugee group. Furthermore the new cultural elements of the host country have not changed the public explanation and meaning given to the sexual violence that women have experienced. Therefore, it is extremely difficult for women who have experienced sexual violence to integrate their personal traumatic experiences into the public narratives of the refugee group they belong to, in order to find a meaning for what happened to them. Some Southern-Sudanese women find some explanation in their religion, but this remains private.

Gossip is a very powerful tool for creating group cohesiveness. This cohesiveness is constricting for women, but at the same time supports them. Gossiping confirms the cultural master narrative of the group and creates both cohesion and detachment or exclusion.

There is, however, another reason why the women feel that it is better to keep silent about sexual violence. Sexual violence has a specific transgenerational effect among the Dinka people due to the habit of giving nicknames to people with a 'dubious' history. If the refugee group knew that a girl was born out of rape, they might stigmatize her. In order to protect her daughter from this, Ajak decided to remain silent.

In closing, much has been written about the relationship between the disclosure of traumatic experiences and the well-being of victims. In the literature on sexual violence, for instance, disclosure is considered a prerequisite for a person's health (e.g. Herman, 2001; Kirkengen, 2001). Experiences that are kept secret can result in physical problems and can reduce the subjective feeling of well-being.

In mental health care for refugees, disclosure is currently not regarded as the sole therapeutic approach. In therapies for traumatized refugees nowadays the emphasis may also be placed on nonverbal approaches, as well as on regaining control in daily life and creating and receiving social support. What we noticed, however, is that many health care workers or therapists do not ask their female clients explicitly about their experiences of sexual violence, on the assumption that the women will bring the subject up when they feel ready. Some women have received therapy without ever having spoken about their experiences with sexual violence. Also, primary health care pays too little attention to experiences of sexual violence. Health care workers sometimes explain that they are afraid of reopening wounds, and that they think they are not able to help these women. At the same time, women stated in interviews that talking has given them some relief. Some women said that they did not want therapy for their experiences of sexual violence, but only wanted to tell somebody so that they could feel some relief. Keeping silent in their own community does not mean that they would not like to talk with an outsider in a confidential setting. However, they tend to stop the therapy if the therapist continues to confront them with their traumatic experiences over and over again.

Many women never come in contact with health care workers. That means that those women never have a chance to tell their general practitioner about their traumatic experiences. This might be partly attributable to the fact that general practitioners hardly make any use of professional interpreters, and communication is therefore poor. When a relative or friend is translating, it is impossible for women to tell their secret. Furthermore, most women will not tell of their experiences without being asked to do so. They feel ashamed, and sometimes it is unclear to them that the general practitioner will keep the information confidential and not tell their husbands. Besides, the doctor will record everything on the computer, which means that it exists there and thus can be revealed, even after their death, and thus can still hurt their children and other relatives.

It was noteworthy that all the women who participated in the research and accepted psychiatric or psychological treatment received vital support from Dutch women to whom they first revealed their stories. These Dutch women, often friends or social workers, informed the general practitioners, who referred the Sudanese women to specialists in mental health. It seems that without the assistance of local women, Sudanese refugee women do not find their way to the health care and the social support they need.

As the case of Ajak shows, the problems women face are multilayered and are both within and beyond the scope of mental health care. Some kind of case manager could be very helpful for the women in finding the support they need in a complicated, unknown, new society with obscure rules and fragmented health institutions. Ajak's life history illustrates that her mental problems cannot be solved without finding a solution for her financial problems. Problems occur simultaneously on psychological, social and economic levels. All these problems are intertwined. A case manager should take all these aspects into account while crossing institutional boundaries. Health care for the women whose predicament we have presented in this chapter should entail more than regular mental health care. It is not only the psychological context but also the social context that determines which interventions and processes are needed.

References

Antze, P., & Lambek, M (Eds.). (1996). *Tense past. Cultural essays in trauma memory*. London/New York: Routledge.

Atlani, L., & Rousseau, C. (2000). The politics of culture in humanitarian aid to women refugees who have experienced sexual violence. *Transcultural Psychiatry, 3*, 435–449.

Becker, G. (1999). *Disrupted lives*. Berkeley: University of California Press.

Bourdieu, P., & Wacquant, L. J. D. (1992). *An invitation to reflexive sociology*. Cambridge: University of Chicago Press.

Daniel, E. V., & Knudsen, J. C. (1995). Introduction. In J. C. Knudsen (Ed.), *Mistrusting refugees* (pp. 1–12). Berkeley: University of California Press.

De Vries, M. (1990). *Roddelen nader beschouwd*. Leiden: Centrum voor Onderzoek van Maatschappelijke Tegenstellingen, Rijksuniversiteit Leiden.

Fentress, J., & Wickham, C. (1992). *Social memory. New perspectives on the past*. Oxford: Blackwell Publishers.

Geertz, C. (1993). *The interpretation of culture*. London: Fontana Press.

Heelsum, A. V. (2005). Afrikanen in Nederland. *Bevolkingstrends* (3e kwartaal), 83–89.

Herman, J. L. (2001). *Trauma and recovery. From domestic abuse to political terror*. London: Pandora.

Jackson, M. (2004). The prose of suffering and the practice of silence. *Spiritus, 4*, 44–59.

Kirkengen, A. L. (2001). *Inscribed bodies. Health impact of childhood sexual abuse*. Dordrecht: Kluwer Academic Publishers.

Kirmayer, L. J. (1996). Landscapes of memory. Trauma, narrative, and dissociation. In P. Antze & M. Lambek (Eds.), *Tense past. Cultural essays in trauma memory* (pp. 173–189). London/New York: Routledge.

Lienhardt, R. G. (1961). *Divinity and experience. The religion of the Dinka*. Oxford: Clarendon Press.

Mahoney, M. A. (1996). The problem of silence in feminist psychology. *Feminist Studies*, 3, 603–625.

Manderson, L., & Allotey, P. (2003). Storytelling, marginality, and community in Australia. How immigrants position their difference in health care settings. *Medical Anthropology, 1*, 1–21.

Mattingly, C. (2000). Emergent narratives. In C. Mattingly & L. C. Garro (Eds.), *Narrative and the cultural construction of illness and healing* (pp. 181–211). Berkeley: University of California Press.

Mattingly, C., & Garro, L. C. (2000). Narrative as construct and construction. In C. Mattingly & L. C. Garro (Eds.), *Narrative and the cultural construction of illness and healing* (pp. 1–49). Berkeley: University of California Press.

Merry, S. E. (1984). Rethinking gossip and scandal. In B. Donald (Ed.), *Toward a general theory of social control. Volume 1: fundamentals* (pp. 271–302). London: Academic Press.

Pol, M. (1998). *We have to sit down. Women, war and peace in southern Sudan*. Utrecht: Pax Christi.

Ramanujam, B. K. (1992). Implications of some psychoanalytic concepts in the Indian context. In D. Spain (Ed.), *Psychoanalytic anthropology after Freud* (pp. 121–133). New York: Psyche Press.

Richters, J. M. (1991). *De medisch antropoloog als verteller en vertaler*. Heemstede: Smart.

Saunders, G. R. (1995). Silence and noise as emotion management styles. An Italian case. In D. Tannen & M. Saville-Troike (Eds.), *Perspectives on silence* (pp. 165–183). Norwood: Ablex.

Saville-Troike, M. (1995). The place of silence in an integrated theory of communication. In D. Tannen & M. Saville-Troike (Eds.), *Perspectives on silence* (pp. 3–18). Norwood: Ablex.

Sheriff, R. E. (2000). Exposing silence as cultural censorship. A Brazilian case. *American Anthropologist, 1*, 114–132.

Tankink, M. T. A. (2004). Not talking about traumatic experiences: Harmful or healing? Coping with war memories in southwest Uganda. *Intervention. International Journal of Mental Health, Psychosocial work and Counselling in Areas of Armed conflict, 1*, 3–17.

Tankink, M. T. A. (2007). 'The moment I became Born-again the pain disappeared'. The healing of devastating war memories in born-again churches in Mbarara District, Southwest Uganda. *Transcultural Psychiatry, 2, 44*(2), 203–231.

Tebbutt, M. (1995). *Women's talk? A social history of "gossip" in working-class neighbourhoods, 1880–1960*. Aldeershot: Scolar.

Walter, J., & Bala, J. (2004). Where meanings, sorrow, and hope have a resident permit: Treatment of families and children. In J. P. Wilson & B. Drožđek (Eds.), *Broken spirits: The treatment of traumatized asylum seekers, refugees, war and torture victims* (pp. 487–519). New York: Brunner-Routledge.

10
Mobilising Social and Symbolic Resources in Transcultural Therapies with Refugees and Asylum Seekers: The Story of Mister Diallo

Gesine Sturm, Thierry Baubet & Marie Rose Moro

Psychotherapies with refugees and asylum seekers are a challenging task for health professionals. Therapists do not only have to face the difficulties of transcultural communication, they also have to confront the omnipresence of social and administrative problems these patients struggle with. They equally have to adapt their technique to the dynamics appearing in therapeutic work with victims of deliberate violence. In this article, we first propose a brief discussion of these problems, their impact on the psychotherapeutic work and our strategies to deal with them. In the following part, we illustrate our approach by a case study.

Talking About Cultural Representations and Emic Conceptions of Distress

Symbolization and the construction of narrations play a central role in psychotherapy. This is why we should think about the way we work with cultural representations patients use as frames in their narrations: theories about the origins of their pain and the possibilities of healing, conceptions of family and social bounds, religious or metaphysical conceptions of the world, ideologies or positions in a field of political conflicts. Anthropology of the last decades has shown that these frames are constantly changing, transformed by globalization, mass media and the dialogue between different symbolic systems (Hannerz, 1991). This means that we have to deal with the dynamic character of collective representations and the interrelation of different symbolic universes. Translation and the shifting between different social and symbolic universes become a central aspect of therapy.

If we insist on the importance of collective representations, this does not mean that patients reproduce them without any transformation. On the contrary, collective representations may be used in a very personal way. They may be commented, questioned or re-interpreted; they may be reorganised in a *bricolage* using different symbolic universes. In any case they play a central role for the process of symbolization in therapy.

Cultural representations provide a frame for the construction of narrations and help to establish connections between the present and the past or to think about the meaning of painful or frightening experiences. Sometimes they may help bridging gaps between disconnected aspects of the patient's life experience. In other cases, they enable to accept the experience of rupture and the impossibility to give meaning to certain experiences. Cultural representations may also help patients to convey their suffering to their social environment, moulding subjective experience into a narration formulated in socially acceptable terms.

By learning how to discuss about cultural representations, we do not only help patients to use their symbolic resources. We also have the possibility to create a dialogue about different symbolic universes, different social environments and different periods in the patient's life. While engaging in such a discussion about cultural frames and contexts, we introduce a double dialogue into therapy. We create a dialogue about the patient's history, his feelings and his inner-psychic conflicts and complete this dialogue with a discussion about the different social and symbolic universes he refers to. French ethno-psychoanalysis has very much insisted on the necessity of such a double dialogue in transcultural therapies (Nathan, 1986; Moro, 1994). In accordance with the propositions made by George Devereux (Devereux, 1985), the two levels of the therapeutic dialogue should not be confounded. This means that we should avoid "psychological interpretations" with regards to collective representations. We should rather consider them as a frame or a container the patient uses in order to think and communicate on his subjective experience. Transcultural therapies are characterised by a constant shifting between a discussion about the social and symbolic contexts patients introduce and the inner psychic dynamics they express in their narrations.

Adapting the Setting: The French Ethno-Psychoanalysis Approach

French ethno-psychoanalysis has developed the idea that cultural representations are no simple explanatory systems for distress or disease (Nathan, 1986). They are considered to be dynamic theories indicating possibilities of symbolization and integration of inner-psychic conflicts. They may also help patients to re-negotiate their social position in socially acceptable terms. Cultural representations may become powerful levers in therapy, permitting insight into social bounds and reflection on emotions and on the sense of present and past life experiences (Moro, 1998).

In order to facilitate the introduction of cultural representations as narrative frames, French ethno-psychoanalysis has proposed inventive techniques and innovative settings. One of these innovations is the use of a multi-cultural group setting (Moro, 2004; Petit-Jouvet, 2003; Real & Moro, 2004; Sturm, 2005). In this setting, a team of therapists trained in culturally sensitive approaches to therapy receive the patient (or the family). Some of them share the experience of migration with the patients, being immigrants themselves or having lived abroad for a certain time in their life. One of the team members assumes the role of the main therapist; therefore he becomes the patient's main interlocutor. The other team members only intervene if they are invited to and all their comments may either be re-interpreted or carried on by the main therapist. The co-therapists formulate their impressions, associations or interpretations in an indirect way, using images, telling stories or talking about cultural representations they are familiar with. This arrangement of the therapeutic dialogue helps to mediate the relation between the patient and the group members and to contain the anxiety their presence may provoke. If an interpreter is integrated into the setting, he is often asked to play the role of a cultural mediator, facilitating the shifting between different social and symbolic universes (Abdelhak & Moro, 2004).

Group setting sessions are not a substitute for other therapeutic interventions. They are part of the psychosocial treatment of the patients. Sessions occur at two different frequencies: a two-hour session per month in the case of extreme trauma and a two-hour session every two months in other situations.

Therapies in the multicultural group setting have proved to be very useful in situations where emic theories about suffering or distress seem to play an important role in the patient's discourse and when patients or therapists feel that it is difficult to discuss these issues in a conventional setting. We also use the group setting when patients seem to have major difficulties to build bridges between different symbolic universes, denying their past or present situation or establishing solid barriers between the interfamilial space and the "outer world" (Moro, 1994). In the context of extreme trauma and deliberate violence, the group setting is of particular interest when trauma has affected the capacity for symbolisation to such degree that elaboration seems to be impossible in a conventional setting. The group setting may equally be helpful when the experience of extreme violence has provoked massive splitting processes.

Working with Victims of Extreme Trauma

In transcultural therapies with victims of deliberate violence we do not only have to work on loss, rupture and bereavement, but also on the experience of feeling oneself "outside humanity", when the victims have lost confidence in others and may carry feelings of guilt and shame. We must also be very careful about the psychic effects of situations patients may be exposed to during the asylum seeking process and to the desperate social situation they often have to face.

The therapies and the psychosocial support we provide to refugees and asylum seekers take root in the work that has been accomplished over the past three decades in ethno-psychoanalytical therapies with migrants in France. The treatment may include therapies in a group setting, therapies in a dyadic setting and therapies with interpreters. The specific dynamics in the therapies with victims of extreme and deliberate violence led us to create a specific group setting for traumatised patients (Baubet et al., 2004; Baubet, Marquer, Sturm, Rezzoug, & Moro, 2005). Most techniques used in the multicultural group setting apply to this group, with some specific adaptations to them. In the trauma group, we pay particular attention to the interrelation between the inner-psychic reality and the social and administrative situation of our patients and we use supervision sessions in order to analyse the dynamics appearing in the therapeutic relationship with victims of deliberate violence. The supervision also proved to be very helpful for the analysis of the specific way in which patients may use cultural representations.

Dynamics in Therapies with Victims of Extreme Violence and Strategies to Deal with Them

In the therapeutic work with asylum seekers, we are confronted to the psychic consequences of extreme trauma and man-made disaster. The dynamics appearing in therapies with victims of extreme violence is sometimes hard to deal with. This is why we consider that it is necessary to reflect on them. In this section we would like to introduce some theoretical frames that proved to be helpful in the work with victims of extreme violence (Baubet, Le Roch, Bitar, & Moro, 2003; Garland, 1999; Lebigot, 2005; Moro & Lebovici, 1995; Rezzoug, Sturm, & Baubet, 2005). This is not our objective to give a review about trauma theory and the different approaches that have been developed in this context. We would like to focus on a presentation of some key concepts and their impact on our work.

Using Object Relations Theory

In the elaboration of our experience, object relations theory proved to be very helpful for the understanding of the specific dynamics we encounter in trauma therapy. Object relations theory supposes that early psychic development is characterised by the integration of different experiences with the first persons to whom one relates. The perception of the other as a person is the result of an extremely complex process that includes the integration of experiences of satisfaction and frustration and the emotional reactions linked to them. These experiences lead to the construction of "good" and "bad" precursors of what psychoanalysts call the object – the inner representation of the relations with the loved caretaker. In normal development these integration processes take place in early childhood, leading to the construction of a solid representation that enables to integrate ambivalence and a relative independence from the caretaker.

Massive traumas destabilise the inner psychic organisation and they may disintegrate parts of the inner psychic object representation. Extremely frightening representations of the relation with the other (the "bad object") may be reactivated. This may lead to the development of a certain number of symptoms we rather know from borderline personalities or psychotics. From a psychoanalytical perspective, many of these symptoms may be understood as a result of early defence mechanisms (splitting, isolation, projective identification, etc.).

In therapy with traumatised persons, the object relations approach may help us to recognise the dynamics we encounter. The disintegration of good and bad aspects of the object relation may undermine the capacity to establish a stable relation with the other and splitting processes may lead to altering attitudes with regards to the therapist. The creation of a stable relation, a relation that may endure aggressive impulses and the appearance of frightening fantasies is of major importance in these therapies. We have to create a *holding* (Winnicott, 1986) that permits the reactivation of positive experiences of early childhood and to reintegrate good and bad aspects of the inner psychic object relations.

In this sense, experiences from therapies with patients suffering from psychotic disorders or borderline personalities may be very helpful for our work. At the same time it is important not to confound the inner-psychic consequences from extreme trauma in adult life with the consequences of deprivation or unsatisfying object relations in early childhood. The traumatised persons we encounter often made satisfying experiences in their childhood that led to a normal development. This means that they potentially have important resources at their disposal; we should try to reactivate these resources in trauma therapy.

Trauma and Fright

Another theoretical conception that seems very helpful to us is the idea of fright, a key concept in Freud's trauma theory. In accordance with this idea, traumatic experience is fundamentally different from other types of inner psychic conflicts because it is characterised by the breaking in of an overwhelming experience into the psychic organism. Images or other memories related to the traumatic experience are not integrated into the system of representations that structures the experience of the subject. They become an alien element that has a profound impact on the inner-psychic functioning.

Interestingly enough, the inner logic of this understanding of trauma comes close to the logic we find in many emic theories about trauma (Baubet & Moro, 2003). Emic conceptions like the *susto* or the *khala'a* contain the idea of fright, rupture and irrevocable change. The discussion about cultural representations related to traumatic experiences may be very useful in trauma therapy because it may help patients to express experiences that are extremely difficult to verbalise. These emic conceptions can also indicate possibilities to represent rupture or the feeling of irrevocable transformation patients often experience.

Emic conceptions may also be used in order to give a new sense to the traumatic experience. Rupture with the past, moments of deliberately created chaos and irrevocable transformation are well-known mechanisms found in ritual practices (van Gennep, 2004; Turner, 1969). These mechanisms are similar to those we find in traumatic experiences, but at the same time there is a fundamental difference between the two types of experiences. Ritual practices may help the individual to engage into a new role and to create a new narration about his life, while traumatic experiences rather destroy the capacity to take over social roles and to give sense and meaning to one's life. Traumatic experiences destabilise the individual and weaken the capacity to represent his experiences and to maintain or create social bounds. Discussing cultural theories of transformation in the conceptual background of therapy may help patients to overcome these destructive processes by the construction of new narrations about their experiences.

In our practice, we often use images or stories that introduce the idea of radical transformation in order to find a way to construct a new narration about the patient's life history. The discussion about cultural representations and practices equally proved to be very helpful when we talk about ways to deal with loss and bereavement or with the feeling of constant menace.

Dealing with the "Outer Reality"

Psychotherapies with asylum seekers confront therapists with patients who live in a very instable situation with many doubts about the outcome of their demand. The asylum seeking process in itself is very challenging because the asylum seeker has to recollect the violence he has suffered from and to defend the veracity of his testimony (Asensi & Le Du, 2003). It can be extremely destabilising and harmful for asylum seekers to be confronted with the doubts the commission members formulate with regards to the veracity of their testimony (Rousseau, 2003). A lot of severely traumatised persons avoid talking about particularly dehumanizing or humiliating experiences they have been through because they do not really feel safe in the environment where they have to make their testimony. In many cases, patients experience the asylum seeking process as a stage of their flight, a condition in between the danger they hoped to escape from and the arrival in a safe country. Somehow they seem to live in a no man's land with the feeling that they have not really escaped yet.

In our practice, we discuss these topics with the patients. In our experience it is important to explicitly distinguish the therapy setting from other contexts where patients have to talk about the violence they have endured. Sometimes patients suppose that their "testimony" in therapy is integrated into the process of asylum seeking and they try to talk in a detailed and convincing way in order to prove the legitimacy of their demand. In these situations, it is helpful to discuss the objective of the therapy and the type of dialogue we propose.

Consequences for the Mental Health of the Asylum Seeker

The outcome of the request for asylum is of major importance for the mental health of the asylum seeker. Depending on the final decision, he may be confronted with fundamentally different social and material situations. More than that, he either experiences the recognition of his testimony and the suffering he has gone through or a refusal that implies the denial of his suffering (Mestre & Moro, 2005).

If the asylum demand is accepted, this decision usually triggers a fundamental change in the inner world of the patient. The acceptance of the asylum application often becomes a turning point in therapy. Many patients express the feeling that they have finally arrived to some place and that their flight has come to an end. The experience to be recognised as a victim of violence and injustice may be extremely supportive. At the same time, the arrival of a positive response may prove to be a delicate moment in therapy. Once the asylum seeker feels that he is at a secure place, he may be overwhelmed with traumatic memories or depressive feelings. Some patients experience strong feelings of guilt and shame with regards to those they have left behind. Being a refugee also means definitely leaving the home country, leaving those who died without being able to see their graves and abandoning those who are alive and in danger without being able to help them. It is often very difficult for patients to share these feelings with others, because their social environment rather expects them to be happy about the positive outcome of their request for asylum.

If the asylum seeker receives a negative response to his demand, he has to face an extremely difficult situation. He does not have the right to receive any social support any more. Sometimes friends or members of the community may help out with food or accommodate him. In other cases he may roam between subway stations, parks and shelters for homeless people. In both cases he becomes completely dependent and extremely vulnerable. Over and above, the asylum seeker has to deal with the memories the present situation reactivates. The fear to be arrested by the police and the feeling of exclusion from the social system may trigger experiences he made before his flight.

In such an extreme situation of social and material suffering, we may ask ourselves if it is of any help for the patients to work on their subjectivity in a therapeutic setting. At the same time, our patients taught us that therapy was crucial to them because it helped them to have the feeling of being considered as a subject, a human being who is able to think about the situation he or she is subjected to. Providing a therapeutic space may also permit the elaboration of astonishing ways to deal with the difficult situation asylum seekers live in.

The Story of Mister Diallo

Mister Diallo is a 36 year-old patient who was referred to our trauma team by a specialist for the treatment of chronic pain. He complained of severe pains that were resistant to pain relieving medication. He suffered from headaches, skin burning sensations and articulation pains in the knees. He had suffered from these pains since his imprisonment in Mauritania where he had been persecuted after engaging in a political organisation defending the rights of the black nomads. He also complained about being irritable, crying without any reason and he was regularly invaded by traumatic recollections related to his imprisonment and persecution during the conflict between the black nomads and the government.

Mister Diallo was imprisoned in the aftermath of the persecution of the black nomad populations of the Soninke, Peul and Wolof groups by official forces of the state of Mauritania in 1989. The government denied the national identity of these populations, pretending that they were foreigners, thus and expelling them and sending them to their "countries of origin". Their passports were destroyed and the members of the black minority groups from the countryside lost all their basic rights as Mauritanian citizens. Years later, the government proposed to those who had left the country to return, but no material compensation or guarantees with regards to regaining their old villages or campgrounds were given. Since that moment, several political organisations defending the rights of the black nomads have appeared. Their activity is severely punished by governmental forces, through intimidations and imprisonment of their members. Violation of human rights and practices of torture in this conflict are well-known (Human Rights Watch, 1994).

Mister Diallo did not mention any psychological problems prior to his arrest. His complaints began after his release, due to the pressure of humanitarian organisations that had been informed about his case. When he finally left the prison after three months of imprisonment, the intimidations and menaces by governmental forces continued. Concerned by this situation, his mother told him to go to Europe in order to find protection and to escape from the political persecution. She also hoped that he might find an adequate treatment for his health problems.

Three years after his arrest, Mister Diallo arrived in France. Mister Traore, a fellow countryman and the brother of his very close friend, accommodated him. Government forces had killed Mister Diallo's close friend after he engaged in the same political movement that Mister Diallo was a part of. Even though there was no direct family bound between Mister Diallo and his host, he was considered as a member of the extended family because of his close relationship to his friend.

Mister Diallo was born in Mauritania as the only son of a nomad of the Soninke group. The Diallo family lived close to the border of Mali, in a settlement where black nomads from the Peul and the Soninke groups gathered. Mister Diallo's father was a shepherd and a wood-carver, while his mother took care of the children and kept the cattle. She was the only wife of Mister Diallo's father and Mister Diallo was their only son. In the therapy sessions, Mister Diallo always talked about his parents with much respect. He insisted on the fact that they commanded respect for their wisdom, their love of justice and their knowledge of the Quran. People would often refer to his father when a conflict arose or for health problems. He travelled in the region, helping out, teaching the Quran and using his religious knowledge in order to heal or to ease the suffering of sick people. When Mister Diallo was a young man in his early twenties, his father died during one of these journeys. Since that moment, Mister Diallo became responsible for his family. He was always very close to his mother whom he described as a very strong woman.

In this period occurred the persecutions and violations of human rights of the black nomads in Mauritania. Being the chief of the Diallo household, Mister Diallo engaged in a political organisation in order to defend the rights of the nomads and the future of his family.

Mister Diallo got married when he was about 25 years old and had four children. His marriage was not arranged, but he told us that his wife was "given" to him as a gift, in order to honour the Diallo family. After the marriage, his wife integrated into his household. Like his father, Mister Diallo lived in a monogamous marriage with his wife. Miss Diallo died in childbed, after the birth of their fourth child and only son. Since that day, Mister Diallo took care of the children with the help of his mother. In therapy it proved to be very difficult to talk about his deceased wife. The particular circumstances of their alliance – his wife being a "gift" made in order to honour his family – and the fact that she was his only wife seemed to have created a very strong relationship between the two of them. At the same time, the monogamous character of his marriage intensified Mister Diallo's fears concerning his children because there was no other spouse who could take care of his children. He entirely depended on the help of his mother.

In Soninke culture, polygamy is a frequent practice. Polygamous marriages may be considered as the result of economic wealth and they provide an important social position to the head of the family (Fainzang, 1988). At the same time, monogamous marriages may be highly estimated because they show the capacity of the husband to confine himself and to respect the alliance with his first wife.

The Trauma Group

When Mister Diallo began his treatment in our outpatient unit, he was referred to a psychiatrist who became his referent. The psychiatrist, a member of the trauma team, proposed regular therapy sessions where he discussed Mister Diallo's symptoms, his present situation and his past. He also proposed a medical treatment with antidepressants. Mister Diallo accepted these propositions and he came regularly to his appointments. He seemed to engage in the treatment and to have established a good relationship to his doctor.

Several months after the beginning of the treatment, the psychiatrist proposed an additional therapy in the trauma group. The trauma group sessions were proposed in order to help Mister Diallo to elaborate his thoughts and feelings in a more adequate way because this seemed to be very difficult in a dyadic setting. Each time he started to talk about his past, he complained about massive pains and tried to defend himself from invading memories and flashbacks by repeating "it's ok, it's ok". The psychiatrist also hoped that the group setting would facilitate the discussion about cultural and religious representations that seemed to be very important for his patient.

In our presentation, we would like to focus on the sessions that took place in the trauma group. During the whole period of the therapy, Mister Diallo attended in turn these sessions and the appointments with his psychiatrist. The trauma group consists of several therapists (psychiatrists, psychologists and a social worker). Some of them have a migration background: Mister Diallo's psychiatrist comes from Algeria, one of the co-therapists is from Morocco, another grew up in an Algerian family in France, the social worker comes from Chile and the main therapist in Mister Diallo's therapy comes from Germany. The other team members have experiences in transcultural therapies and therapies with victims of extreme violence in the context of humanitarian interventions. The therapy sessions are proposed at a frequency of one session per month. As in the transcultural group setting, the main therapist leads the therapeutic conversation and decides when the other team members may intervene. In response to the feelings the patient expresses with regards to the group, he may decide to include them at an early moment or only at the end of the therapy session. In the trauma group, we often use images and stories in order to help the patients to elaborate their situation. We also may discuss collective strategies of healing that were used in other countries in the aftermath of war and extreme violence.

Course and Outcome of the Therapy

When Mister Diallo began his treatment, he had just submitted his request for asylum. A few months later, he received a negative response from the government agency. His objection to this decision was not accepted. Mister Diallo's psychiatrist proposed to ask the authorities to allow Mister Diallo to stay in France for medical reasons. When we started the therapy in the trauma group, Mister Diallo was waiting for the response to this demand.

Getting Started

In the beginning of the therapy, Mister Diallo often complained about the pains he suffered from. It was difficult for him to talk about his past or about the feelings he had with regards to his present situation. He often started to cry and repeated to himself "It is ok, it is ok" in order to maintain his composure. Mister Diallo never explicitly shared the traumatic situations he experienced. The only way he talked about them was by saying "My knees ache because they shackled me and forced me to stay on them for days" or "My head aches because they hit me". His narrations about the past and his description of the present situation of his family in Mauritania were characterised by a feeling of insecurity and menace. He was worried about his mother's health and wondered who would be there to protect his children when she would no longer be able to take care of them. He also felt guilty because he could not be with the family. He often insisted on the fact that his duty was to be with them because he was his mother's only son.

In the beginning of the group therapy with Mister Diallo, we did not introduce an interpreter because our patient seemed to speak French well enough to engage into a therapeutic dialogue. We decided to discuss this issue only after he attended a few sessions, with the idea that the introduction of the Soninke language into the therapy would facilitate the discussion about cultural representations and his past in Mauritania. Mister Diallo agreed to work with an interpreter, but after a short time, his social situation became so difficult that he started to come very irregularly to the sessions. Therefore, it became difficult to arrange an appointment with the interpreter. We continued to work without an interpreter and it took us several months before we could re-introduce the interpreter into the sessions.

A great difference was observed between the sessions with an interpreter and those without. When the interpreter was present, Mister Diallo talked a lot more and in a different way. He took the time to tell different stories about his family history and his religious instruction appeared more clearly in the interpretations he made of his situation.

In the sessions where we had to work without an interpreter, it was extremely helpful that two of the co-therapists had North African backgrounds. For Mister Diallo these co-therapists were important interlocutors when he conveyed religious concepts, or when he wanted to introduce a story referring to the Quran or the Sunnah. The co-therapists had some knowledge of the Quran and they could introduce images or stories coming from an imagery developed in Muslim societies. They were also familiar with the family organisation in cultures with a strong influence of Islam. They could use their contextual knowledge in order to talk about religious obligations and the different ways to adapt these obligations to one's life situation. The use of this contextual knowledge enabled Mister Diallo to overcome rigid conceptions of the religious and cultural context he referred to, and offered opportunities for re-interpretation and adaptation of his religious obligations.

The discussions with these co-therapists also helped the other group members to perceive Mister Diallo's interpretations of his culture and religion and the inner conflicts that appeared in these interpretations. He experienced feelings of guilt and shame and the feeling of not being able to pay his duty. These feelings appeared when he talked about his incapacity to take care of his mother and his children, but also when he evoked his debt with regards to Mister Traore, who accommodated him since his arrival in France. Being an adult man, he considered that he should contribute to the expenses of the Traore household. His incapacity to help them on a financial level put him into a position of dependence and raised the question of his capacity to assume his role as a man and head of the family. The feelings of guilt equally appeared in his relation to the trauma group, when Mister Diallo told us that he felt uncomfortable because he was not able to "give" anything in return for the help he received.

Creating Images

In the trauma group, we often use images or stories in order to create frames that may help the patient to reengage in a process of symbolization. In the beginning of the therapy, patients often avoid to use collective representations. The absence of images and collective representations is due to the effects of trauma on the capacity to symbolise. Over and above, this is linked to the fact that these representations remind patients of their former life before their flight and the suffering related to loss and bereavement. In our trauma group, patients may first just listen to the images suggested by the co-therapists. Later on, they start to introduce their own representations, or to use cultural representations that have been put forward by other group members, and which they are familiar with. Sometimes they also create their own representations as a creative mixture of different symbolic universes.

This process was very tangible during the therapy with Mister Diallo. For instance, at the end of a therapy session that took place in the first months of his therapy, the group members were looking for an image they could use to close the session. When the main therapists asked the group members for an image, Mister Diallo surprised us by saying that he had one. He introduced the image of a mango tree, saying that this tree needs much time to grow and much care during its growth. Once its branches are large it will give delicious fruits, nourishing the people who took care of it while it needed it the most. Through this image, Mister Diallo was able to talk about his deepest feelings as well as his wish to pay his duties as soon as he could. Later on, we sometimes reminded Mister Diallo of this image, especially in times when he was overwhelmed by his social situation and the dependency he was experiencing.

A Letter From Bamako

During the first months of the therapy, Mister Diallo was waiting for the authorisation to stay in France for medical reasons. He had no permission to work and depended entirely on the Traore family, who was accommodating him. Since his flight from Mauritania three years before, he had not received any news from his family and he had been very anxious about their situation. Some months after the beginning of the therapy, Mister Traore left for Mali. Mister Diallo hoped that his friend would be able to bring him some news from Mauritania. He was excited but also afraid about the news he might receive.

When Mister Diallo finally received a letter from his friend, it did not contain the news he longed for. Mister Traore asked him to leave his household as soon as he would return from his journey. Mister Traore explained that he and his family were no longer able to support him, and that he should ask the doctors for help and accommodation. Evidently, Mister Traore's letter brought our patient into a very delicate situation. The Traore household was the only secure place he had in France and Mister Traore was like a brother to him. He felt that he was losing the only place that he could call home in France.

At the same time, Mister Traore's letter also proved to be challenging for the therapeutic team. We knew the precarious situation of our patient, but somehow we had hoped that the Traore family would be able to support him, giving him a place to sleep and something to eat. We felt powerless because we could not find a satisfying solution to improve his social situation. The places for homeless people were regularly booked out and we were also concerned about the violence he might encounter in such an environment. Without the possibility to influence his desperate social situation, our attempts to help our patient to recover seemed helpless.

The discussions in the team and the supervision sessions helped us to understand that our desperate feelings were also an echo of the ambivalences and fears our patient experienced. For Mister Diallo, the arrival of Mister Traore's letter was extremely menacing. Not only did it show to which degree his social situation was instable, but it also seemed to threaten the positive image he had of his friend.

During the following weeks, Mister Diallo waited for the Mister Traore's return. He tried to find a way to preserve the positive image of him and to understand why he did not want to accommodate him anymore. Finally he explained to us that his friend did not have any other choice, because his wife did not agree with his presence in the Traores' home anymore. This explanation certainly reflected a true aspect of the Traores' current situation. Mister Diallo had to share the room with the children and Miss Traore was afraid that they could be scared by his behaviour, his absent-mindedness, especially at times when he was visibly depressed. At the same time, Mister Diallo's understanding of Mister Traore's behaviour allowed him to preserve the positive image he had built up of his friend and helper and to attribute the "bad" image to the wife, using the psychological mechanism of splitting.

Leaving the Traore Household

When Mister Traore came back from his journey, he explained that he would not turn down his friend without any alternative accommodation. At the same time he expressed his expectations with regards to our team: he hoped that the health professionals could take over the responsibility for the social situation of his friend. We started to feel as if we were being designated to take over a role that we could not play, because we had no satisfying solutions to propose. During this period, Mister Diallo's depressive symptoms had worsened severely. His psychiatrist considered the possibility of a hospitalisation in order to give some rest to his patient and to adapt the medication to the present situation. But at the same time, the idea of a hospitalisation seemed to be risky. Wouldn't it mean that the team accepted the designation received by Mister Traore? It seemed necessary to explain that we were not able to find a solution for Mister Diallo's social situation. Mister Diallo's psychiatrist decided to discuss the situation with Mister Traore. Mister Diallo agreed with this idea and finally the conversation with Mister Traore proved to be very helpful. It helped Mister Traore to construct a realistic image of the help health professionals can offer and it was reassuring for our team because Mister Traore explained that he would not leave his friend alone in case he was hospitalised.

From the Local Mosque to the Junk Room Next to the Garbage

Mister Diallo stayed for three weeks at the hospital. The hospitalisation permitted him to regain some strength, but his mental health state remained unstable. When he left the hospital, his friend had found a new accommodation for him: Mister Diallo could sleep in one of the local mosques, together with a group of other people in equally desperate situations. Later, Mister Diallo told us that his friend had to pay a fee for this accommodation. In the therapy sessions during his stay at the local mosque, we often discussed his perception of this place, the conversations he had with the local imam and his disappointment with the fact that the latter had accepted money in return for his help.

A few months later, Mister Diallo had to leave the mosque. His friend found a new place for him, a tiny room without heating next to the garbage-containers shelter, in the huge building the Traore family lived in. Meanwhile, Mister Diallo seemed to be completely destabilised by his social situation. He often missed his appointments with the group or with his psychiatrist, or arrived several hours or even days later. Sometimes he told us that he had not eaten for a whole day or that he had not managed to sleep in his shelter because it was too cold. During that period, the members of the trauma group often had severe doubts about the sense of a therapy under such extreme social conditions. At the same time Mister Diallo insisted on the importance of the therapy, regularly asking his Doctor when we would "group" again. Looking back to this painful period, we consider that our role was to be with our patient, not to abandon him but to support him at times of helplessness and despair. We had to be more flexible with regards to our role and to the group setting. We would for instance offer him something to eat and accept that he sometimes sleeps for a couple of hours in our waiting room.

Regaining Social Status

Mister Diallo's situation and his mental health changed entirely when he finally received the authorisation to stay in France for one year as well as a working permit. With the help of Mister Traore, he found a part-time job and a modest accommodation, which he shared with a compatriot. He proudly brought his first wage packet to the therapy session. Even though his job did not pay well and he was still dependent from the help of his social environment, he regained some confidence. He finally felt as a man, contributing the needs of the community.

Heading for Bamako

During this period, Mister Diallo and Mister Traore set up a plan for a journey to Mali where Mister Diallo could meet his mother and his children. Mister Traore had contacted them with the help of friends who travelled regularly to Mauritania. He invited Madame Diallo and the children to stay in Bamako, at his mother's house. This plan would allow the Diallos to organise a family reunion at a secure place. At the same time, this meeting would reinforce the strong relation the two friends had build up in the meantime.

Evidently, the plan for a trip to Mali was only possible because Mister Diallo had received the authorisation to stay in France. In fact, he was able to leave the country legally and to return to France after the trip.

The preparation of the voyage to Mali and the hopes and fears with regards to this trip had an important impact in the following therapy sessions. Eventually, Mister Diallo left and stayed for about two months in Bamako. The therapeutic team was impressed by the organisational effort Mister Traore had made in order to help his friend to see his mother. We were full of hope with regards to the positive effect of this reunion.

Back in Paris

When Mister Diallo returned from his trip, he told us how much he enjoyed meeting his mother, receiving her advises and spending some time with her. But meeting her also meant having to leave her once again and this proved to be extremely painful. The return to France seemed to reactivate souvenirs of his flight and some of the feelings he had experienced when he first arrived in France. During one of the sessions, Mister Diallo related how the government forces came into the village, killing and mutilating the villagers. This was the only moment in the therapy where he directly talked about the traumatic events he had experienced in Mauritania.

In this period, Mister Diallo seemed to be very destabilised. He was not sure anymore whether his decision to return to France was the right one. This time, his mother had not advised him to leave, and she seemed to be afraid that they might not meet again. Without the benediction of his mother, the return to France seemed to be senseless and in disharmony with his destiny.

A short time after Mister Diallo's return, his authorisation to stay in France expired. Once again, he had to wait for several months for the renewal of his residence permit. He lost his work and his accommodation and once again he found himself in an extremely precarious situation. This time, he could stay at the Traores' place because one of their daughters had left the apartment to go to Mali for a few months time. Still, Mister Diallo knew that this was an unstable and short-term solution. He had the feeling of being at the wrong place, far away from his family, who needed him.

During this period of doubt and insecurity, frightening news arrived from Bamako: the Traores' house in Bamako had caught fire. Mister Diallo's mother and his children, who were still being accommodated at the Traores' place, had been hospitalised for several days.

These news reinforced Mister Diallo's feeling that his family was in danger and that he should be with them. More than that, the news seemed to justify his feeling of constant menace and the idea that the destruction he had experienced could be dangerous for the people who were close to him. The frontier between the frightening fantasies of his inner world and the events in the outer reality seemed to blur.

In the following sessions, Mister Diallo often expressed his fears about his mother's health. Once, he related a dream about an airplane that crashed into the sea. According to Mister Diallo, this dream announced the death of an important person, someone who was not only dear to him but also of public interest. He was terrorised by the idea that his dream might announce his mother's death.

A Sudden Death

A short time later, Mister Diallo came to our unit and insisted on seeing his psychiatrist urgently. He was very agitated. He explained that his host, Mister Traore, had been killed in a robbery. Mister Traore lived in a humble place and did not have much money of his own, but he was responsible for collecting money that community members sent to their villages in Mali. Some days before, a TV documentary about the communities of African origin in Paris was broadcast. The documentary presented Mister Traore. Two robbers, learning about Mister Traore's function in the community, surprised him when he was about to send the money to Mali. He was shot and died immediately.

This event was extremely frightening for our patient. To him, Mister Traore was not only a very close friend, but also a protector and a paternal figure. The sudden death of Mister Traore reactivated his feelings of insecurity and menace. It also seemed to increase the fear that the destruction he had experienced continued to accompany him and was even harmful to his environment. Once again, the barrier between "outer reality" and frightening fantasies seemed to blur in a very destabilising way.

When Mister Diallo came to our unit in order to tell us that his friend had died, we improvised a group session with some of the therapists. The therapeutic group was also shaken by the news of the sudden and violent death of Mister Traore. Even if the group members never met him, he had become an important interlocutor for us. He was in the centre of Mister Diallo's social environment and we were afraid that this microcosm would collapse again, leaving our patient in a social situation we cannot influence. We were also very much concerned by the dream that Mister Diallo had shared with us earlier. Would he feel that he had transgressed by telling the dream or worse, would he think that the announced "death of an important person" became true because he had spoken out about the dream? During the session, Mister Diallo told us that he thought that his friend's death was the dramatic event his dream announced. He was shocked and surprised, but he did not feel guilty for talking about the dream. However, he rather felt guilty because he had survived and he asked himself: "Why did they choose him? And why not me?" For the first time in therapy, he revolted against destiny, talking about his anger and the feeling that there was no divine justice in life after all.

Emerging Again

In the following weeks, the team proposed to Mister Diallo to attend several sessions in a small group in addition to the appointments in the trauma group and the sessions with his psychiatrist. To our surprise, Mister Diallo proved to be less fragile than we thought. Gradually, he regained a certain confidence and the capacity to project himself in the future. We learned that in the meantime our patient had taken over an important role in the Traore family. He had become close to Mister Traore's children and in this period, he became an important counsellor for them. Sometimes his mobile phone rang during the therapy sessions and he, who had been in tears a moment before, would talk with a soft and reassuring voice to one of the Mister Traore's children calling him for a minor problem or just to hear his voice.

We also found out how much Mister Diallo's position in the family was respected by the members of the Mauritanian community in Paris. They invited him to accompany Mister Traore's body to the funeral, which was supposed to take place in Bamako. The community members would pay for the expenses of the journey.

But once again, we were confronted to the problems relating to his administrative situation: Mister Diallo was still waiting for the renewal of his authorisation to stay in France. We felt helpless because we considered that it would be extremely helpful for our patient to attend the funeral, but we also knew that he could not take the risk to travel without a residence permit.

Finally, the funeral was held at the Muslim cemetery of Paris, due to the requirements of the French law in case of a murder. The therapy group received a formal invitation to attend the funeral. We discussed the issue in our group and decided to express our condolences to Mister Diallo and to ask him to transmit them to the Mister Traore's widow.

In the following week, Mister Diallo did not come to his appointment. He was so much involved into the re-organisation of the Traore family that he did not have time to come. Some days later, he suddenly appeared at the hospital, wearing a beautiful dress as if he was about to participate in an event of major importance. He told us that he had received the invitation to collect his residence permit at the police office. Our social worker had offered to accompany him because we had been informed about some fake invitations that had been used as a mean to get hold of immigrants without legal residence permission. Even though he knew about the risk he was taking, Mister Diallo decided to go by himself and to inform us about the outcome as soon as possible. Later, he told us that he had not been afraid of going alone to the police station because he had dreamt of Mister Traore, telling him not to worry, and that he would get his papers. For Mister Diallo, this dream was reassuring and it helped him to control his fear of being expulsed from the country. It was also a dream that helped him to deal with his feelings of debt and guilt with regards to his deceased friend. Somehow the dream seemed to prove that he had the right to survive and to stay in France and maybe even to stay in the close environment of the Traore family. For us, the dream proved that Mister Diallo had regained a certain stability that helped him to keep a positive representation of his friend, despite the violence of his death and the ambivalent feelings it provoked.

Mister Diallo's therapy has not come to an end yet and we still accompany him in the struggle for a new balance in his inner world and in his efforts to create acceptable social circumstances in his life. We consider that the therapy helped Mister Diallo to regain the capacity to think about his situation and to negotiate his position in the social environment – within the community in France, within the Traore family in Paris and in Bamako, and within his own family in Mauritania. Our goals are at the same time very modest and quite ambitious. Even though we know that we are not able to resolve the social problems of our patient because we depend on the immigration laws as much as he does, we know that we may help him to act as a subject, and to think, despite all the obstacles.

Diagnostic Formulation

Using the DSM classification (APA, 1994) of mental health problems, we may consider that Mister Diallo suffers from post-traumatic stress disorder provoked by complex trauma together with a strong depressive component. We find symptoms as flashbacks of the traumatic events, nightmares and emotional instability. We also find more non-specific symptoms as the chronic pains that our patient is suffering from.

From a psychodynamic perspective, we can conclude that Mister Diallo suffers from symptoms related to the breaking in of the traumatic event into the psychic organism (all the symptoms related to repetition), but also from symptoms that may be interpreted as a result of a disintegration of "good" and "bad" object representations (the feeling of constant menace, the difficulty to accept ambivalent feelings with regards to his close friend). The traumas Mister Diallo was subjected to activated strong feelings of guilt and shame, feelings that were often in the centre of our psychotherapeutic work.

Societal Dimension

If we try to understand the inner experience of our patient and the strategies he uses in order to negotiate his social position, we have to consider the different societal contexts and cultural norms he refers to. Some of these references may be defined as elements of the "Soninke Culture", as the narration about the Egyptian origins of this group, source of pride about the glorious past of the Soninke. Other elements of Mister Diallo's "Native Culture" are less specific because they are shared by many West African societies, like the particular role the eldest son is supposed to have in the family or the reliable relationship someone may establish with a "brother" without direct family relations. We also find many references to Muslim religion and family organisation as the duty to accept one's destiny or the wish to pay a trip to Mecca to his mother. At some moments, and in a more implicit way, our patient also made allusions to cultural practices that are rather anchored in pre-Muslim societies of West Africa. When he talked about the sudden death of his father during one of his journeys, he evoked the jealousy of the people and the dangers related to practices of sorcery or "maraboutage".

All these different elements of Mister Diallo's "Native Culture" and their interactions have to be considered when we try to understand his conception of his duties and his strategies to negotiate his social position. They are the expression of the profoundly hybrid character of West African societies (Amselle, 1990).

But considering the "Native Culture" of our patient equally demands to consider the political context of his life experience and the conception of a cultural or ethnic identity he developed in response to this experience. The conflict between Mauritanian government and the black nomads was accompanied by discourses about ethnic affiliation and national identity. Ethnic barriers between black populations and the moor society and the question of "colour" were of great importance. Our patient seldom talked directly about these issues. At the same time, we felt how important the question of "colour", ethnic and religious identity was for him. He often insisted on the fact that coming to the group sessions was a particular experience for him, because we could be together and understand each other, even though we were not of the same colour. The presence of the "white" North African group members was particularly important to him, not only because they could introduce contextual knowledge about Muslim societies, but also because he could experience a non-violent dialogue between "black" and "white" Muslims and an acceptance beyond racial barriers.

Considering all these different elements, we have to state that our patient's "Native Culture" is quite a complex one. But there is more than that. We do not only have to consider the cultural contexts he lived in before his migration, but also his relationship towards the "Host Culture" in France and the interaction between these two sociocultural and political contexts. Finally, we have to understand the particular representation our patient has developed with regards to his "Native Culture" and the "Host Culture".

For Mister Diallo, the encounter with "French Culture" was above all the confrontation with French asylum policy and its consequences for his social position. The refusal of his demand for asylum and the social exclusion he experienced were probably particularly violent for him because they reactivated frightening memories of exclusion, denial of his citizenship and the basic human rights in his home country.

On the other hand, the "French Culture" was related to the sociocultural microcosm Mister Diallo was part of in Paris, in the Traore family and among other people at the Mosque. This context was at the same time familiar and strange to our patient. For example, the Traores tried to preserve religious and cultural values from Mauritanian society, but they also had to adapt to the requirements of daily life in France. In this context, the conditions of housing and the organisation of family life limited their possibility to accommodate guests. The specific situation of the Traore family may also be interpreted in the context of the recent changes in French welfare politics. Recent restrictions with regards to welfare transformed the life of immigrant communities, putting an important strain on the solidarity amongst them. Looking for different accommodations for his friend was part of Mister Traore's strategies to adapt cultural practices such as hospitality and taking care of a "brother" to the life situation in France.

Collective Self and Social Roles

In the beginning of the therapy, Mister Diallo mainly talked about his incapacity to take over the roles he was designated to in Mauritanian society: the one of a good and reliable son who takes care of his elderly mother, the role of the only adult male and chief of the family, and the role of a good Muslim. In the periods when he went through extreme dependence and social suffering in French society, he also talked about the roles he was attributed to in France and their contradiction with regards to those he wanted to take over. He was rejected as a refugee, excluded from the social system, considered as someone who should not construct any long-time project for a stay in France. After a certain time, a third field of roles appeared in the discourse of Mister Diallo. He started to consider himself as someone who had certain knowledge and some dignity, despite all. This feeling permitted him to negotiate and invest a socially acceptable role in the Traore family. It also encouraged him to develop a critical position with regards to authorities, as the local Imam who had accepted money for his accommodation. The role he decided to take on when Mister Traore died showed how well Mister Diallo succeeded in overcoming the role of a petitioner and a powerless victim.

Conclusion

Transcultural therapies with asylum seekers confront therapists with an extremely complex field of interrelations between different cultural and political contexts. Therapists should consider these sociopolitical and cultural contexts and try to understand the unique way their patients try to deal with them. Accepting the impact of "outer reality" on their subjectivity is an imperative in therapies with refugees and asylum seekers. At the same time, we should also insist on the importance of subjective experience and the unique way in which the individual perceives and transforms the reality he or she encounters.

References

Abdelhak, M. A., & Moro, M. R. (2004). L'interpréte en psychothérapie transculturelle. In M. R. Moro, Q. De La Noë, & Y. Mouchenik. (Eds.), *Manuel de Psychiatrie Transculturelle. Travail clinique, travail social* (pp. 239–248). Grenoble: La Pensée sauvage.

American Psychiatric Association (APA). (1994). *Diagnostic and statistical manual of mental disorders* (4th ed.). Washington, D.C.: American Psychiatric Association.

Amselle, J. L. (1990). *Logiques métisses. Anthropologie de l'identité en Afrique et ailleurs*. Paris: Payot.

Asensi, H., & Le Du, C. (2003). Savons-nous accueillir les réfugiés en France? In T. Baubet, K. Le Roch, D. Bitar, & M. R. Moro (Eds.), *Soigner malgré tout. Vol 1: Trauma cultures et soins* (pp. 241–251). Grenoble: La Pensée Sauvage.

Baubet, T., Le Roch, K., Bitar, D., & Moro, M. R (Eds.). (2003). *Soigner malgré tout. Vol. 1: Trauma cultures et soins*. Grenoble: La Pensée sauvage.

Baubet, T., & Moro, M. R. (2003). Cultures et soins du traumatises psychiques en situation humanitaire. In T. Baubet, K. Le Roch, D. Bitar, & M. R. Moro (Eds.), *Soigner malgré tout. Vol. 1: Trauma cultures et soins* (pp. 71–95). Grenoble: La Pensée sauvage.

Baubet, T., Abbal, T., Claudet, J., Le Du, C., Heidenreich, F., Lévy, K., et al. (2004). Traumas psychiques chez les demandeurs d'asile en France: des spécificités cliniques et thérapeutiques. *Journal International de Victimologie* 2(2): [1 screen]. Retrieved April 16. 2004 from: http://www.jidv.com/BAUBET, T-JIDV2004_%202(2).htm.

Baubet, T., Marquer, C., Sturm, G., Rezzoug, D., & Moro, M. R. (2005). Un dispositif original, le "groupe trauma". *Rhizome, Bulletin National Santé Mentale et Précarité, 21*, 33–36.

Devereux, G. (1985). *Ethnopsychanalyse complémentariste*. Paris: Flammarion.

Fainzang, S. (1988). *La femme de mon mari*. Paris: L'Harmattan.

Garland, C (Ed.). (1999). *Understanding Trauma. A Psychoanalytical* Approach. London, New York: Karnac Publications.

Hannerz, U. (1991). *Cultural Complexity. Studies in the Social Organisation of* Meaning. New York: Columbia University Press.

Human Rights Watch. (1994). *Mauritania's Campaign of Terror: State-Sponsored Repression of Black Africans*. New York: Human Rights Watch.

Lebigot, F. (2005). *Soigner les troubles psychotraumatiques*. Paris: Dunod.

Mestre, C., & Moro, M. R. (2005). Comment sommes-nous devenus si inhospitaliers? *L'autre, Cliniques, Cultures et Societé, 3*, 411–415.

Moro, M. R. (1994). *Parents en Exil*. Paris: Presses Universitaires de France.

Moro M. R., & Lebovici, S (Eds.). (1995). *Psychiatrie humanitaire en ex-Yougoslavie et en Arménie. Face au traumatisme*. Paris: Presses Universitaires de France.

Moro, M. R. (1998). *Psychothérapie transculturelle des enfants de migrants*. Paris: Dunod.

Moro, M. R. (2004). *Enfants d'ici venus d'ailleurs*. Paris: Hachette.

Nathan, T. (1986). *La folie des autres. Traité d'ethnopsychiatrie clinique*. Paris: Dunod.

Petit-Jouvet, L. (Executive Producer). (2003, October 16). *J'ai rêvé d'une grande étendue d'eau*. ARTE: Abacaris Films.

Réal, I., & Moro, M. R. (2004). La consultation transculturelle d'Avicenne. In M. R. Moro, Q. De La Noë, & Y. Mouchenik. (Eds.), *Manuel de Psychiatrie Transculturelle. Travail clinique, travail social* (pp. 217–237). Grenoble: La Pensée sauvage.

Rezzoug, D., Sturm, G., & Baubet, T. (2005). Le traumatisme psychique en situation transculturelle. *Psycho-Média, 4*, 59–62.

Rousseau, C. (2003). Violence organisée et traumatismes. In: T. Baubet & M. R. Moro (Eds.), *Psychiatrie et Migrations* (pp. 148–154). Paris: Masson.

Sturm, G. (2005). *Les thérapies transculturelles en groupe "multiculturel". Une ethnographie de l'espace thérapeutique*. Unpublished doctoral dissertation in Psychology and Cultural Studies. University of Paris XIII (France) and University of Bremen (Germany)

Turner, V. (1969). *The ritual process. Structure and anti-structure*. Chicago: Aldine.

Van Gennep, A. (2004). *The Rites of Passage*. London: Routledge.

Winnicott, D. W. (1986). *Holding and Interpretation*. London: The Hogarth Press and the Inst of PSA.

11
Lost in the Desert – from Despair to Meaningful Existence: A Chechen Refugee Family Crossing Borders

Nino Makhashvili & Lela Tsiskarishvili

"Can your medical center help me in selling my kidney?" These words, which caused a shock-like state of several colleagues sitting around the table in our treatment center in Tbilisi (Georgia) belonged to Kazbeg, a man of 40 years, refugee from Chechnya. This was his first visit to our center.

Kazbeg's grandfather was a participant of 1944 Chechen rebellion against Soviet Regime and by Stalin's order, together with his family (Kazbeg's 7 years old father among them) and some 1 million Chechens has been deported to Central Asia stuffed in railway car for cattle. The itinerary from Chechnya to Kazakhstan was extremely long and full of suffering. After 6 weeks of journey, only half of the million Chechens managed to survive. However, that did not break their spirit. As Alexander Solzhenitsyn describes in his Archipelago Gulag:

The Chechens never sought to please, to ingratiate themselves with the bosses. As far as they were concerned, the local inhabitants and those exiles who submitted so readily belong more or less to the same breed as bosses. They respected only rebels. And here is an extraordinary thing – everyone was afraid of them. No one could stop them from living as they did. The regime which had ruled the land for thirty years could not force them to respect its laws. (as cited in Baiev, Daniloff, & Daniloff, 2003, pp.3–4).

In 1957 Chechens were allowed to return home and start over a new life, however they were not rehabilitated formally. During years of living in extremely harsh conditions in exile, Kazbeg's grandfather and 2 uncles died alongside many others under forced labor. Kazbeg's father refused to leave Kazakhstan, and the family separated. Kazbeg's pregnant mother, older sister and grandmother returned to their native town of Grozny in 1963, the year that Kazbeg was born.

He and his sister were growing up in caring family, among loving women, mother and grandmother. From those years of his childhood and adolescence, Kazbeg developed deep respect of women and belief in their power and outlook.

After graduation from the secondary school, Kazbeg became a student of civil engineering department in Moscow. During one of his holidays back home, he met Khava, a beautiful Chechen young girl of 18, fell in love with her and soon they married. The couple went to Moscow, where after graduation from the university Kazbeg started to work. Their family was quite wealthy. They gave birth to three boys. After Chechnya declared independence, the family decided to return to homeland. Their fourth child, a baby girl was born in Grozny.

When the first Russian-Chechen war broke out (December, 1994–August, 1996), Kazbeg's family seriously suffered, like many others. Bombardment damaged his house, the walls came apart, caught fire and his elder son, who then was 13, burned his legs. There was no place to hide 3 infants (2-year-old twin boys and a baby girl of 10 months). In the following year, during continuous bombings, Khava had a miscarriage of twins because of stress.

One day soldiers of Russian federal troops broke into Kazbeg's house. He was severely beaten (especially on his head) with feet and guns, and threatened that his wife and children will be executed. The assault lasted for more than an hour. The soldiers were demanding "information", money and gold. "It was the hardest when they pointed a gun at my wife and asked if I could see her killed and still say nothing," told us Kazbeg. Khava too has undergone physical and psychological abuse (mocking, threatening).

After that, he was arrested and held in custody in the basement of the Gudermes Prison. They interrogated him about the Chechnyan Resistance and since he "did not know anything", he was subjected to a severe torture. They tortured him for 10 days and he ended up with a broken collarbone and perforated appendix. Then they threw him unconscious out into the street where he spent all frosty night.

Upon termination of the first Russian-Chechen war, Kazbeg together with his wife and children left for Ukraine. In Ukraine, he met a Tibetan lama, who determined Kazbeg's further life outlook – a philosophy of active non-violence. The Tibetan lama preached that a human being had to resist injustice with all his spirit and energy. One has to be free, although not through war and brutality, but through active nonconformity and non-violence.

Kazbeg was so fascinated by this concept that he started introducing this philosophy to his fellow Chechens in Ukraine. He created a forum for non-violent struggle and organized a conference for promotion of non-violent vision of resolution of the Chechen conflict. For majority of his compatriots this philosophy was unacceptable, since "historically, Chechens are fighters". Unfortunately, violence reached his family again. Before the outbreak of the second Russian-Chechnyan war (in 1999), Khava, together with her elder son and little daughter, returned to Chechnya to visit her family.

One night, during a regular "Zachistky[1]*"* the Russian soldiers burst into their house and arrested her 26 year old brother. "They did not even allow him to put on his clothes" remembers Khava. All this was happening in front of the family members, accompanied by physical and psychological abuse. The soldiers

---

[1] "Zachistky" – a periodic cleansing carried out by Russian Federal Troops aimed at arresting resistance fighters, however in many cases peaceful population, including women and children, were subjected to torture and ill-treatment

pointed a gun at Khava's head and at her small daughter threatening them with execution. Khava was crying, trying to defend her brother and was seriously beaten, especially on her head. Finally, soldiers took her brother and after that, nobody has ever heard of him. That night many men were taken away from their homes.

Khava later described that "despite the summer heat, I froze and I was shivering". She could hear how her daughter was weeping and begging to be taken away from the house. After that incident, whenever her daughter saw uniformed people, she always tried to hide, starting crying and asking for help. That time Khava's psychological state deteriorated. She developed a fear of being left alone, a fear of darkness and uncontrolled shivering. Her daughter started to suffer from night enuresis. Since it was not possible for Khava and her little daughter to leave for Ukraine, Kazbeg with his sons immediately returned to Chechnya, but soon upon his return he was taken by Russian soldiers to a filtration camp[2], where he spent 10 days kept in waist-deep water. He has again undergone insults, threats, beating. He was released only after his relatives had paid the ransom. After having witnessed all this terror, Kazbeg's elder son, despite his father's arguments and reprimands left the house and joined the resistance fighters.

In autumn 1999, Kazbeg moved with his family to Georgia, and left his mother, who refused to leave Grozny, behind.

In 1999, the Georgian Government declared its readiness to accept refugees from Chechnya and settle them in Pankisi Gorge, a place populated by ethnic Kists. Historically Chechens and Kists have the same origin, they speak the same language and share common customs and traditions. The refugees were granted a group refugee status, meaning that they did not receive individual documentation and were restricted in their traveling within the country. The State did not take any responsibility to provide refugees with shelter or material assistance and addressed international humanitarian organizations to support the refugees. However, those refugees who would leave the Gorge and settle somewhere else in Georgia would not receive any assistance whatsoever. Nevertheless, a certain number of refugees chose to live in Tbilisi, the capital of Georgia instead of being trapped in Pankisi Gorge. Kazbeg was among those refugees. The family lived in harsh circumstances and poverty. Very often they did not have money to pay their bills and were left without electricity and gas. After spending two years in Tbilisi Kazbeg learnt about our center, which provided medical and psychosocial assistance to refugees from Chechnya.

---

[2] Filtration Camp – military camps where Chechens were gathered by federal army soldiers for identification of resistance fighters. Often these camps served as punitive prisons – big majority of refugees were severely tortured there. See Baiev, et al. (2003) for additional information.

The First Meeting

"Can your medical center help me selling my kidney?"

"Sell your Kidney?!"

"Yes, this is a very expensive organ; I'm selling it for cheap, for transplantation."

Kazbeg said that he was in urgent need of money, in order to leave Georgia, since he and his family were in danger.

He described how he found out about the center through several Chechen refugees, who were our clients already. When Kazbeg saw their psychological state improving, he decided to "check us out, pay a visit and see what kind of work we are doing". That is why he asked a friend (a client of the center) to accompany him during his first visit.

At our first meeting, he and his friend Said were sitting around the table with gloomy faces. Said remained mostly silent. Kazbeg was telling the story of his family – how they lived in extreme poverty in Georgia, how his children, who were 10 and 8, did not attend school because they couldn't speak Georgian, and how he refused to take them to a Russian one out of his principles.

As Kazbeg explained, one of the main reasons why he wanted to leave Georgia for any European country was to give his children proper education. Since he had not received from the authorities any answer to his requests to transfer him and his family to the third country, he decided to sell his kidney, and considered this as the only way to earn money for the trip and save his family.

After the "kidney story", the center's lawyer was invited to join the meeting, in order to persuade Kazbeg that selling the kidney was illegal and that nobody would be willing to help him. We tried to convince him that he should forget this option. He seemed convinced, and gradually dropped the issue.

Then we[3] explained to Kazbeg what services the center is offering to our clients, what kind of assistance he and his family could receive from the team, and what was the concept of "psychosocial and medical treatment and rehabilitation". We also offered him to involve his children in therapy group at the center, as this might be useful for them. Kazbeg refused these offers, though he continued the conversation. He spoke of Chechnya, he recalled the history of his people, mentioned the Georgian-Chechen unity stressing that both nations belong to the culture of the Caucasus, sharing similar history, traditions, etc.; spoke of the hard lot of the refugees, as "most of them feel endangered in Georgia and would like to seek asylum in the West."

At the end of our first meeting, our lawyer offered Kazbeg his assistance in preparing documentation for submission to relevant official bodies that deal with transfer of refugees to the third countries. Kazbeg accepted this offer and we set the next appointment date.

---

[3] This article is written by Kazbeg's psychotherapist and the child therapist who worked with his children. By using the "we", authors pay tribute to the colleagues, center's multidisciplinary team members, who were involved in Kazbeg's and his family's treatment/rehabilitation process at various stages.

This meeting gave the onset to our long-term relationship with Kazbeg and his family. Presumably, during the first meeting we managed to gain some trust of Kazbeg and from that day on, slowly, over the following two years, he became our client, friend, partner and one of our main contact persons with the Chechen community in Georgia.

The Next Visit

At the second visit, Kazbeg came with his three children, but not at the appointed time, we had previously agreed with him. He did not consider it necessary to explain why he had not come to the appointment on time. As we eventually learned, there was no use to set appointments, neither with him, nor with other refugees from Chechnya. The only time category that worked was "first half of the day or second half of the day", however even this often was not respected either.

At the second meeting the center's lawyer helped Kazbeg in writing a statement for granting asylum. Kazbeg engaged in the discussion on the legal procedures with great interest. Meanwhile, his children were informally talking with a psychologist. They were drawing pictures and viewing other kids' paintings that were hanging in the office.

After finishing the affairs with legal documents, Kazbeg remained at the office. It was obvious that he wanted to continue the dialogue, so he was invited to the psychotherapy room. He talked about what was going on among the Chechen refugee community in Pankisi Gorge, what was happening in Chechnya and how people lived there. Suddenly he took out his mother's letter and started to read it. Mother was informing Kazbeg about the deaths of several relatives and about frequency and horror of "Zachistky". Kazbeg could not finish reading the letter, as his voice started to tremble, his breathing became uneven, and he stood up and started to walk in the room nervously. When he calmed down, he remembered how he was leaving Grozny, and spoke of his journey from Chechnya to Georgia. Together with other refugees, he and his family crossed the Georgian-Chechen border through steep and mountainous areas, the route was difficult, especially for little children, who had to walk and climb for hours. Then he briefly recalled their short stay in Pankisi and hard days in Tbilisi. "Now I don't know who I am any more", he said, while he kept smoking, felt restless and slightly shivered. He mentioned that his family did not suffer that much, and that there were hundreds of thousands of other Chechens who experienced worse things. Their family members have died or disappeared. "At least I see my kids running in front of me", he added. Once again, he was offered to engage his kids in group therapy sessions, but he refused it again.

However, several days later Kazbeg called the centre saying that his children really wanted to come and asked when this would be possible. He started bringing his children to the group sessions.

Children

Records of the Child Group Therapists

Twin Brothers Musa and Abek (10 years old)
and Their Sister Zara (8 years old)

All three children had a high level of anxiety, sense of insecurity, fears; little girl had sleeping disturbances with nightmares. She had witnessed the violence of the soldiers, saw the kidnapping of her uncle and beating of the mother, blood and despair; she had night enuresis, could not stay in bed alone and slept in one bed with her parents. Apart from group work, she was engaged in individual psychotherapy course with a child-psychotherapist; the sessions with her and sometimes together with her mother proved to be successful.

Children engaged in group work with great enthusiasm. They showed interest towards different activities and topics. They were smart, though there was an observable gap in their education. Sometimes group work was impeded by the fact that all three were from the same family. The brothers often made fun of their little sister, and she always reacted with crying.

Children had a brother who was a Chechen resistance fighter and they have not heard of him for over a year. They talked very often about the brother. While recalling him their narration became incoherent and fragmented, as they got upset. Little girl's breathing became uneven and difficult.

During discussions, they overtly expressed revengeful attitudes, saying that all Russians, including little babies, should be punished. Their parents were very concerned about this disposition.

At some point, children stopped attending the group sessions. As we learned, due to material poverty, the parents took the twin brothers to Medresse, an Islamic boarding school, where they were given shelter and food and taught Koran. Although, several weeks later parents realized that this school would intensify enmity of the boys towards the surrounding world and took them out.

After returning to the group, the younger twin brother was very happy whereas the elder one was stiff, and unwilling to communicate. He declared that he preferred to be in Medresse where he was taught how to pray.

Children remained in the group for one year. In the beginning, the group sessions took place 2 times a week for 1.5–2 hours. Afterwards the meetings were less frequent.

The primary aim of the group work was mainly to support the development of children and the correction of disturbances – high level of anxiety, fears, aggression, etc. Another intention was to engage the whole family into the treatment and rehabilitation process via children.

First sessions of the group process were devoted to creation of safety, offering some routine and recurrent experiences, trust-building exercises, and fairy-tales. Therapists tried to structure their day, offering very simple home tasks, like "draw the tree that is seen from your window", "produce the best day story".

The work was mainly implemented through art-therapy techniques (painting, drawing, using clay, etc.), developmental games and expressive methods. Later they were offered exercises in effective communication and conflict resolution. Special attention was given to the topics "acceptance of subjective realities", tolerance-building through stories, etc. We tried to teach them how to identify emotions and manage them. Later on, we focused on processing the enemy image.

In the beginning of the intervention, their drawings were full of blood, killings, and shootings. Children used much red color. Gradually the content of the drawings changed and centered on family, nature, heroes from the books that we were giving them to read. Regularly, we exhibited their paintings at office walls and organized exhibitions for staff and office-attendees.

As the treatment process unfolded, the children became more joyful and open, their anxiety level significantly reduced and mistrust and enmity was transformed into positive attitudes towards their immediate environment. They showed their regained confidence in many ways, but most obvious was the touch[4] – they started to allow others to cuddle them and they were spontaneously hugging others when greeting or leaving. In case of Zara, her enuresis stopped after 6 months, she gradually was able to sleep separately from parents, her self-esteem raised and became clear that she reacted adequately to jokes and teasing.

Khava

After 1.5 months from the initial meeting, Kazbeg brought his wife to the center. Khava presented mainly with somatic complaints – headaches, nausea, periodic vomiting, pain in the waist area and in the lower abdomen, difficulties in movement. She was mainly visiting a GP of the center, though she counseled with a psychiatrist and other specialists as well.

---

[4] Touch is the cultural taboo among Chechens; men and women are not allowed to touch each other; it is impossible to form the cycle while playing or doing the exercise as girls and boys can not hold each others hands.

Record of the Psychiatrist

Khava, 39 years old

The client complained about persistent insomnia, inner tension and increased irritation. She could not name the cause of her problems, because "there are so many reasons and it's impossible to track them". During conversation, her voice trembled and her eyes became tearful. Before recalling something that was particularly painful, she made a long pause, closed her eyes and took a deep breath. General anxiety, depressed mood and impaired attention were observable.

Client required medication, but refused to take them. "Due to the lack of food, I can't take the pills", she says. Client was willing to get medical assistance, although it was difficult to persuade her to keep appointments with a psychiatrist or attend psychotherapy sessions.

Khava was referred for consultations to a neurologist, gynecologist, and psychologist. She underwent laboratory and clinical examinations and was assessed by PTSD, depression and anxiety questionnaires. She was diagnosed with chronic PTSD, residual effects of cranium trauma, intracranial hypertension, angiothrophic neurosis and some other somatic diseases.

Khava was prescribed a course of poly-vitamins to regain strength. Afterwards she went through a medication treatment for somatic symptoms and physiotherapy with medical massage. Her careless attitude towards health was alarming; she repeatedly said, that when her brother and son are missing, when her children are so malnourished and pale she could not possibly think of her health. She was missing the appointments with the doctor and was taking medicines irregularly.

The family atmosphere was very loving. Kazbeg and Khava had mutual understanding and were very affectionate towards the kids. As for children, the elder twin brother was slightly thorny and always reprimanded his younger brother for his softness.

Kazbeg

Increasingly the trust towards the center and the team working with his children and his wife was growing; Kazbeg was visiting the center systematically, the meetings with various colleagues were becoming regular. The sequel of his trauma was becoming evident also.

Kazbeg gradually started to open up and talk about his concerns. He said that he had a constant feeling of danger. He feared that one day he would be "stopped in the street and imprisoned", suspected that he was under constant observation. He could not walk alone. 'I have to be accompanied by at least one of my kids, in order to tell the family afterwards what has happened to me in case that I get arrested". He was afraid that Georgian security forces together with Russian FSB (Federal Service of Security) would capture and eliminate him. When, in the therapy process, rationality of his fears was discussed, he told about friends and acquaintances that have simply disappeared. Kazbeg's feeling was that one day, he too, could just disappear, vanish. Thus even taking his little daughter with him might have prevented this, or, as he said, he could at least have a witness.

Because of this on-going, permanent feeling of threat, Kazbeg was careful, he was checking the street out of the center's window, selected time of leaving the building. Often his actions seemed incoherent and reckless, he was impulsive; might leave the room on the mid sentence, was easily irritated.

On various occasions Kazbeg mentioned that he "doesn't believe in anyone or anything", "doesn't trust anyone", "entire world and surrounding reality contains danger", "world is an enemy", "we are surrounded by enemies." Sometimes he was in complete despair – "with this attitude I am not able to bring up my kids properly", "I know that it is damaging for their development to be growing up in the atmosphere of such hatred". That's when he asked us to help him in bringing them up.

Kazbeg had difficulties communicating, he was afraid of leaving his house. Officially, due to a refugee status, he was not allowed to work, although sometimes, "when luck was on his side" he managed to earn money by working as a loader at the railway station. However, because of his physical weakness he had difficulties working. In the beginning of the treatment, he seemed rather lonely, disconnected from others despite the fact that he had some close Chechen friends.

Apart from a psychotherapist and lawyer, Kazbeg was referred to the medical doctor as well. He was complaining about itching pains in the heart, general weakness, asthenia and dizziness. Doctor assumed that he was malnourished; once he was not able to finish the cardiac test – became weak, dizzy and finally he fainted.

We realized that very often the family did not have enough food and gradually, very carefully and politely, began offering them a lunch at the office. This could probably be considered as a turning point in their treatment. We started offering something to the entire family. At first, it was just a cup of hot tea, and later on, we invited them to the office kitchen to share a meal with us. We were trying to convince them that we just had lunchtime as they arrived. Half a year later, while having a meal with her, Kazbeg confessed to our medical doctor that his dream was to treat himself one day with lot of roasted beef and a half a liter of vodka.

Meetings with Kazbeg were not "formally" named as psychotherapy. These were just his "visits" to the center and conversations with me, but also with other members of our team – psychologist, lawyer, medical doctor, child therapist, social worker, nurse, and others. Topics discussed concerned problems of his community, family, politics and general philosophical issues. Sometimes he was agitated, impulsive, talked much and associated freely. From time to time, he was engaged in "Socratic dialogues" or was listening silently to the explanations about the trauma psychology, human behavior and power of the mind. There was a time when he told me that those conversations were "as rain to the dried out soil of the desert".

On several occasions, Kazbeg repeated during the sessions that these conversations "make him weaker, softer. He looses strength". Despite these reprimands, he continued individual "meetings". "I am regaining my internal world that had vanished," told he.

Our team was giving him a frame to understand his complaints and pains, providing some structure in daily routines and guidance in reorganizing his life.

His visits to the center went on for many months, and never had he come alone. He was accompanied either by his children, by his wife, or by other Chechens, but most frequently he would come with his little daughter.

The psychotherapeutic process was directed at deepening a secure and trustful relationship. On the other hand, the work was directed at re-structuring trauma and identifying his values and principles, meanings that he was giving to the events and situations. We also worked on channeling his visible interests and skills – working on the community problems, leadership. Much time was spent in helping him to identify his problems, prioritize them and play with options to resolve them positively. This process turned out to be very fruitful.

Gradually Kazbeg's social inclusion was increasing. This involved caring for others, his fellow Chechens. He articulated to us their problems and addressed the center's lawyer, psychotherapist, social worker or doctor to help him in solving them. One thing was apparent – in all his activities, he wanted to engage either the center, or particular professionals to back him up and support him. This was related to his lack of confidence and insecurity. In order to compensate these feelings, Kazbeg established safe relationships with the center and tried to rely on us.

Slowly Kazbeg managed to channel his energy in activities such as writing petitions regarding various problems of the Chechen community in Georgia. He advocated for refugees living in Tbilisi who did not receive humanitarian assistance, kept pressing relevant organizations to increase the food ration for refugees and to provide them with at least tea and milk and to give additional aid to families with infants.

At our center Kazbeg organized several meetings with a relatively large group of refugees, who shared with us the problems of their community, like absence of medical assistance, lack of proper education for children, having a group refugee status and, most importantly, disappearances and extradition of various refugees living in Georgia.

These large group meetings, for long time, stayed very chaotic and repetitive in content. The group was all heavily emotional, irritated and frustrated. Most of the times these men, inhabitants of Tbilisi and Pankisi Gorge, talked about entrapment – "Georgian government offered us a refuge, but imprisoned us in Pankisi Gorge and use Chechens as a tool for bargaining with Russia". Sometimes we too were objects of their rage, as Georgians, representatives of the country with above-mentioned double standards of behavior. On several occasions they recalled the Georgian-Abkhazian war[5], which is the main reason of hostility towards the Chechens in Georgia. They were mentioning that only mercenaries fought against Georgians in that conflict, and that all the hired soldiers from the Northern Caucasus were wrongly labeled as Chechens. "How can't you understand this, we forgave you Stalin!" they once said. They were recalling the 1940s genocide and deportation of Chechens by Stalin's order and that Stalin was of Georgian origin.

They were going even further back in history and talking about Imam Shamil[6] and the 40 years of war with Russia-"That's when Ichkerya[7] was devastated. In that conflict, Georgians were on the Russian side, against Shamil and freedom!" These accusations came up on a number of occasions. These were unconscious articulations of their doubts towards our team's intentions and motives and, at the same time, their hope for help. Together with the lawyer and other colleagues, we tried to facilitate meetings, summarize speeches, and conclude with small steps to the direction of improvement and justice.

Kazbeg was an obvious leader during these meetings. He was respected, was being listened to, he always managed to calm down the heat in discussions, but he could also be very strict, uncompromising and demanding. He was very grateful for our support. During one of these meetings he declared – "We considered entire Christianity as our enemy, but now, after getting to know you, we realize that we were mistaken".

Gradually, Kazbeg took up a role of an informal leader within the community. He revived the Chechen Human Rights Committee, although he did not occupy any formal position there. He became the main organizer of a hunger strike, a well-organized action that took place simultaneously in Tbilisi and Pankisi Gorge, which lasted for a month. The aim of the action was to bring to the attention of the Georgian Authorities, International Human Rights organizations and Mass-Media, the problems of Chechen refugees and to publicize the facts of disappearances and extraditions. With the center's facilitation Kazbeg organized a round table that was held at the Public Defender's office, where the voices of Chechen refugees were heard for the first time. Kazbeg opened the meeting. The presentations of Chechens were well-structured, succinct and very clear. This was the first dialogue of the refugee community with various stakeholders, a meeting where they were perceived by others as equals. After that event this dialogue has been continued with unstable success and regularity until now.

---

[5] After becoming independent in 90's, Georgia started a process of transition to democratic State, characterised by the long-term political-social-economical crises, accompanied by the internal ethnic conflicts with Abkhazians and South Ossetians. After these conflicts Georgia lost its territorial integrity – two important regions, Abkhazia and Shida Kartli, became cut off from the rest of the country and approximately 272 000 persons (nearly 5% of the country population) were displaced.

[6] Imam of Dagestan who ruled for 25 years and united Dagestan and Chechnya in struggle against the Russian rule

[7] Historical name of Chechnya

Later on, Kazbeg became a respondent of various international human rights organizations. He gained fame; he strived for protection of the rights of Chechen refugees and incessantly revealed facts of different human rights violations. On the behalf of Chechen community, he participated in the pacifist action against war in Iraq. He continued being in touch with the center, however his visits became rarer. Whenever he came, he tried to express his gratitude to us. On one occasion, he donated a part of humanitarian assistance, which he had received, to the center. "You know people who might benefit from these things", he explained.

Unfortunately, Kazbeg's feeling that he was endangered continued to intensify. He was mentioning several suspicious, threatening phone calls from the side of Georgian law enforcers that he had received. His wish to leave Georgia was becoming stronger. Although he always assured us that he preferred to stay in Georgia, among friends and, most importantly, close to Chechnya and his mother, he also thought that his children should be brought up differently. "Our nation requires a new generation – well educated and civilized. Freedom is not reached only through war, but through civilized means, through bright mind" – he would add. Finally, Kazbeg and his family managed to cross the Georgian border illegally. Only after his departure, we realized that the refugee community lost its main drive, its unifying force.

Soon after he left, he called. He was in one of the refugee camps in Slovakia. He enquired whether it was possible for us to consult the young psychologists working with the refugees in Slovakia. "They don't know how to work with our people here", he added.

Kazbeg is now, after 6 years since his escape from Chechnya, a citizen of one of the European countries. He still keeps in touch with us. During one of the phone calls, his little daughter Zara asked to talk with her therapist. "I have changed, I am a big girl now," she said happily.

Multilevel Trauma

In Kazbeg's case we are dealing with several levels of trauma – with the individual trauma, inflicted to him during two wars, and entailing his physical and psychological abuse; with the secondary trauma, related to insults and abuse suffered by his wife, intimidation of his children and disappearance of his eldest son; and with the large group traumatic experience associated with defeat, collective extermination and humiliation of his ethnic group. Moreover, he is still subjected to on-going, stressful and severe social-economic living conditions mixed up with a strong feeling of intimidation and threat.

Although Kazbeg is a refugee, his life is still in danger. There is a significant difference in how refugees are treated in western countries and what they have to confront with in developing countries like Georgia. Apart from the scanty food, lack of education and proper housing, and absence of work opportunities, these people often fall victims of political manipulations. Any new event on political arena, a diplomatic meeting or a statement can easily intensify their sense of insecurity.

Periodic bombings of the Pankisi Gorge by Russian air force, and Georgian Police checkpoints with machine guns at the entrance of the Gorge, where they check the refugees' documents, make their old traumas feel more painful.

Due to the abovementioned multilevel traumatic experience, Kazbeg was diagnosed with PTSD. However, his after-trauma sequel can be fairly described within the category of complex Posttraumatic Stress Disorder (Herman, 1992; Van der Kolk, Roth, Pelcovitz, Sunday, & Spinazzola, 2005). Apart from 'classical' PTSD symptoms, he suffers from changes of **basic assumptions** (Janoff-Bulman, 1983; McCann & Pearlman, 1990), feeling despaired, hopeless and unable to trust. He presents **alterations in affect and regulation of impulses** (affect regulation, modulation of anger), **somatization** (fatigue, pains in chest, respiratory problems, and headaches), **alterations of self-perception** (crisis of I-identification) and **alterations in perception of abusers** (Enemy image formation).

The last two phenomena – Identification crisis and Enemy image – are strongly linked with the post-traumatic societal dynamics of Kazbeg's community. These are not just his, as individual's, traumatic features, but represent the large group's after-trauma processes that greatly influence the individual responses, are insep-arable and interrelated.

Identification crisis and Enemy image formation portray well the individual and societal domains of complex trauma and should be taken into consideration while addressing the traumatized individuals and traumatized groups. These processes will be specifically described below.

Who Am I?

The most evident aspect related to Kazbeg's traumatic experiences is connected with his self-esteem, identity and inability to ascribe meaning to things. This was verbalized at the first our meeting, when he said "I don't know who I am any more, what do I represent". A symbolic externalization of the loss of identity was manifested in the fact that angry Kazbeg has torn his Russian passport into pieces. He no longer needed an identification document, a card verifying his name, place of birth and residence, since he has lost all of these. Therefore, Kazbeg demon-stratively destroyed his ID. On the conscious level he explained his action as a protest against being a citizen of Russia, the country which is responsible for tor-turing his people and being its worst enemy.

His inaction, a sense of guilt (towards his family that is unprotected and vul-narable), his humiliation, helplessness and uncertainness about his present and future have deepened Kazbeg's deprivation of self perception. In Chechnyan mas-culine culture, a man is the leader and decision maker, and his helplessnes is per-ceived most dramatically. It is noteworthy that many young Chechen men, who were clients of our center, had complaints of impotency of a psychological nature. This, of course, was related to a type of torture they have been subjected to (severe beatings in genital area, kept in waist-deep water for many days in a row, cases of male-rape), however in *all cases* clinical examinations showed that these men did not have any organic disturbances of their genital apparatus. After a course of psychotherapy some of these men overcame the problem, got married and had children. This syndrome mirrored the internal psychological state of the defeated men, their self-perception and attitude towards the oposite sex. The psychological impotency portrayed the loss of basic capacities, like the reproduction and satisfaction. This was a metaphor for the lost future and reflected a profound existential crisis among the defeated, insulted and traumatized men. Kazbeg shares this sense of dishonour and loss of self-respect that affects his core personality.

Subsequently, Kazbeg felt himself hunt down "driven into a corner", entrapped in Georgia, sticking deep in his memories of wartime, and his trauma. He was unable to change anything, to help, to persuade, to earn, to escape. A feeling of inescapability has being described as one of the most critical features of a severe trauma (Saporta & van der Kolk, 1998).Inescapability is a feeling that all the ways to escape are cut off and a victim can not do anything to eliminate a massive threat. Victim's coping ability is shattered. While facing repetitive and uncontrollable stress, humans and animals develop the phenomenon of "learned helplessness", a syndrome characterized by a behavioural deficit (Maier & Saligman, 1976). One develops:

• Deficit to learn avoiding new stressful situations
• Low motivation to learn response outcome relationship
• Low ability of exploration and learning
• Signs of chronic subjective distress

Learned helplessness affects and modifies the perception of the "Self" as competent, capable, and being in control. The "Self" perception is damaged and gradually transformed into an "I-concept" that is negative, helpless, and full of guilt.

Kazbeg's self-esteem and self-perception are damaged. "I was a strong person, but I lost every bit of myself", confessed he to me. He has difficulties making decisions, since he does not know what he is capable now of. "I can't identify what I can do" "I can't even bring up my kids", he admitted. He has no confidence toward himself and therefore does not trust others either. When he starts up something, he feels a strong necessity of help and "others", since his "I" identity is helpless and impotent. This leads us to discussion of his attachment to his daughter which is very remarkable. This relationship bears the signs of mutual traumatic bonding. The two helpless souls reciprocally support and strengthen each-other. The little girl needs to be protected, especially during the night, when she feels frightened and has to sleep with her parents, next to her "protector" father. On the other hand, Zara, the scared child who is often crying without any reason, gives Kazbeg enough strength to walk in the streets in her company. Both, Zara and Kazbeg use these traumatic rituals in order to diminish their anxiety caused by obsessive fears. This happens through a silent agreement between the two of them.

Being in a "lost" and defeated position is unbearable for Kazbeg. At one point, he tries to make an unconscious sacrifice in order to overcome his sense of vulnerability. He wants to cut out his kidney – a part of his physical body, if it only could help him to recover his confidence that he is the head of his family, able to support them, secure their future and regain freedom, and at the same time hoping that his self-perception might be liberated from the burden of helplessness.

"I am . . . Them"

One of the Kazbeg's main defenses throughout his personality crisis is his identification with his own group – the Chechen people, the refugee community, its shared problems and the common history. He finds strength in the "We-ness". The "Ethnic Tent" (Volkan, 1997) gives him a shelter, a sense of belonging and security, and eases his search for the lost "pillar" of identity.

An individual's core I-identity, a persistent sense of sameness within the self (Erikson, 1956), also includes the large-group, the We-identity, that links a person to the others within an ethnic, national or other large group (Volkan, 1999). When I-identity is shaken, We-ness is often actualized, especially in collectivistic cultures.

Collectivistic cultures are regarded as societies where the groups' interests prevail over the individual ones. In collectivistic cultures, people share strong "We-identity" feelings. The impact of massive or repeated trauma on these societies is different from societies where individual freedom and parity among group members are highly valued and individuals are not "tightly tied" by large groups' norms and traditions. Chechen society belongs to the collectivistic culture, where special importance is given to the group interests in general and to extended family interests in particular.

The need to attach to others increases during stress or exposure to danger. Stable and close attachments help in limiting overwhelming physiological reactions of distress. The presence of "others" also helps validating the individual experience and making sense out of what has happened (Bowlby, 1969, 1973). "Ethnic tent" and the We-identity help Kazbeg in mobilizing his efforts and coping with internal anxiety and personality crisis. Kazbeg openly identifies himself with a large group, with a refugee community. He always speaks on behalf of the "we" (the group of refugees) and struggles for the common goals, realizing that these activities are directed at wellbeing of his family, too. The collective "self" gradually manifested itself in increasing Kazbeg's social liveliness and, as it later appeared, this was his successful strategy of coping with traumatic experiences.

I Versus Us

There is yet another, very important, aspect that definitely deserves attention – the interaction of the developed "I" concept with the "We"-ness. Traumatic experience often contributes to regression of a person and causes one's declination from personal values and beliefs in order to maintain the "we" identity. In case of

Kazbeg, his conscious and moral achievement, the Tibetan non-violence concept, is in conflict with the large group's traditional concept of revenge. In the attempt to portray Kazbeg's psychological features, this internal fracture and the subsequent path towards synthesis might be the most essential aspect.

Kazbeg has an identity of a follower of Chechnyan Sufi Islam. He prays, pays tribute to traditions and customs. He is a son of his nation. This is the basic, core part of his We-identity, which largely evokes during the time of his exile, while identifying with his ethnic group. However, after some time from the first traumatic experience, he has found a new meaning through the concept of non-violent resistance. This attitude is alien to his culture. Confrontation and struggle are acceptable, but a "peaceful way" is a strange option, as people who had been in battles for over the centuries have become accustomed to aggression and revenge. These have become inseparable parts of their identity.

Kazbeg put lots of efforts and energy in interiorizing and gradually introducing his non-violence belief system, a system, which is in conflict with his "We" identity. His non-violent "I" has to either "pass away", has to be denied and suppressed, or Kazbeg has to say no to his "ethnic tent" – a frame that gives him strength and confidence in these difficult times of his life. Therefore, Kazbeg is going through a deep internal conflict; he is ambivalent and faces aversive choices. His identity is loosing its coherence and energy, it becomes fragmented. This resembles the metaphor for the fracturing of the soul, self, and identity – the broken spirit (Wilson, 2004).

It is no surprise that his anxiety level is high, that he is incongruent and unconsciously sending double binding, conflicting messages to his children. This is why, despite his conscious non-violent and peaceful choice, his twin boys are full of revenge on their enemies. "They should all die", – as one of them mentioned. An evident illustration of Kazbeg's incoherent actions is his decision to take his boys to Medresse, an Islamic boarding school. There they are brought up together with other Muslim boys, which will foster their "We" identity. However, as soon as Kazbeg realizes this and notices increasing aggression in his children, he immediately takes them out, and brings them back to the rehabilitation centre – a place where his non-violent "I" feels more secure.

His ambivalence towards the therapeutic process can be explained by this internal splitting, too. Under the "tent", Kazbeg's collective identity allows him to act aggressively for the sake of his people. He mentions the "white rage", which is rising in him when he is looking at the suffering of his people. He is unstructured, impulsive, and often full of destructive ideas, but gradually he gathers around him a group of refugees. On the other hand, during the therapeutic process, his hidden values and beliefs are revealed and emphasized. Here, his mindful "I" looks for explanations and arguments, to justify and explain why the Chechnyan path should be peaceful. This is the voice of his individual "I". It is perceived as weak and vulnerable, since it lacks the protection of the "We" shield. That is the reason why Kazbeg sometimes keeps repeating that psychotherapeutic conversations are making him weaker, though he keeps attending these meetings because they emphasize his "I" and prevent him from becoming completely merged with the

"We-ness". This is why he does not discuss his non-violence theory with Chechen groups, and never mentions his elder son who was fighting in Chechnya and is missing. He tries to draw a line between his two inner worlds.

Only after a certain time, Kazbeg manages to "reconcile" these two parts of his identity. This is the beginning of his integration and inner synthesis. Kazbeg discovers the concept of human rights, which allows him to lead an uncompromising struggle, using non-violent, peaceful methods. He manages to overcome his non-authenticity. Together with maintaining his "We" identity, his individual, unique traits become more distinctively outlined.

Societal Trauma

In order to understand the basis of Kazbeg's uncompromising struggle and, as he himself calls it, "power", it is important to discuss the psychological dynamics of large "we" ethnic groups. Description of this phenomenon leads us to the concept of societal trauma. The "large group" of Chechen refugees is going through a crisis itself. The group has been severely traumatized, and subsequently thrown into an alien culture, a different religious and linguistic environment.

To begin with, it should be mentioned that this society is bearing a historic trauma. A brief overview of the late history of the Chechen people illustrates at least two deliberate attempts of destroying this nation. First in the beginning of the nineteenth century, when the Chechen people struggled for liberation from the Russian rule for almost 40 years and almost lost all its male population, and in 1944 when the entire ethnic group was accused of cooperation with the Nazis and deported to Central Asia. These traumatic memories are alive in the society and their burden exacerbates the severity of more recent events. These mental representations are mixed with the memories of the current traumatic events – a lost war, torture experiences. They add and magnify each other and outline a perception of a group's role, its mission and place.

After prolonged and/or repetitive traumatization, the whole community develops a complex constellation of shared feelings, attitudes and behaviour patterns. It forces a group into the role of a victim. "We –representation" of the victimized group correlates to a passive, unskilled, unable and unsure image. The large group of refugees experiences threatening of its identity. A role of victim is unbearable and offensive for Chechen fighting community.

The group tries to maintain the positive "We –concept". One of the basic mechanisms used for this purpose is projection. The group projects all bad, non-human, non-tolerated affects to "others" in order to "clean up" its own victimized and negative identity.

Formation of the Enemy Image helps the group of refugees in defining their collective identity and promoting a sense of "We-ness". Aggressive attitudes towards the "Enemy" give them the strength to "assemble" themselves and achieve an inner cohesion between community members. Aggression becomes a powerful weapon for keeping the group mobilized and fighting back the enemies.

Kazbeg is full of a sense of danger and mistrust, he is afraid of the entire external reality – the city, the people in the city, etc. "Entire world is an enemy," he says. Kazbeg tries to cope with this fear through non-violence, in order to compensate destructive tendencies and his longing for revenge. However, the "Enemy Image" is a phenomenon that we consider an important marker for his psychological portrait, as well as the portrait of the other Chechen refugees.

These feelings and attitudes are spread around and passed down to future generations through the processes of interpersonal and intergenerational transmission. These feelings are contagious. "Enemy Image" is easily generalized beyond the real adversary, exaggerated and transferred to immediate but different neighbours, other ethnic or religious groups, or international organizations. Sometimes, as we observe in the case of Kazbeg, the whole world represents the enemy.

The transgenerational transmission of the enemy image is well illustrated by Kazbeg's children (especially his elder son), who are developing a traumatic identity and becoming reservoirs of hate and aggression. This has a great impact on their development. The only responsibility and mission they uphold in their life is revenge:" We will grow up and pay back the Russians, Christians and other people who betrayed us."

Core Elements of the Intervention

The case of Kazbeg and his family helped our team to get insight into the individual and community problems of refugees from Chechnya living in Georgia, and create an integrated, culturally sensitive intervention approach.

Explaining core elements of the approach will outline the strategy of intervention with Kazbeg and his family and clarify the process and the goals of working with the Chechnyan community in general.

The first, basic and broadly accepted element is ***creating an atmosphere of trust***. One of the consequences of complex trauma is a loss of trust – when one cannot trust and does not feel safe and secure anymore. Kazbeg, Khava and many others have difficulties believing that others "hear" and understand them. In the beginning, they trust neither our organization, nor the team. They think that the world is full of enemies. We are required all our professional patience, openness and a non-formal attitude to shorten the distance between us in interpersonal contact, in order to gradually change this attitude and persuade the client that he/she can share the pain with us. Therapeutic intervention requires a long-term relationship, which can only be built on trust.

We realize that we are dealing with complex trauma in complex and difficult circumstances, so general treatment schemas are discarded. The length of initial meetings is not limited; sometimes they last for 2–3 hours, as in case of Kazbeg. We allow the client to ventilate his emotions, listen to him empathetically and give him our time. The most important thing is our solidarity, eagerness and delicacy to recognize the person with his/her needs, aspirations, etc. This core element of the approach is ***non-neutrality and empathy***. Therapist's emotional availability and engagement creates the framework of healing.

A safe environment contributes to a formation of feelings of trust and safety. The interior of the center plays an important role here. The office is located in a regular apartment building, which already creates an informal atmosphere. At their first visit, after the intake interview, we show the clients the office, its different rooms, in order to "identify the territory" for them, reduce their anxiety level and explain how the center functions.

To reach inclusion of clients into the treatment process we often ***start working with children***. As we mentioned earlier, caring for the family is characteristic to the cultures in the Caucasus region. Well-being of children is given the primary importance. Improvement of children's psychological and physical condition increases trust towards the therapeutic process as well as our organization. Simultaneously, in the course of the treatment we try to engage other family members as well. Apart from caring for their individual health, this is aimed at studying the functioning of the family and selecting further intervention strategies. Therefore, the following important element is the ***emphasis on the family***.

The next important element is bearing a message – "***Be flexible and pursue the uniqueness of each client***." Kazbeg did not accept his role of a patient, neither consider himself a "victim of trauma"; nevertheless he was willing to continuously visit the center and receive indirect assistance. He wanted to be more than a client, rather a friend. My colleagues and I allowed him to have this role. We did not try to bring his visits under a somewhat strict schedule of psychotherapeutic sessions (e.g. your appointment with the therapist will be held on Tuesday at 12:00). We tried to get him "invited" inventing different reasons, like therapy of his children, appointment with a lawyer, or just a conversation. A turning point in our relationship was when Kazbeg started to accept our invitations for a meal. One usually shares a meal with a friend. This is a demonstration of hospitality and closeness. Since that moment, he actually started to believe that we accepted him as a friend and happily took up that role. As a result, he became our center's contact person and advanced in his role of a "friend-client-collaborator". He had identified and referred to us many severely traumatized Chechen refugees. He has also become an active advocate of their rights, knowing that we are backing him up.

Providing a structure is one of the central elements of intervention and entails introducing a structure into the chaos that traumatized victims suffer from.

The traumatization is very vivid in the attitude towards time. A group of Chechen refugees is attached to their Past, that is brighter than the present, which is interlaced with it filling with new emotions. At the same time, the Future is unclear, vague and full of uncertainty. For many of them the future is lost, since they do not have any hopes. Nobody is making any plans for Future, while being deprived of the Present too, containing danger and humiliation. The time line of Yesterday-Today-Tomorrow is confused and mixed up. Time is disregarded and given hardly any attention. We can judge about such attitude towards time by Kazbeg's and others untimely visits to the Center. The community is lost in time and space.

Routine tasks for children or routine appointments are necessary for "improving" a sense of time and fostering feeling of regularity, a rhythmic order. Sometimes the clients do not know what day or which month it is. Marking the "mental" calendar arranges days, and helps planning. Continuity of relationship and offering care contributes to organizing one's future and forming the feeling of safety.

The next element of our approach *"goals orientation instead of symptoms orientation"* is defined by the social-political, economical and cultural reality of the refugee community. To justify this approach we need to analyze the complex context of refugees' life.

Traumatic symptoms of traumatized refugees are aggravated by the uncertain, troubled and alert reality. In the beginning, when we heard their stories of living in Georgia full of fear and danger we thought of delusional nature of such thoughts. However, we soon learned that these fears were quite realistic. Refugees living in Georgia were suddenly disappearing. There were other numerous facts of deportation and illegal extradition of refugees to Russia. Kazbeg's feeling of constant danger was, perhaps, an overreaction, but the external reality was indeed threatening[8].

When the reality is so forbidding, the treatment and rehabilitation process goes extremely hindered and blocked. Any efforts to alleviate the trauma symptoms are futile and ineffective. Orientation on goals implies to strive for ensuring the clients maximal desirable and achievable quality of life and a maximal health potential within given circumstances. Our main goal was to facilitate the development of the optimal functionality and personal potential of Kazbeg, his family and his community. On the long run, we tried to achieve mobilization of his resources, enabling factors that would help him to cope with the contextual and personal threats.

The process of intervention often follows a route *"from periphery to the center,"* with the traumatic experience as the "center" and resources – the knowledge, the experience, and the skills – as the "periphery." Strengthening the resources, we can subsequently deal more efficiently with the trauma. In some cases, similar to that of Kazbeg, it might seem that no direct work on trauma experience took place, and that we only build up the "periphery", his self-esteem and social engagement. In his treatment, our attention was mainly focused and the most time spent on strengthening his ability to concentrate on his problems, identify possible ways of solving them, and increase his skill to make decisions independently, to revitalize the interests and motivation to act and to overcome the feelings of helplessness and inescapability.

---

[8] For more facts see reports issued by organizations as Amnesty International, Human Rights Watch, etc.; especially the most recent report by Human Rights Documentation and Information Center (2006) *Situation of Refugees from Chechnya.* retrieved October,10, 2006, from http://www.humanrights.ge/eng/files/Chechen%20Torture%20in%20Georgia%20-%20JZ%2011-04-06.pdf

Much attention was paid to his social domain, which seemed more important for him than just physical and psychological health improvement. Thus, sometimes working on client's social domain is the only opening into the therapy – it is required by the client's disposition, interests and by the community needs and evidences (e.g. deprivation, injustice, etc.).

Kazbeg's case showed that it is not effective to work on the problems of an individual or a family if we are not familiar with the general tendencies of the person's community and its psychosocial patterns. One has to ***involve community as much as possible*** and be aware of how the individual relates to the community and what feelings are reinforced by the large group's We-attitudes. Both, individual and community define and characterize each other. In case of Kazbeg, we are dealing with individual and societal consequences of trauma that are interrelated. Because of that, we combined the individual and family tailored therapy with community directed psychosocial interventions.

Dealing with the Enemy Image is a central part of our strategy developed for addressing the Chechen refugee community at individual, family and societal levels. "Enemy image" formation is a survival strategy for the community, because this process fosters inter-group attachments, prevents identity crisis by maintaining positive self-image and gives the meaning to the community members' life – that is seeking the justice and revenge! However, this survival strategy soon grows into destructive and negative attitudes and lifestyle. It drains the psychic energy from the community/group, imposes fragmentation within the group and deteriorates the functioning. This phenomenon is so dominant in Chechen refugee community that it becomes crucial to tackle it at all levels and in all formal and informal institutions, including kindergartens and schools.

For addressing the Enemy Image, it is important to operationalize the concept and "translate" it into concrete feelings, stances, attitudes, behaviors, etc. These characteristics of the Enemy Image can be called the secondary "derivative toxins" (Makhashvili & Javakhishvili, 2005).

The "secondary toxins" of the Enemy image in traumatized communities and individuals are:

• Mistrust and alienation
• Feelings of betrayal and hatred
• Intolerance and prejudices
• Rigid stereotypic interpretations of events, world order, etc.
• Low self-esteem and self-confidence (sometimes hyper-compensated in exaggerated, false self-esteem)
• Aggression, violence outbursts
• Destructive behaviors – towards oneself, others, environment
• Not taking responsibilities

All these "derivatives", sometimes hidden and silently poisoning the society for a long period, should be considered and targeted during psychosocial intervention. We deal with a closed cycle – on one hand, these "toxins" are rooted in the

Enemy Image and on the other, they themselves reinforce and strengthen the Enemy Image phenomenon. After the identification of "derivative toxins", we had the targets for intervention on individual, family and community level. Each of them are addressed systematically, repeatedly and on the long-term run by different therapeutic means, exercises and techniques; the promotion of creativeness is much used as an "antidote" to rigidity and intolerance.

To summarize the intervention strategy it should be emphasized that using metaphors, as therapeutic tool, appeared to be very fruitful during all levels of the treatment process. The Chechen culture is very open towards metaphoric thinking. An explanation and argument is better understood when it is proposed in a condensed way, through fables, parables, sayings. The metaphoric arguments work with individuals, as well as groups.

They are especially successful with children who are main targets of intervention when dealing with the Enemy Image (as victims of its transgenerational transmission). Metaphors help children to comprehend basic values (friendship, love, and faithfulness), to generalize personal experiences and to develop forgiveness and tolerance. They offer models, which can be internalized during the process of personality development and promote the children's ability to conceptualize an empathetic understanding, a caring attitude towards others, and some strong ethical principles (Sarjveladze, Javakhishvili, Makhashvili, Beberashvili, & Sarjveladze, 2001).

To close with, we would like to tell a story, a parable, which helped Kazbeg, as he told us several months after having heard it, in overcoming his identity crisis.

The River Story

One day a rapid river reached the sands of the desert. For some time the river continued to flow carelessly, but gradually, because of heat, it started loosing its water and slowed down its pace. After some time the river could not flow any more, it started to dry out and became lifeless. The desert sands tried to soak it up and the river struggled for its survival. Then, a hot desert wind blew through and told the river: "Follow me, I will take you on my wings, lead you through the desert and then return you back to the earth". The river responded: "I can not come with you; I don't know what will await me there, high in the sky. I won't be myself any more; I do not want to loose myself". The wind repeated: "You should better follow me, you have only two more days to live, what do you have to loose?" The river preferred to stay in the desert, although the next day it realized that it is loosing all its strength and was in anguish. The desert wind came back again and this time took the river to the sky. The river became a cloud and a companion of the wind. After having crossed the desert, it returned to the earth as rain. Then it transformed into a small stream that was slowly getting stronger. The river thanked the desert wind: "I am still myself, I survived and also I discovered so many interesting things during my journey.

The story of Kazbeg resembles the story of this river and trust in wind. He allowed us to join him on this interesting journey and enriched us with new impressions and ideas. While we share them, we hope to follow the path that leads out of the desert.

Acknowledgment.   We want to thank Mr. Michael Nishnianidze for his speedy, delicate and crucial editing of the text.

References

Baiev, K., Daniloff, R., & Daniloff, N. (2003). *The Oath: A Surgeon under Fire* (pp. 3–4). New York: Walker & Company.

Bowlby, J. (1969). *Attachment and Loss.* (Vol. I), Attachment. New York: Basic Books.

Bowlby, J. (1973). *Attachment and Loss.* (Vol. II), Separation. New York: Basic Books.

Erikson, E. H. (1956). The Problem of Ego Identification. *Journal of the American Psychoanalytic Association, 4*, 56–121.

Herman, J. L., (1992). *Trauma and Recovery.* New York: Basic Books.

Janoff-Bulman, R. (1983). The aftermath of victimisation: Rebuilding shattered assumptions. In: Figley, C. R. (Ed.), *Trauma and its wake* (Vol. 1, pp. 15–35). New York: Brunner/Mazel.

Maier, S. F., & Saligman, M. E. (1976). Learned helplessness: theory and evidence. *Journal of Experimental Psychology (Gen), 105*, 3–46.

Makhashvili, N., & Javakhishvili, D. (2005). Overcoming Trauma: Special Focus on School Context. In B. H. Johnsen (Ed.), *Socio-Emotional Growth and Development of Learning Strategies* (pp. 193–214). Oslo: Oslo Academic Press.

McCann, L., & Pearlman, L. A. (1990). Vicarious traumatization: A framework for understanding the psychological effects of working with victims. *Journal of Traumatic Stress, 3*, 131–149.

Saporta J. A., & van der Kolk, B. A. (1998). Psychobiological Consequences of Severe Trauma. In M. Basoglu (Ed.), *Torture and Its Consequences* (pp. 151–171). Cambridge University Press.

Sarjveladze, N., Javakhishvili, D., Makhashvili, N., Beberashvili, Z., & Sarjveladze, N. (2001). *Psychosocial Rehabilitation of Internally Displaced Persons* (pp. 49–51). Istanbul: TUTU Publishers.

van der Kolk, B.A., Roth, S., Pelcovitz, D., Sunday, S.,& Spinazzola, J. (2005). Disorders of Extreme Stress: The Empirical Foundation of a Complex Adaptation to Trauma. *Journal of Traumatic Stress 18*(5), 389–399.

Volkan, V. (1997). *Blood Lines: From Ethnic Pride to Ethnic Terrorism.* New York: Farrar, Straus and Giroux.

Volkan, V. (1999). The tree model: a comprehensive psychopolitical approach to unofficial diplomacy and the reduction of ethnic tension. *Mind and Human Interaction, 10*, 142–206

Wilson, J. P. (2004). The Broken Spirit: Posttraumatic Damage to the Self. In J. P. Wilson & B. Droždek (Eds.), *Broken Spirits: The Treatment of Traumatized Asylum Seekers, Refugees, War and Torture Victims* (pp. 109–157). New York: Brunner-Routledge.

12
Survival As Subversion: When Youth Resistance Strategies Challenge Tradition, Religion, and Political Correctness

Cécile Rousseau & Déogratias Bagilishya

A clinical assessment relies first and foremost on a story told within a particular cultural and political framework: what is said and what is unsaid, whether expressed nonverbally or silenced.

The goat rejoiced because she was expecting a baby, but just as she was giving birth, she realized she had twins and was overwhelmed because it was too much for her. She went all through the village lamenting. Some time later, one of the kids died and once again the goat was totally distraught, this time because of her loss. She told everyone what had happened, and the whole village became concerned. As everybody was worrying with her, listening to her story and retelling it, the goat felt some relief.

This African story evokes the trauma which can be caused by too much or too little, or a loss, and describes trauma transmission as an inherent part of the reconstruction process, which is seen as social. In the goat story, time is the great healer.

In this chapter, we will present the story of Agrippine, a young girl from the Great Lakes area of Africa, focusing on the intertwining of cultural and political signifiers, in both trauma and the reconstruction process. To demonstrate the importance of time in the clinical encounter—the time needed for disclosure, for building meaning, and for establishing trust—we have chosen to present her story linearly, as it unfolded, and to examine how different layers of understanding emerged over time. This article extends the clinical process as a dialogue between the two main clinicians involved, illustrating the convergences and divergences between their voices and the images they represent: African and Canadian, black and white. These differences in the team provided a space where the patient and her family could negotiate meaning and take action.

An Adolescent Refugee Newly Arrived in Canada Who Challenges her Stepmother's Parenting Skills

Agrippine arrived in Canada at the age of 15 as an unaccompanied minor. She comes from a polygamous family of four children. She is the first-born of twins, and is thus considered the eldest. Her twin's status is that of "little brother."

She also has two younger half-sisters, the daughters of her stepmother, her father's second wife. She was born and raised in Kinshasa, the capital of what is now the Democratic Republic of Congo, until she fled to Angola when she was about 13 years old.[1]

Agrippine's life in utero and birth were unremarkable, as was her early childhood, of which she has good memories. When Agrippine was 6 or 7, her parents divorced. Her mother left the family and had no opportunity to maintain contact with Agrippine, who went to live with her stepmother. Despite that, Agrippine has positive memories of the atmosphere in the family. Her stepmother, who was very fond of her and her brother, devoted her time and energy to household tasks and to taking care of her own children as well as those of her former cowife (Agrippine's mother).

Agrippine reported that she and her father were very close and he considered her, as the eldest daughter in the paternal line, to be a model of family virtue for her younger siblings, especially her little half-sisters.

Agrippine's family was very close to ruling families of the old régime in Congo, and these ties to the family of the former president were apparently what led to the extraordinary events that adversely affected Agrippine directly and through her family. When she was 12 years old, her father was killed in cold blood by the members of an armed rebel group that had just seized power. She was at school when it happened and could not be present at his burial because she had to hide out. In her memory, the death of her father seems unreal and she still sometimes wonder if it has really happened. After his murder, Agrippine's stepmother was sent out of the country with her two children, while the twins were left in the care of a paternal uncle who had held a government position under the old régime.

With the aid of his military-political-administrative connections, the uncle fled to Angola with Agrippine and her brother. After two years of living in exile in Angola, the two children left Africa for Canada, thanks to a nun who obtained travel documents for them. She rapidly obtained her refugee status and did not have to go through the angst of a lengthy and difficult determination process (Rousseau, Crépeau, Foxen, & Houle, 2002).

Shortly after her arrival here, Agrippine managed to find her stepmother, who had been living in Canada with her daughters, now aged 12 and 14, for about a year. As is the family custom in some parts of Africa,[2] Agrippine and her brother went to live with their stepmother, who again took on the role of substitute mother. A few months later, Agrippine's stepmother brought her in to the transcultural psychiatry outpatient clinic at the Montreal Children's Hospital for a consultation at the request of child protection services, which had been alerted by

---

[1] To respect confidentiality, names and details of the story have been changed; we have however tried not to alter the cultural logic of the story.

[2] We are using the expression "some parts of Africa" to refer to customs, traditions or beliefs common in Central and Western Africa, though there is obviously significant heterogeneity throughout African societies.

the school. The teachers were originally concerned about Agrippine's frequent absences. Then rumors began to circulate: Agrippine was going out with older men, she received gifts. The school soon started talking in terms of prostitution, conduct disorder, possible delinquency.

This was the background to our meeting with Agrippine and her family. The stepmother complained about Agrippine's increasingly inappropriate behavior: for some time, she had been seeing an African boy she did not want to introduce to the family. She was worried about Agrippine's persistent promiscuity, which in her opinion violated basic ancestral values that should serve as a code of conduct for girls. For example, a girl cannot date a boy without her family's approval. She should also keep her virginity until she gets married (some rituals allow to verify that). According to the stepmother, Agrippine exhibited recurrent behavior that was negative, provocative, and disobedient. She got angry at her stepmother at the slightest frustration, argued with everything she said, actively opposed or refused to comply with her requests or house rules, deliberately did things to annoy her, blamed her for her own mistakes or misconduct, and was mean or vindictive towards her.

Since she had been going out with this boy, Agrippine had been upsetting the established family order by coming in late and even staying out all night without telling her stepmother. The relationship between Agrippine and her stepmother was becoming a real trial. Agrippine insulted her under her breath and answered back impulsively and without respect for either her age or hierarchical status within the family.

Agrippine was informed that her promiscuity was giving her a bad reputation and causing the entire family to lose face. But she seemed indifferent to the warnings, and appeared bored at home and more concerned about attracting boys than about her image in the community.

She interpreted her stepmother's attempts to interfere with her sex life as aggressive and unjustified. Agrippine's stepmother was worried about the potential effect of her behavior on her half-sisters for which she should have been a role model, even if at the time, there was no indication of a direct impact on the younger siblings. Agrippine's behavior was so disruptive and unacceptable that she thought she might have to put Agrippine out of the house. She said that since fleeing her homeland, she had felt anxious, but not to the point that it had a noticeable effect on her parenting abilities; however, for three months now, she had been feeling agitated and tense most of the time. The stepmother spoke only reluctantly of the school and child protective services. Offended by the investigation, she felt both humiliated and angry at this institutional intrusion into the family's life.

Background on Congolese Refugees in Montreal

In 1990, under growing pressure from international community, members of the political opposition and the local population, president Mobutu was forced to allow multiparty elections after 23 years of a single-party system. This attempt at democracy led to extensive organized violence. Mobutu reformed the Civil Guard and the President's Special Division (DSP), elite forces intended for the "maintenance of order", which repressed popular movements. The opposition media were silenced, and opponents and their families were persecuted. Thousands of opponents were assassinated, tortured, raped and/or "disappeared", as were thousands of other civilians. Starting in 1994, the genocide in the Great Lakes region exacerbated existing ethnic and political tensions. Laurent Desiré Kabila, the next president, then exploited the situation to gradually topple Mobutu and set up the Democratic Republic of Congo (DRC), which at first gave rise to great hope. The change ran out of steam, however, and the violence continued. According to (Lomomba & Otshudi, 2000), many factors explain the stagnation of the situation: the ambiguous, to say the least, role of the international community, the redistribution of neo-colonialist subcontracting roles on the regional chessboard, and national despotism, all combined with confusion among political opponents and civil society.

This is the backdrop against which Agrippine and her family escaped. Immigrants from the DRC who settled in Quebec are mainly from Kasai, Bandudu, Bas-Congo and Kivu; ethnically, most of them are Luba, Kongo, Mbala, Hunde and Nande. From 1994 on, the influx of Congolese refugees to Quebec increased. Approximately 60% of those who applied for refugee status were accepted. The families who were turned down were nevertheless allowed to stay in Canada thanks to a moratorium on expulsions to Congo because of the ongoing war. Nearly, 80% of the refugees from the Democratic Republic of Congo to Canada have settled in and around Montreal.

A Victim of Incestuous Sexual Abuse and Child Prostitution Associated with Witchcraft

The initial assessment took place at the Montréal Children Hospital, a university institution with a long tradition of adapting services for a culturally diverse population. The clinical team consisted of a male Rwandan psychologist and a female French-speaking child psychiatrist perceived by the family as belonging to the host society. The interview took place in French, a language that Agrippine and her mother mastered very well since their schooling was in French and belonged to well to do families. They sometimes spoke to each other in Lingala, their mother tongue, a language that the African therapist does not understand.

They categorically refused the presence of an interpreter because of potential breach of confidentiality within the community. Agrippine had no spontaneous complaints, although she acknowledged being sad. She did not however consider that state as being symptomatic, but rather as an essential part of her life experience. She disclosed reluctantly her repeated nightmares and alluded to dark male figures and blood, but without wanting to describe them further. She was not suicidal and only thought about it when placement was mentioned by youth protection authorities. The behaviors reported by both her stepmother and the school: promiscuity, runaway, blatant opposition to adult authority, rude language, suggested a diagnosis of oppositional defiant disorder with conduct symptoms. Her own story coincided rather with a post-traumatic stress disorder diagnosis. Neither of these diagnoses offered an adequate understanding of the central issue: the conflict between Agrippine and her stepmother. To the African therapist, the crisis between Agrippine and her stepmother, as presented, was somewhat puzzling. Immigration and adolescence could not really explain the intensity of the family conflict. She has been in Canada for less than a year and, while in school, appeared to have few links with the host society. She did not have stable friends and hanged around with some boys although she favored dating older men. In some ways, her stepmother was more acculturated than Agrippine. She had more information on Canadian institution and on what were the politically correct things to say to health and education professionals.

Indeed, over the course of clinical appointments with Agrippine and her stepmother, Agrippine seemed to be a model girl who appreciated African ancestral traditions. She was reserved and calm. She showed no emotion. She fit the image of what she used to be like, a girl who had at a very young age developed habits of respect, submissiveness, devotion to the family, even to the point of self-denial and sacrifice—the opposite of the provocative and disturbing behavior reported by her stepmother.

So what was the cause of her many transgressions, from lack of respect to dating patterns? At the second appointment, the stepmother answered this question without hesitating, but in a barely audible voice: "She likes opening her legs for men, that's her choice." Agrippine's sole response to this was silence, probably expressing her disagreement with her stepmother's answer.

To the African therapist, the stepmother's answer was at odds with the way many Africans look at life's events, whether traumatic or not. She was alluding to personal responsibility as an explanation of the crisis for which the consultation had been requested. It rang false, because it seemed foreign to the system of thought that organized this family's understanding of the world.

The African therapist then said: "As an African, there is something I don't understand. Agrippine is barely 15 years old and she already has the reputation that she likes to open her legs to men. What's going on?"

Agrippine began to weep silently. After a long sigh, her stepmother replied in a voice filled with sadness and terror: "You can't understand . . . She's a twin, the elder twin . . . It all started in Angola . . . It was her paternal uncle . . . She was sacrificed, offered to the spirits . . . "

That is how we learned that as a result of traditional beliefs about twins in some parts of Africa, Agrippine had been sexually abused many times by her paternal uncle. In many African countries, twins have a diverse range of very special attributes. For example, they can have healing and divination gifts that are used for good or evil purposes. Sometimes when the twins are of opposite sex, the second one might be considered to be a curse (to the point of being sacrificed in certain cultures). In other cases, the boy will be strongly favored over his twin sister even if she was born first.

For about two years, she had lived in constant fear of being sexually abused by her uncle, and was punished harshly when she refused to comply with his demands. These incestuous practices were organized around witchcraft, which attributes significant power to twins that is transmissible through sexual intercourse. Taking this power is a mean of ensuring victory over one's enemies.

Although this practice provides power it is considered as harmful witchcraft and illegal. According to traditional laws in some parts of Africa, relatives who engage abusively in this practice are hunted down and punished as criminals. Against tradition, Agrippine seemed to have been chosen by her paternal uncle (substitute father in traditional law) as protection against the ill wishes of the living and the dead, a worker of inner peace, a fetish who crushes the enemy and foils the plans of those who are jealous. In some African culture, jealousy and envy are very dangerous. One should first try to avoid eliciting these feelings, but if in a prominent positioning, one need to look for protection from the destructive projects toward the family and the community.

Her brother knew about his big sister's abuse, but was forced to keep it secret for fear of reprisals. The two children were also tormented daily by hunger, because their uncle, whose financial situation in Angola was precarious, neglected them. To survive, Agrippine and her brother often begged in the streets. It did not take long before prostitution, which Agrippine practiced without her uncle's knowledge, but with her brother's complicity, became the solution to their hunger. Agrippine's prostitution and the children's dire straights eventually attracted the attention of a nun working with an NGO helping young war victims. She managed to obtain travel documents for the children, so they could escape to Canada.

With this second explanation of Agrippine's traumatic experiences, the stepmother was much more in line with the way many Africans view life's events. In many African societies, God is thought to be responsible for various social conditions, for the unequal distribution of good luck and bad, for birth defects and for accidents of every kind. Ruin, illness, loss, premature death, and accidents may all be punishments of an offended God, but more often they are attributed either to the anger of ancestors or to the witchcraft of living people. The former attracts the attention of their neglectful descendants by constant annoyances or plagues them with misfortune out of pure spitefulness; the latter uses spells and curses to harm their adversaries. Agrippine's stepmother did not mention divine malediction as an explanation of the trials suffered by her stepdaughter. The fact that she was in Canada was, to her, a sign that she was still under divine protection. Instead, she explained Agrippine's experience as a form of traditional possession which the uncle thought would allow him to take over the power she possessed as an elder twin, thus putting an end to the misfortunes that had befallen the family since the beginning of the armed conflict and recovering his lost privilege. The stepmother nonetheless viewed the possession as an assault.

The choice of such a ritual is often the result of a complex consultation by specialists (animist priests, keepers of tradition) of the spirits of deceased ancestors, in particular those who have held notable positions or have been senior dignitaries within the community. Once the consent of the spirits has been obtained, the designated girl is informed of the honor bestowed upon her: ensuring the protection and success of a dignitary. This is usually revealed on the occasion of a traditional feast and cannot be appealed, because any refusal would be an insult to the spirits of the ancestors involved in the decision. The chosen girl leaves childhood to become a woman who meets the needs of the members of her family. In the case of Agrippine, this procedure had not been followed both because of the family disruption induced by the war and the exile to Canada. This displacement did not allow this ritual to take place and partially transformed her relation to traditional beliefs and practices.

Even in therapy, any mention of witchcraft is associated with fear and threats. In this case at hand, the therapist then asked, "If the problems persist, does that mean that the witchcraft is still at work here?" Quite unexpectedly, Agrippine was the first to answer, her voice full of emotion: "She's the witch." This answer expressed her great ambivalence towards her stepmother.

A witch is perceived, ideally, as someone to whom God has given knowledge of and power over the things of the invisible world, and someone who is more skilled and powerful than ordinary human beings. This type of witch uses his or her skill for good, only going on the offensive to prevent an attack. But the popular concept of witch has taken on a starkly contrasting negative connotation. A witch is seen as a caster of curses, a maker of potions and spells, the author of machinations aiming to cause death or to force love.

After a long silence, the African therapist suggested: "Sometimes in Africa, stepmothers are considered to be spiteful, unfair and heartless, but they are rarely called witches. I wonder if your daughter Agrippine might not have something in her heart that should not go beyond her neck." This African proverb, "what is in the heart should not go beyond the neck," means "you must know how to keep a secret." The stepmother answered then, her voice cracking with emotion:

"Agrippine has hated me ever since she found out that I went to a fertility clinic to see about artificial insemination. Since my husband died, I've wanted to have a child. Three months ago, I went to the artificial insemination clinic . . .

Since then, nothing has been the same between Agrippine and me. She won't listen to me . . . She hates me . . . She's trying to drive me crazy . . . I can't kick her out. My home is also her father's home . . . I don't know what to do anymore . . . Since then, our relationship has just kept getting worse."

Now that we knew about the fertility clinic, the answer "she's the witch" and the family crisis opposing Agrippine and her stepmother made sense. In the teenager's imaginary world, only a witch could have the power to penetrate a woman's body and deposit the seminal fluid necessary for fertilization. While the clinical team saw the stepmother's action as a way of refusing to grieve for her husband, Agrippine experienced it as a direct extension of her own trauma. To her, such an intrusion was unthinkable, totally unacceptable.

The Family Council as an Institutional Framework for Moving From Witchcraft to Therapy

In our context of a Western psychiatric unit, a wide range of therapeutic models was available, but the fact that witchcraft was involved meant that an overall clinical perspective that would take into account the cultural universe of Agrippine and her family was required. Indeed, witchcraft became a clinical instrument that made it possible to talk about things that might otherwise have remained taboo: Agrippine's loss of her father (and the stepmother's loss of her husband), sexual abuse, the necessary prostitution, the dissolution of the protective nature of the family.

In reply to the question, "If you went back to Africa with your family, what would you do to make Agrippine better?" the stepmother replied, "You're African, aren't you? You should know: the family council, at the request of Agrippine's father, that is, my husband, . . . but without him, as now, it has to be someone from her father's family, . . . but someone who knows what to do in such cases would have to be consulted." So we discussed with her whether there was anyone from the paternal line whom the family could talk to about ways to repair the damage Agrippine had suffered and help her regain trust in her family and take her rightful place in it once more.

Agrippine's stepmother named a brother-in-law in the United States. She was very comfortable with the idea of a family council, as it appeared to be an appropriate institutional framework for helping children and adolescents struggling with the symptoms of witchcraft perpetrated by a relative. In the case of sexual abuse within the family, a family council could be called. It would have a therapeutic effect (and in a traditional setting, also a legal effect), in that its purpose is to help the victim and her family to make sense of the assaults and to express their disapproval of the abusive relative without making the family feel too guilty and upset about failing to prevent the incestuous abuse. One particular function of the council is to restore differences between generations that have been denied by the incestuous relationship and to offer the child victim an alternative parental image to the one discredited by the violation of the incest taboo. It also makes it possible to get the family involved in the process of symbolically making amends to the victim.

Traditionally, the family council meets after an adult lodges a complaint with the person who has the status of family patriarch. The council is composed of family elders (men and women) known for their wisdom and experience. The family council may decide to consult a witchcraft specialist for help in identifying and treating the problem suffered by the family member. Although this was never evoked in Agrippine's case, in some parts of Africa, the incestuous sexual abuse of a minor is held to be the result of a curse by deceased members of the family, angry at having been prevented from reaching the world of their ancestors.

These deceased outsiders—between the lands of the living and the dead—may act by taking over the identity of a close relative for a specific purpose, such as joining the ancestors upon the death of the relative they have possessed. The identification of hostile spirits who have taken possession of the person is a complex operation requiring the establishment of physical communication with the spirits in question through an animal intermediary (bull, goat, ram, rooster, etc.). The communication begins with a ritual to transfer the abusive family spirits from the body of the victim to that of the animal intermediary. During this ritual, the witchcraft specialist opens the jaws of the animal intermediary and drips some of the victim's saliva into its throat (in the language of witchcraft, the saliva is designated by the term for semen). This transfer by way of saliva seems to obey the law of similarity and analogy: the name pronounced produces the thing expressed, the action conjures up the intended reality, the theatrical representation of a death may cause it, the symbol influences the thing it evokes. Identification of the hostile spirits is followed first by a purification ritual for both the victim and the community taking part in the family council, and then by a few more sessions of complementary rites for the victim as an individual to help her rebuild herself internally and become invulnerable. The final stage of treatment of an intrafamilial assault or possession is a ritual meal presided over by the head of the family council in the victim's home. It is a feast of reconciliation (called messenger of peace) between the various family members (living and dead) affected in different ways when a loved is a victim of witchcraft. This ritual feast is a highly social event, the purpose of which is to maintain group cohesion and solidarity. The feast has two high points: an offering, to the ancestor who founded the victim's paternal line, of a few mouthfuls of food and a few drops of drink and of requests by the head of the family on behalf of everyone to eradicate this type of abuse within the family; and an offering to the victim of gifts from each household to symbolically make amends for the harm suffered. At the end of the ritual meal, the victim of the assault or possession finds inner peace and family peace because the curse at the root of the problem has been expelled from her body and family environment.

When victims are in exile in a country like Canada, the family council cannot call in a witchcraft specialist to help remedy a past trauma. An exiled or foreign therapist can, however, involve the institution of the family council in assessing and treating African refugee children who have had exceptionally traumatic experiences. Through the family council, the child finds support within her family, who take steps to overcome the repercussions of the trauma. This therapeutic institutional framework attenuates the feelings of isolation, often exacerbated by the misunderstandings and doubts expressed by friends and family in cases of incestuous sexual assault. In Agrippine's case, her uncle sexually abused her many times and she had no one in the family to turn to for protection. Through the family council, Agrippine's family could play a legitimate supportive role.

To enable Agrippine to put together the pieces of her past, to find herself in the present and project herself hopefully into the future, we suggested that she and her stepmother take part in a therapeutic process in the form of a family council comprising themselves, Agrippine's paternal uncle living in the U.S. and his wife, two therapists from the transcultural psychiatry team (a Canadian woman and an African man) and a social worker of Somali origin. The make-up of this reconstituted "family council" thus included the legitimate traditional authorities for Agrippine (paternal uncle and stepmother), the African therapist in his role as an elder and mediator, the social worker, who represented both a host society authority with considerable power over the family (child protective services) and their home continent, and the white child psychiatrist, who could speak on their behalf to the school and other host society institutions, but also offered implicit protection against the dangers of witchcraft.

We organized monthly 90-minute conference calls among all the members of this council, with the goals being to transform the relationship between Agrippine and her stepmother by legitimating the latter's position and shoring up her role as a protector, and redraw the boundaries between the generations that had been severely damaged by the trauma, as well as to bring Agrippine's feelings of rebellion under control to prevent her from reliving her trauma and acting out in various ways (especially prostitution). While organizing a conference call in North America is a trivial event, it becomes a challenging task when the participants are in different war-torn zones and often with no access to a personal phone. To the technical obstacles, we should add the psychological and cultural ones in a context where the organizing institution is a western "white" hospital having to deal with a problematic alluding, even indirectly, to witchcraft. The role of the African therapist in making this happen was central. Lengthy negotiations with the different family members involved took place before the calls could be made.

The family council conference calls were preceded by three sessions of individual psychotherapy. This individual therapy consisted in working on representations associated with the family council process, the goal of which was to reestablish the bond between Agrippine and her family and to create a special space in which the suffering she had experienced could be talked about in another way. The search for meaning could then depart from the meanings proposed by the family or the culture of origin, and strengths that the family might not have acknowledged could be emphasized.

Gradually, through what parental figures had to say, the family council enabled Agrippine to find her place within the family and regain a degree of respect for her stepmother. Gradually, the traumatic experiences of the different family members (the horror of the transgression by a parental figure, the loss of the father, the impossibility for the stepmother to grieve, were no longer things that kept them apart, but instead bound them together. After eight months of conference calls (eight sessions), the therapeutic process initiated with the family council wound up with the arrival in Montreal of Agrippine's paternal uncle, accompanied by his wife and three children, for a final therapy session. His eldest son brought a video camera to immortalize this significant moment in the family's life (and perhaps capture the strengths present, as video and photographs are often used for witchcraft or to protect against it). At this meeting we discussed the process of identity transformation of young Africans in a foreign land and the ability to create social connections to replace those lost through migration and the trauma of war. It is important here to underline that the identity transformation provoked by the losses of migration, although a very common reality for young migrants, was not the central issue for Agrippine at the time of the therapy. However, evoking it provided a common, relatively non-threatening, metaphor to address the identity transformation secondary to unspeakable traumas and the need to recreate the family network. This use of migration as an explanatory model is often very useful for both families and clinicians since the external attribution of the problem to the migration process protects the family and the therapeutic relation from more sensitive issues and provides a common meaning for the hurt. It may however become an obstacle if underlying conflicts, within the family or between the family and the team, are totally ignored. We also discussed reestablishing bonds within the African family after a long period of separation and the meaning of losses and trauma, but avoided any direct mention of those difficult memories. In individual sessions with Agrippine, after this meeting, she referred many times to the family reunion presided over by her uncle and the gifts she had received from every member of her family. The family regained its rightful role, gradually, and the family council became an alternative institution that strengthened the bond between Agrippine and her stepmother.

In parallel to the family council, another process was taking place. This was a process of negotiating the case plan dealing with Agrippine's risk behaviors. Initially the child protective services social worker had considered out-of-home placement for Agrippine. That would have solved the family conflict and stopped her prostitution-like behavior, but raising this possibility had been associated with increased suicidal ideation. Agrippine would rather die than be locked up; she could not contemplate the idea of her life being controlled in that way. While helping protect Agrippine against sexually transmitted diseases and AIDS as much as possible by referring her to a physician specialized in the treatment of adolescents, the child psychiatrist tried to convey the team's perception of Agrippine's behavior to child protective services. Prostitution had enabled Agrippine to save her twin brother; it had become a survival strategy, a sacrifice for those she loved. The temporary persistence of this behavior should not be interpreted as a sign of delinquency. Agrippine needed to have her strengths recognized and to be guided as she learned that other strategies were possible in her new environment. Child protective services agreed to delay her placement, and then, seeing that the family situation was improving, closed the case.

Discussion

Agrippine's story illustrates the frequent entanglement between political and cultural signifiers in traumatic experiences in Africa and the tensions between therapeutic and institutional-political issues in the host country. Within the assessment and intervention process three elements appear to have played a key role.

First, the dyadic work of a black African psychologist and a white Canadian child psychiatrist throughout the process allowed us to constantly modulate proximity and distance, us and them, security and threat. Both of us were in different ways a source of comfort and fear. The African therapist was seen as a protector against racism and discrimination and as someone who could understand what was going on. Yet his capacity to understand was a source of ambivalence: it was clear from the beginning that both Agrippine and her stepmother preferred to frame things within a Canadian individualistic perspective to avoid traditional issues, which were much more threatening. But the African therapist was also suspect because of his real or potential knowledge of witchcraft and, at that level, the Canadian psychiatrist was seen as a naive bystander whose presence partially protected the family from a possible curse. Nathan (1994) explains how the dyadic patient-therapist relationship can sometimes represent a danger to African patients and he advocates a teamwork approach, in part because of its protective role. The white therapist, however, also represented the power of the majority, the negative perceptions of refugees and of blacks in mainstream society, and the terrible threat of the health, school, and child protective systems, which could legally but, from the community viewpoint, illegitimately, remove children from their families. The joint work facilitated a simultaneous representation of both worlds, the here and there, and a negotiation of meanings and treatments within a relatively safe environment. At the time of the intervention, the two therapists had been working together for about 8 years. In the early years of their collaboration, there was a tendency for the Canadian psychiatrist to wish to appear, or become, as knowledgeable as possible of cultural specificities in order to be more sensitive. The African therapist, on the contrary, felt he should display mainstream professional qualities in order to be accepted and considered by the institution. With time, the Canadian therapist discovered that her ignorance could sometimes be useful, and the African therapist learned to utilize his powerful cultural knowledge in ways which did not betray the families (by reducing them into western therapies under false premises) nor fragilize him within a professional setting. We both learned about our respective fears: the white fear of being again in a colonizer position, the African respect for witchcraft which should not be evoked in trivial ways or out of voyeur curiosity. This enabled us to work delicately around the others' blind spots and anxieties and to use our respective strengths and weaknesses as therapeutic tools. In spite of this long familiarity and common work, we both acted out at some point of the therapeutic process, forgetting appointments or important calls. These were key moments to reconsider our global therapeutic plan and adjust it to our unspoken (but acted) uneasiness.

Second, the therapy would have been fruitless without concomitant work within the child protective system to avoid out-of-home placement of Agrippine and court involvement in her case. The condemnation of Agrippine's prostitution-like behavior by host country institutions lent weight to the stepmother's blame, resulting in Agrippine's despair and suicidal ideation. Without in any way romanticizing strategies like prostitution, it is nevertheless important to recognize their key role in survival in many war contexts and the ways in which they also represent a mature (and often almost parental) self-sacrifice. These strategies may not only ensure physical survival, but they also often constitute, in spite of the shame and trauma, a shift toward an active stance, an agency that empowers the youngster over her own life. Once in a safe environment, these strategies do not automatically disappear. Stripping a youngster of her sense of empowerment, blaming her for what allowed her heroically to sustain her loved ones and to survive, can have disastrous consequences. While it may be politically correct to try to "save" girls from a life of prostitution, we must be very careful to consider the potential violence of well-intended protective intervention. An understanding of the significance of "deviant" behavior of children of war is necessary and precedes the difficult negotiation of a case plan with institutions, which are inherently against risk taking.

Third, therapy combined traditional, systemic, and psychodynamic modalities. The specific time and space dimension of the therapy should be explained. In terms of space, the therapy mobilized the family's transnational networks, recreating shared spaces through telephone conferences, which brought people together despite the geographic distances between them. Interestingly, during the actual family reunion, the video camera may have both represented the need to maintain a certain distance and symbolized the connection with other networks. The creation of transnational networks by means of new technologies has helped refugee families become less isolated and maintain connections to their roots, introducing the possibility not only of reestablishing but also actively transforming family interactions and of involving the extended family in the healing process even at a distance.

In terms of time, disclosure happened over time, and only when trusting relationships were established with the team. In our experience, pushing families to disclose traumatic experiences prematurely during the assessment process can be very painful and often counterproductive. Creating a holding environment is a priority and therapists should negotiate the pace of the intervention with their patients.

References

Lomomba, E., & Otshudi, O. (2000). *Le changement en panne au Congo/Zaïre: De Mobutu à Kabila.* Montréal: Éditions les 5 Continents.

Nathan, T. (1994). Les bienfaits des thérapies sauvages. Thérapie scientifique et thérapie sauvage. *Nouvelle Revue d'Ethnopsychiatrie, 27,* 37–54.

Rousseau, C., Crépeau, F., Foxen, P., & Houle, F. (2002). The complexity of determining refugeehood: A multidisciplinary analysis of the decision-making process of the Canadian Immigration and Refugee Board. *Journal of Refugee Studies, 15*(1), 43–70.

13
"I Think He is Still Inside Me": Mother/Child Psychotherapy and Sandplay with a Kosovar Woman and Her Infant Son

Elizabeth Batista Pinto Wiese

" . . . a world where broken spirits abound and surround us with their silent cries and unspoken loneliness"

Wilson (2004, p. 109)

The psychotherapeutic process of a Kosovar adolescent asylum-seeker mother exposed to violent traumatizing experiences is described and discussed in this chapter. The effects of these experiences, especially in the vulnerable period while she was pregnant with her first child, resulted in severe consequences in the mother/child interaction and brought extra complexity to the case. The description of this psychotherapeutic process was enriched in the text by theoretical elements relating clinic to theory.

In the therapeutic process of the client here described, conducted in a center for child and adolescent mental health care in the Netherlands, we made two different modalities of psychotherapeutic interventions with Sara, the adolescent mother: the first intervention, after the beginning phase (in which her partner was also present), was an individual psychodynamic psychotherapy, while the second intervention was a mother/child psychotherapy, with Sara and Denis, her one-and-a-half-year-old child. During both psychotherapies, the Sandplay method was eventually used to help the client to project and elaborate her inner world and conflicts.

Considering the fact that asylum-seekers, refugees and immigrants are high risk populations for psychiatric disorders, the Reinier van Arkel Groep, in 's-Hertogenbosch, in the Netherlands, developed the *Transcultural Problems Program – BTP*, a specialized service for these infants, children, adolescents and their families. Since January 2007 this service was integrated with the service for adults in the new Psychotraumacentrum Zuid Nederland – PTZN, International Centre for Victims of War, Trauma and Political Violence. The *PTZN* consists of a multidisciplinary team which includes psychiatrists, psychotherapists, health psychologists, system therapists, physicians, social-psychiatry nurses, creative therapists and others. In addition to the outpatient treatment, the PTZN provides, if necessary, in-patient treatment (in a short-term closed setting) and a day-hospital treatment. The children and adolescents whose mental conditions do not allow them to attend a regular school, may attend a special school affiliated with the clinic, while participating in the clinical or day-hospital treatment.

The diagnosis and treatment process for infants, children and adolescents in the *Transcultural Problems Program – BTP* (Wiese & Burhost, 2004, 2007) and recently in the PTZN starts with an initial interview with the child and his/her parents, and results in an individual treatment plan, established by the multi-disciplinary team. The treatment plan may include medical and/or psychiatric assessment, psychological assessment, system assessment, anamnesis, play ther-apy, individual group or family psychotherapy (including ethopsychotherapy), art therapy, parent counseling etc. After three months the assessment and treatment evaluations take place, followed by further three-monthly follow-up evaluations.

I work as a psycho-dynamically oriented psychotherapist and treatment coor-dinator at the PTZN, with children and adolescents, as well as with babies and infants (in parents/child psychotherapy). Love brought me to the Netherlands and my life changed suddenly when I married a Dutchman. Prior to this, I was a psy-chologist, born in Rio de Janeiro, with extensive professional clinical experience, who was for many years a lecturer in the Clinical Psychology Department of the Institute of Psychology of the University of Sao Paulo, in Brazil. My knowledge of languages and my experiences of living abroad in different countries during various periods of my life also help me with the challenges of my clinical work in the Netherlands.

The fact that I am not Dutch myself, but from South America, makes it easier for many clients to identify themselves with me (also a foreigner) and this iden-tification seems to help them to develop a positive transference and a therapeutic bond. For the asylum-seeking clients in particular, the fact that I am a foreigner helps them to regard me as someone who is disconnected from the very strict asylum policy of the Dutch government.

It was in this context that I saw Sara for the first time. She was referred to me by a *BTP* colleague, because of my experience in parents/child psychotherapy (Batista Pinto, 2000, 2004; Wiese, 2004).

The Encounter with Sara

Sara came to the outpatient clinic, brought by her partner Andre. When they entered the consultation room he had Denis, their seven-months-old baby, sleeping in his arms, to whom Sara did not even look during the first interview. Sara was eighteen years old and Andre was twenty-six years old at that time. The couple was from Kosovo, from an Albanian ethnic group, and Sara's family had a Muslim background.

Andre requested treatment for Sara because he was worried about her psychological condition, her depression, isolation and inability to take care of herself and of their child. He attributed Sara's condition to traumatic experiences, including rape, she had suffered in Kosovo, shortly before they left the country.

Considering the importance of the attachment to the mother for the baby's development, Sara's treatment coordinator in BTP asked my intervention as a psychotherapist, aiming to improve the mother/child interaction.

Kosovo is a small province in Eastern Europe, located in southern Serbia, with a majority population of Albanians. Kosovo has had a long-running political and territorial dispute with the Serbian authorities. During the twentieth century, the Kosovo population had six different government systems, ranging from a dynastic monarchy (until 1918), a constitutional monarchy (1918/1941), fascist occupation (1941/1945), a communist one-party government (led by General Tito from 1945/1990), a nationalist dictatorship (1990/1999) to a United Nations administration (1999 to present). During the period of nationalist dictatorship, an unequal gender and ethnic policy was imposed, resulting in a bloody ethnic-cleansing campaign against non-Serbians ethnical groups (United Nations Development Fund for Women War Peace, 2006).

In Kosovo, in 1996, an armed conflict started between the Serbian and Yugoslav army, security forces and the Kosovo Liberation Army, an Albanian group seeking independence for the province. Following this conflict, in 1999, a war started between Yugoslavia and the North Atlantic Treaty Organization – NATO. From 1996 to 1999, thousands of Kosovars were killed and approximately 1 million people were forced to migrate (United Nations Interim Administration Mission in Kosovo, 2004).

This period was experienced by the Kosovar-Albanian women in various ways: a few of them took up arms, but the majority lived through this conflict as civilians, and experienced traumatic situations. During this period, the Kosovar-Albanian people were internally displaced, with work and school interrupted. Many of them had their properties destroyed and their belongings robbed; they were threatened and they witnessed or underwent sexual violence and other human rights violations on a large scale. These experiences caused extreme traumas, with posttraumatic stress symptoms in many persons (International Helsinki Federation for Human Rights, 2000).

The United Nations Population Fund – UNFPA (2006) report of May 1999 (Fitamant, 1999), described accounts of rape, abduction, detention and torture of women refugees in Kosovo. According to the same report, young women, including pregnant ones, were abducted in groups, were threatened and raped by scores of men.

During our first consultation, in the presence of an Albanian/English interpreter, Andre told me that, in 2004, he and Sara had fled from Kosovo to Sweden when she was seven months pregnant. Sara was very disturbed at that time because of the recent traumatic experiences she had in their country.

Denis was born in Sweden, where the family stayed for a few months. Although very important in her culture, Sara refused to breastfeed her baby.

After the birth of Denis, Andre decided to come to the Netherlands to ask for asylum, because their asylum procedure in Sweden was not going well (after the killing of the Swedish foreign minister Anna Lindh by the son of Serb immigrants) and because he did not like the medical treatment Sara was receiving there.

In 2004, the worst ethnic violence (since 1999) happened in Kosovo, when houses and cultural sites were destroyed, people were killed, injured and displaced. In this displacement, women and children were the first group to be evacuated from their communities, and relocated in refugee camps, without knowing whether they would ever be able to return to their homes (United Nations Development Fund for Women War Peace, 2006).

The effects of these traumatic experiences were enormous, long-lasting and shattering to these women's inner and outer worlds. This was worsened still by religious and cultural attitudes. In the Muslim culture, the honor of a woman for example, reflects upon her entire family. Therefore, a rape victim of Muslim faith may believe that the rape was a punishment for some sin she had committed. Even if she does not blame herself, she may feel such a strong cultural responsibility to protect her family that she remains silent about the rape (National Center for Posttraumatic Stress Disorder, 2006).

The family had been living in the Netherlands for the past four months, in a reception center for asylum seekers, and Sara's mental health problems prevented her from taking even fundamental care of herself and her child.

From our first contact, Sara made a strong impression on me: she avoided eye contact and seemed to me frightened, weak and hopeless. Even though she was a beautiful young woman she did not look well: her facial expression was sad, closed, and she had wrinkles in her forehead. She was disoriented about time, space and about her actual life context. She was afraid of and she was very confused towards new places, new people, the present and the past. She almost could not talk, not even with the help of an interpreter, and when she tried to answer a question or to say a few words, her voice was so low that it was very difficult to hear and to understand her. Sara's self-esteem seemed very low and she did not seem capable of any basic independence.

Sara was suffering from the basic symptoms of Posttraumatic Stress Disorder (PTSD) combined with depressive symptoms and psychotic hallucinations which repeated the traumatic events in flash-back. She also had a remarkable lack of attachment to her child. She would talk to Andre, her partner, when she did not understand one of my questions, but she avoided any physical contact with him. During the first session, it seemed to me that the presence of Andre was important for Sara to feel safe and to build the foundation of her relationship with me.

Sara already was been treated by a psychiatrist and taking psychiatric medication (for anxiety, depression and psychotic symptoms), and she and her husband were being supported by a colleague, a system therapist.

After the exposure to traumatic events a victim may have heterogeneous and complex manifestations and symptoms (APA, 1995). Yet, in the etiology of trauma, it is also necessary to consider the person's mental state at the moment of the traumatic experience, when several affective impressions were agglutinated.

Freud (1917,1992) postulated that in trauma there is an indirect relationship between two factors: one being the *predisposition* of the person and the second being the *fantasy* about the event and the gravity of the event itself. Therefore, in the trauma, the terrifying feelings (as experienced by the victim) are frequently more important than the fact or situation itself.

In the first consultations, Andre did most of the talking, describing the day-a-day difficulties with Sara in the dealing with her frightened and dependent behavior. I gave them support and understanding in order to develop their adjustment to this new period in their lives.

After a few consultations, Sara slowly started to talk about her fear. It seemed to me that she wanted to tell more about her past experiences, but that it was difficult for her to do so in the presence of her partner and of the interpreter. I understood that her need to talk to me was also related to her need for female support and for a more flexible and benevolent "mother figure" with whom she possibly identified me.

Although Sara would still deny the presence of her child in the sessions (and in her life), she slowly started to take care of some of the child's possessions, for example, bringing his bag to the consultation room, or arranging his toys when I gave them to her at the end of the sessions. These were the first signs of her acceptance of her child's presence in her world. However, Sara's psychological condition was very vulnerable and unstable and the mother/child relationship was at high risk.

To bring a child into the world, especially the first child, is, for the immigrant woman, a very important step in her own immigration history, because it is through this child that, in general, she will have more contact with the host society, its culture and demands. Besides pregnancy and birth being very vulnerable periods for a woman, for immigrants these periods can be affected by several influences, for instance by the migration project itself (reasons, conditions, experiences, feelings, hopes, etc.), the number of years spent in the new country, the cultural differences between the country of origin and the new one, the social and economical conditions, and the support from partner, family and community.

When the birth of a child occurs during the migration process, it exposes the parents to the paradox of being *parents between the others and for the others* (Sayad, 1999). The immigrants are torn from their original group, what can be very disturbing, especially when they were used to belong to a rural collectivist society, in which the community bonds were very strong. They must also assimilate into their host society which requires them to be like the people in their new country. This injunction, in the case of occidental western societies, includes the consideration of a more individualistic culture.

Mestre (2003) pointed out the importance for a new mother of the presence of her own mother and of close female relatives at the moment of the child's birth and in the first period hereafter. On top of this, we know that loneliness is not an exclusive experience of the immigrant woman. The loneliness of the mother in occidental societies is a cultural constant, but it can constitute a real trauma for immigrant mothers, especially for the ones who came from a more traditional environment, where the culture supports the circulation of the child between relatives in the family (Rabain-Jamin & Wornha, 1990). As a consequence, loneliness in the absence of partnerships with other women of the same family can be a real threat.

Therefore, a woman who gives birth to a child in isolation frequently forgets the rituals of her own cultural group, and this makes the child more vulnerable to and dependent on the mother's personality and competences. The presence of elements of the mother's cultural group can, as a result, be important to support cultural transmissions to the child. Besides, the immigrant mother can be burdened by the responsibilities in raising a child that must achieve more individual goals and values, as expected from a *good mother* in the occidental culture.

To better understand this process, Mestre (2003) conducted a survey among immigrant women in France, and observed that all of them spoke about the absence of their own mother with sadness, fear, pain and stress. However, these feelings depended on the quality of attachment the woman had to her own mother and on her competences to take care of a child, as she developed in her own childhood. This survey showed that good attachment to the own mother can provide a basis to be more competent in the care for her child and to build a harmonious relationship with her child.

The resources of the mother's own culture are also very important, to give to her a sense of her role as a mother and, in case of psychological or psychiatric disorders, the culture can provide an *envelope* to support mother and child in their interaction, especially in critical periods.

Considering culture as a transgenerationally transmitted system of shared beliefs, values, customs, behaviors and artifacts that members of a society use to cope with their world and with one another (Schwimmer, 2006), the *cultural envelope* brings to the person magical components of his/her group. These components can assure the maintenance, the countenance, the inscription and the transmission of the basic elements in the mother/child dyadic and mother/child/father triadic interaction.

Therefore, the parents' migration brings a vulnerability factor for the child, because being *in between* different cultures, with conflictive values and beliefs may result in considerable risks for the child's psychological development. This vulnerability can be apparent in the child's less resistance to traumas in comparison with children who are raised within their own parents' culture. About this matter, Lebovici (1989) stated that the same circumstances and situations can have many different effects in infants.

Denis was a pretty, blond, healthy and active baby. He received ample attention from his father, with whom he had a secure attachment, but he avoided any contact with his mother. Denis had just started to go to créche once a week. During the first sessions with the family, I observed that Denis had good cognitive and motor development but emotional difficulties in the attachment with his mother.

The mother/child emotional communication, since the early period of the child's life, is based in the rhythmic and dynamic frames of their affective interaction (Golse, 2004). Therefore, at a very young age, the child is, in general, competent to decode the modality and interactive style of the mother (or her substitute), and to adjust to it.

The babies of traumatized mothers perceive, directly or indirectly, their mother's traumas, as they leave strong traces in their relationship. These traces are written in a developmental line, in the present of the child, but also in his/her future as an adolescent and an adult. We can hypothesize that these traumas modify the child's perceptions of his/her past and history (Moro, 2005).

When the parents are traumatized, it can result in direct consequences to the child's life and development, because traumatized adults are often unable to deal with the child's needs.

The Video of the Mother/Child Interaction

After a short period to establish good rapport with Sara, her treatment continued with the regular procedure for mother/child psychotherapy and a video recording of Sara and Dennis in a free play session was made.

This video recording technique aims to have a detailed assess to the mother/child and father/child interaction (Batista Pinto, 2001; Piccinini et al., 2001).

In the mother/child video-interaction, when Denis was 12 months old, Sara did not give him any spontaneous attention. The child did not want his father to leave the room during the session and he seemed to be afraid of staying alone with his mother and me. While Denis cried, Sara did not look at him, she did not touch or approach him. My intervention in the situation was necessary, so I took the child and helped him to sit in his mother's lap and, very slowly, she could accept to hold her child by herself.

The qualitative analysis of this video-interaction concluded that Sara did not show sensitivity to her child, even when he was reacting in a disorganized way. She did not give him any structure in the play. Sara was not intrusive in her behavior, on the contrary, she avoided interaction most of the time, and showed a covert hostility towards the child. Dennis showed moderate responsivity to Sara (for example looking at her and taking a toy from her hands), but very little involvement in the spontaneous interaction with her (he neither looked for physical contact, nor did he give signs of pleasure in the interaction).

Several factors can affect the parent/child interaction, and it is very important to assess them in an early stage of the child's life. This helps to plan interventions that can prevent and/or treat functional disorders and psychopathology. It is important to consider the patters of attachment and the dynamic of the interaction in the parent/child interaction.

In this phase of the treatment it was difficult for Sara to start to talk. It seemed to me that her thoughts were empty, far away from reality and from the therapeutic encounter. She could not recollect memories about her past or even talk about the present. She said that it was very difficult for her to talk about her family and even more difficult to talk about what happened to her and to talk about her child. I made an interpretation, establishing a connection between these three subjects, telling her that because of the difficulties in the relationship with her family and because of what happened to her in Kosovo, she had difficulties in the relationship with her child at present. She listened to my interpretation but did not have any direct reaction to it.

At that stage in the psychotherapeutic process, as an attempt to give Sara a mean to express herself in a non-verbal way, I proposed to Andre and Sara to do a Sandplay.

The Sandplay

Sandplay is a non-verbal psychotherapeutic method created by Dora Kalff (1980), a Swiss Jungian analyst. The method (Batista Pinto & Franco, 2003) consists of inviting the client to create a scenario, in a standardized box filled with sand, using miniatures at his/her disposition, which broadly represent elements of the world (persons, animals, trees, houses, cars, food, sacred objects, instruments of war, etc.).

The sand-box constitutes a field in which the client can use his/her creativity to project elements and conflicts of his/her internal world. Therefore the client can be taken by images or sensations that the sand and the miniatures elicit in him/her, turning fantasy into an actual scene, which he/she leaves in the sand-box with the psychotherapist (Mitchell & Friedman, 1994).

At the end of the Sandplay activity, the psychotherapist asks the client to give a title to his/her scene, and if the client wants, he/she can also explain the scene he/she has created or comment about his/her feelings while doing it. The psychotherapist subsequently takes a photograph of the scene and asks the client to close the box.

The basic function of the Sandplay method is to challenge the client to express, in a non-verbal way, the conscious and unconscious contents of his/her internal world and, by doing so, to develop the psychological function of self-regulation (Jung, 1935/1991).

In the Sandplay method the contents and interpretations of the scene are not discussed with the client in the same session, but eventually this can be done after a continued period of psychotherapy, when the psychotherapist can bring the photographs of the scene and discuss the material with the client (Batista Pinto & Franco, 2003). This way, the client's non-verbal projection in the Sandplay is preserved, but at another stage of the therapeutic process it is possible to talk about it enhancing the understanding of the client's conflicts and psychological mechanisms.

Andre started the first Sandplay scenario by putting the figure of a (Dutch) country man and, next to it, the figures of a (Dutch) country woman and child. Although Sara was very depressed and inactive in that period, she started working persistently on the scene. She was very focused on the activity. Immediately, surprised by her motivation and initiative, Andre withdrew and let her do the scenario alone. Sara created a very detailed scene in her first Sandplay scenario which she named "War and rape".

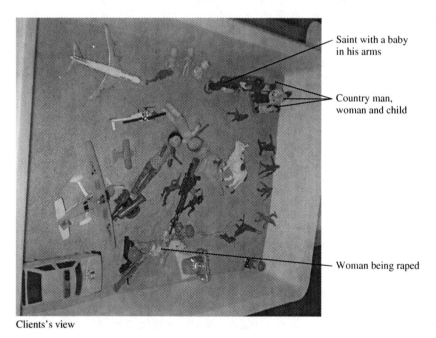

Saint with a baby in his arms

Country man, woman and child

Woman being raped

Clients's view

FIGURE 13.1. The first sandplay scene: *War and rape*.

The first figure that Sara chose was the saint which holds a baby in his arms. She put it next to the family that Andre had placed in the sand, projecting the wish for protection for her small family. Then she made a disturbed scene of an armed conflict, with several dead people, especially children and women, and also with some dead animals. There were soldiers with guns everywhere.

The scene is divided in two parts: one representing the war and violence with all its elements – soldiers, guns, people immobilized watching, dead people, women being raped and threatened; in the other part some other elements emerged: the police car, airplanes and helicopters. This part of the scene possibly illustrates that the only way out of the chaos, the suffering and the fear of death, is to run away. But we also see in the scene a small separation between the elements of chaos and the possibility to escape, to move and run away, showing that Sara realized some possible solutions for the situation in her mind.

Sara projected herself directly in the scene, pointing out to me that she was the young woman being held by two men and being raped. She was alone, powerless, facing strong armed men and unable to defend herself, paralyzed by the trauma.

Through the Sandplay, Sara was able to express her recent traumatic experience during her pregnancy. The presence of her partner in the room, his knowledge of the facts and his unconditional support to her, seemed to comfort Sara.

Sara projected a weak and vulnerable image of herself in the scene and of women in general, as victims who cannot protect themselves nor their children. The men in the scene were mainly aggressors.

In this scene there were only few elements, such as the "Dutch" country family, which could be related to her present life. The trauma seemed to take up all the psychological space in her mind. Nevertheless, the making of the scene showed Sara's possibilities to recover traumatic memories and to express them, with fear, grief and sorrow.

Andre, by way of the only figures he chose – a Dutch country man and a Dutch country mother holding the hand of a child – projected the strong maternal figure he had preserved in his internal world, making it easier for him to be identified with her and to also be a maternal figure to his own son. He also showed confidence in me and in Sara's treatment, as well as his hope for their future as an integrated "Dutch" family.

In this first Sandplay scenario, Sara was able to express her trauma in a non-verbal way. The method helped her to open a door to her past.

The analysis of the Sandplay scenarios shall consider, besides the photos of the scenes, also the notations made by the psychotherapist, including the free-association, comments, attitudes and behaviors of the client during the activity. It must also take into account counter-transferential elements from the therapist. For a better categorization of the scene a Sandplay Categorial Checklist (SCC) as the one proposed by Grubbs (1995) can be very helpful. For a qualitative interpretation of the scenario, Mitchell & Friedman (1998) created some criteria of analysis of elements related to *psychological wound* (aspects in the scenario related to: chaos, emptiness, division, threat, wound, hiding, tension and block out) or *indicative of cure* (aspects in the scenario related to: journey, union, energy, birth, profoundness, reconstruction, centralization and integration)

From the moment Sara made her first Sandplay scenario onwards she started to share some of her memories.

As a child and adolescent she lived in a very big house with her family and her uncle (her father's brother) and aunt, in a remote rural area close to a small village in Kosovo. She could not remember whether her uncle and aunt had children who would live with them in the same house. Sara remembered that she and her parents, her brother and sisters slept together in a very big bedroom. She did not remember her bed . . .

These memories were from the period during the war, when the family was afraid all the time, because Serbians lived behind their house. They could not have electricity in their house, so at night they stayed in the dark, and Sara could see the neighbors in their lit houses. The family received anonymous written messages stating that Albanian children would be kidnapped. So Sara, her brother and sisters could not play outside the house, and they could only leave the house in the company of an adult man. They could not go to school anymore either, because the schools were closed for Albanians when Sara was about twelve years old, and in seventh grade.

The descriptions above gave us the thread to follow fragments of her memory and recall experiences from her childhood. I could interpret Sara's current passiveness and her dependence, in relation to her war experiences, when she was dependent on others and had to stay at home. It seems that in Sara's mind the streets and paths were still closed and she needed Andre to be her protector and guide. This interpretation provided an explanation for Sara's fear towards unknown people and her neighbors in the asylum-seeker center, whom she perceived as dangerous enemies.

At that stage, I thought that Sara needed individual attention and space to talk about herself, before being able to include others in the sessions, especially her child. I proposed to her to continue the treatment in individual psychotherapy.

At that point, I knew more about Sara's psychological functioning, her Posttraumatic Stress Disorder – PTSD, with depressive and psychotic symptoms – and her behavior difficulties. I hypothesized that her psychiatric problems were a result of several related factors: an attachment disorder from childhood; a war trauma, which included displacement and the witnessing of violence in her community, a trauma of the rape she experienced during pregnancy, a trauma of forced immigration and the lack of safety in her current asylum situation.

In the individual psychotherapy, Sara was able to talk about herself, to answer questions, and her attention span was longer. She seemed to have a good understanding of the interpretations that were made in the sessions, but she also said that she very easily forgot about them. She was still weak, and she left all initiatives to others. I realized that Sara had a positive, but very dependent, relationship with me and with her partner. Sara's behavior was very passive and she was depressed.

It was during this period in her individual psychotherapeutic process that Sara created her second Sandplay scenario.

She had difficulties starting the activity, but after a few minutes she was able to do it independently. She also worked continuously and was very focused. She named the scene "Big graves".

The second scenario expressed again a very traumatizing event for Sara. It is a disturbing scene of an armed conflict, with several dead persons – including many children – and animals. There are armed soldiers all over the scene. It expresses the power of the army towards people, who were impotent and immobilized in the situation. It also showed Sara's suffering and fear. In this session Sara shared with me yet another of her many traumatic memories.

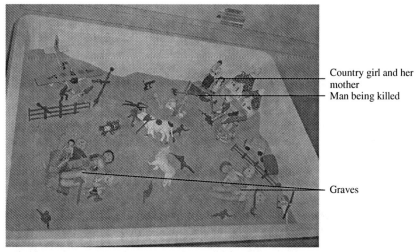

Country girl and her mother

Man being killed

Graves

Clients's view

FIGURE 13.2. The second sandplay scene: *Big graves*.

Sara projected herself directly in the second Sandplay scene, as the small (Dutch) country girl with her mother (placed close to the house), relating it to a traumatic scene she witnessed during the war, when she was about twelve years old and when her uncle was killed by Serbs. The mother figure, who could have represented an element of protection, was not effective, and both she and the child figure (representing Sara herself) were only able to observe the terrible event. It is possible that Sara, identifying herself with her mother's attitude, was also immobilized and unable to give protection to her own child.

In the scene there are no elements related to her present life, as the past and the traumas probably still took most of the psychological space in her mind. The direct projection shows the strong physical and psychological violence to which Sara was submitted.

Nevertheless, the making of this scene showed Sara's possibilities to express her memories and feelings in a coherent way.

While in the first Sandplay scenario Sara expressed a recent trauma, in this scene she expressed traumatic experiences from her childhood.

In the following sessions, Sara continued to talk about her memories of the war in Kosovo, when she was around twelve to thirteen years old. This was the framework that Sara provided to start to talk about the trauma which she expressed in the second Sandplay: her uncle had his head chopped off by the enemies in front of her and her mother. It was a terrifying experience which paralyzed Sara's emotional development: she even today still behaves as that young twelve year-old girl.

In the following period Sara again suffered great emotional instability. She re-started having hallucinations (visual and acoustic), re-experiencing the traumatic events, which frightened her very much. In this period she was able to talk to me and to answer questions about her present and day-to-day functioning, being extremely focused only on herself and her own needs, and unable to pay any attention to her surroundings and the needs of others. In addition, the difficulties in the family's asylum procedure caused her great fear for their present and future.

Sara's passive and very dependent behavior started to affect me, especially because she seemed to perceive it as normal. For me, a Brazilian who had immigrated to the Netherlands less than one year before and who was also facing many cultural differences and changes in life to adjust to the Dutch system, Sara, with her extreme passivity, mirrored the opposite behavior of mine and challenged me to understand and accept her slow adjustment rhythm.

During the subsequent period, Sara recovered some psychological stability and she did not have hallucinations, although she was still very frightened. When asked about the beginning of her relationship with Andre, Sara did not at first remember how she met him. After a while, she could remember that his sister was married to a man who lived in her village. Andre sometimes came to visit his sister's family and that was how they met. They started a secret relationship because of the background of Andre's family, especially because of his father (who had already died) who had worked for the Yugoslav police, something which was condemned by her family.

A short time after the beginning of their relationship, Sara and Andre decided to live together and she left her family and moved with him to his mother's house in the city. Sara's family did not accept their relationship and broke off contact with her. Sara and Andre were very afraid of her family's reaction, especially of her father's and uncles' possible revenge. Sara was pregnant and she and Andre made plans and dreamt about having the child.

One day, when Sara was seven months pregnant, she was alone at home and the house was invaded by two men who sexually abused her, using violence. These men had guns and they spoke another language, which Sara could not understand. From this moment, Sara was shocked, terrified and immobilized. During the short period they continued to live in Kosovo, she and Andre received anonymous threats by telephone to kill her, Andre and their future baby.

After these traumatic experiences, Sara's psychological development and the emotional interaction with the child who was growing inside her belly were frozen. She was extremely afraid and panicky when she saw or heard other men, especially if they communicated in other languages.

It seemed to me that Sara established a perverse link between her rape and her pregnancy, with the notion that the unborn child was contaminated by elements of the men who had raped her during her pregnancy.

Pregnant women who were raped can have feelings that, in addition to themselves, their child was also abused. To touch an unborn child with violence has a very strong symbolic meaning which includes elements of today and tomorrow, present and future, leaving important consequences in the transmission of the trauma and the risk of a secondary trauma for the child. As Moro (2005) reminded us, the family can have a Biblical curse with a heritage of suffering for *seven generations*.

To talk about traumatic experiences was still difficult for Sara but at the same time, slowly, it enabled her to start moving away psychologically from the "frozen state" she was in. To share these experiences with me was very important, also because of her parents' refusal to have any contact with her. Sara also had fantasies that the rape could have been ordered by her own father as revenge for the fact that she was pregnant and she went to live with Andre.

For Sara the fact that I, as well as being her psychotherapist, was an older woman, who could accept her story and support her in her grief, anger and sorrows, helped her in starting to let go of the weight with which these traumatic experiences and thoughts had burdened her.

When facing concrete problems, Sara was still very passive and incapable of finding ways to solve them. Her fear of a man physical proximity brought her great difficulties in medical and other treatments, but also in her relationship with Andre. She systematically refused any physical or sexual contact with her partner, who accepted her behavior with resignation.

During the psychotherapy, Sara was able to communicate better than before (we had been assisted by a female interpreter via the telephone). Sometimes she was able to bring up some special subject by herself, but she was very passive in her actions. Nevertheless, a change started to occur because she began to bring up themes related to her difficulties in the relationship with her child.

Through the way Sara spoke about Denis, describing his behavior when they were together, I understood that her interaction with him was developing, but more so in her mind, in her fantasies, than in her behavior or in practical aspects. She was still not able to interpret his actions and intentions, nor was she able to give him the attention and care he needed. She did not feel responsible for him, not even for his basic needs or his safety.

At one point in treatment, during my vacation, Sara had a relapse and was admitted to a closed ward for a few weeks. It was an attempt to provide her with more intensive treatment in a closed and protected setting, where she might have felt safer. She was having acoustic hallucinations again with male voices demanding she kill herself. She also replied to these voices, saying: "I will not kill myself because I am not guilty", referring to the rape. Upon discharge from the closed clinic, she said that the men's voices were still in her mind during our consultation, and they talked about the rape and sometimes she felt that these "men", who "talked" to her, would also touch her shoulder.

We worked in the sessions on the possible sources of Sara's guilty and ambivalent feelings, but she did not have memories of her parent's moral values in her education nor did she know what they would think about subjects such as pregnancy out of wedlock, rape and immigration. I gave Sara an interpretation in which I related her guilty feelings to the fact that she had left her family and was being punished by them. As a consequence of the conflicts and dilemmas related to her relationship with the parents, she seemed to be also punishing herself with isolation from those who were close to her – Andre, her partner, and Denis, her child. I also pointed out that a possible meaning of her hallucination could have been roused from ambivalent feelings about being "touched": in one way a desire for a loving sexual touch, and in another the fear for it, which perhaps made her produce the specific hallucination of being "touched" in a threatening way.

It was, in general, difficult for Sara to develop her thoughts and insights when the interpretations were given, but she listened to them, and slowly she started changing her behavior, showing that she had integrated them.

During the following period Sara started to feel calmer. She was able to tell me about her daily life: she liked to do embroidery and to help Andre in the kitchen. They sometimes prepared dinner or sandwiches together, but she could not help cut vegetables, out of fear of cutting herself with the knife. We worked on her fantasies about knifes, which were related to aggression. We also brought to light some memories related to food: her mother used to cook for the family and Sara did not usually help her; her mother made a good goulash and Andre also made a very good one.

In these sessions we helped Sara to recover some balance in her day-to-day activities. She also spoke about the birthdays: in her family they were not used to celebrating birthdays. She talked of a date in July when she would be twenty years old. She remembered that they had celebrated Denis's birthday, but she did not know when it was. She did not know the year in which she was born, Andre's birthday nor month or year in which Denis was born. She also did not know which date or month it was; she only knew the year correctly. This lack of memory can be understood as Sara's effort to keep herself distanced from reality.

At this point in her treatment, Sara made a third Sandplay scenario, which she gave the name "Problems of my dead".

Sara did not want to comment on or explain the scene. I understood her refusal as being related to the sexual elements present in the scene, in which several figures, representing men and women, old and young, mostly at home, were engaged in sexual intercourse. Considering the title of the scene, we can also suppose that for Sara these figures represented dead persons. Therefore the scene establishes a relationship between sexual intercourse and death, and is a direct reference to Sara's traumatic sexual experiences and her psychological "death".

At the same time, the fact that she had created this scene and left it closed in the sandbox in my care, could represent her liberation from this psychological "death".

As Sara started to be more aware of her day-to-day life, it was arranged for her to have a female home help coach three times a week, aiming at structuring her life and helping her to raise the child. Frequently the coach went out with Sara and Denis for a short walk and some play with the child, but in her absence Sara did not know how she could play with him. Sara also thought that it was difficult to play with him because he was agitated and she liked to be quiet. She told me that Denis did not have "good behavior", because

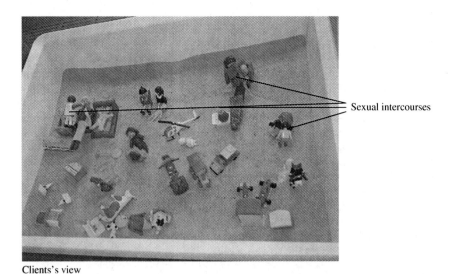

Clients's view

FIGURE 13.3. The third sandplay scene: *Problems of my dead.*

he did not "play nicely alone" as she would like him to do. She only wanted him to stay quiet and when Denis screamed it would make her afraid.

Sara seemed to me like a little girl when she said about Denis's behavior: "I do not know what to do." I interpreted to her that on the one hand she loved him and worried about him, while in the other hand, she did not want to talk to him, play with him or educate his behavior. At that point Sara expressed the following wish: "When I am alone I think he is still inside my belly", relating this thought to the rape during her pregnancy.

With this affirmative Sara expressed her wish to stay physically attached to Denis but to avoid bringing him into the world, with all the responsibilities of raising the child and promoting his development. Sara also showed that she wanted to postpone her role as his mother.

At that time, Sara told me that Denis was starting to talk: he would call "Mamie" and "Papie". It seemed to me that Sara's fear for Denis could be related to the fact that he only spoke baby language, a mixture of Albanian, Dutch and German (which he heard in TV cartoons). Sara said that she could not understand what he wanted to communicate nor the words he said. I spoke about his command of language, which was adequate considering his age and the bi-lingual development. I also spoke about his need to listen to their language, Albanian, and how important it would be if she could speak to him, stimulate his communication and have verbal interactions, teaching him simple words. After some time, I understood that Sara was afraid for Denis to learn Albanian, afraid of him relating to her country and culture. This was an important point to understand in Sara's conflict in her role as Denis's mother and in helping her to overcome it.

After several months of individual treatment Sara was felling better. She told me that she was having problems with Denis, and that she was worried about their relationship. It was the first time in the psychotherapy that she spontaneously considered her child from the point of view of a mother, bringing up her worries about their interaction. She said that he would beat her, throw his toys at her and cry when he was left alone with her. Through these talks Sara opened another door in her mind for her child.

Sara's increasing interest in the child gave me the opportunity to propose to re-introduce the child in the psychotherapeutic setting. So, six months after the beginning of the individual psychotherapy, I proposed to Sara to re-start the mother/child psychotherapy with her and Denis together.

Dennis came to the first mother/child psychotherapeutic session, holding his mother's hand. He started playing with the baby doll and putting it in the stroller. In this play he was reproducing the previous situation when he came to the consultations and was put in a stroller. He tried to include his mother in the game but she did not join him.

Sara could not understand the meaning of his behavior. She had some attention for concrete aspects of it, but she did not get the symbolic meanings and this made it very difficult for her to play with him.

After a short period of mother/child psychotherapy, Denis, who was about twenty months old at that time, showed me that he enjoyed the sessions very much. He included both his mother and me in his play. He was very serious, but also curious. He explored his surroundings and played constructive simple games. He was also able to imitate me, which he enjoyed. Sara stayed seated close to him, but frequently she seemed to be bored.

When the session was over, Sara would help me to re-arrange the room. Denis, often, did not want to leave the room but he would accept it when I would take him by the hand and hand him to his mother. They would walk away together. My feelings were that these were very good sessions where mother and child were starting a positive interaction. I also felt that it was necessary to continue the treatment at a very slow pace.

As their psychological treatment progressed, Sara and Dennis developed a routine in the sessions. Denis would say good-bye to his father and take Sara's hand to enter the play room. He would go straight to the toys and start to play. Sara was starting very slowly to get used to his play and to follow him in some of it, when he asked her to.

In the mother/child psychotherapeutic sessions, Denis was usually calm and he played well for his age. He sometimes needed guidance which Sara was not able to give to him. We divided the sessions in periods during which we would talk and periods that we would play with Denis. Trucks and cars in a noisy garage were his favorite toys at that time.

Denis was frequently kind and friendly to his mother: he would take her by the hand and smile up at me, as if showing his understanding that I was there to help him and his mother. At that time, any negative behavior by Denis during the sessions had disappeared.

Sara called the forth Sandplay scenario "Difficulties".

In this fourth Sandplay scenario, the elements of war and rape are still present (especially in the right-hand side section of the scene), but there are also several elements in the left part, where we can see a country house and animals. So, we can see elements representing Sara's former life in her own country as well as other figures, such as the windmill and the winter house, which possibly represent her current life in the Netherlands.

At this same time a new situation arose: the family was granted asylum in the Netherlands on medical ground (due to Sara's mental problems and necessity of the treatment). At first, after receiving this information, Sara had difficulties understanding what it was all about. It fueled fear of changes in her life: the family was to move from the asylum-seeker center to a house. She was also afraid of going to live far from the clinic, and perhaps having to stop the mother/child psychotherapy, which was so very important to her. This was a difficult period for Sara and her condition worsened for a few weeks, with more somatic complaints and an exacerbation of depressive symptoms. However, this time she did not suffer from psychotic symptoms at all.

At night Sara could not sleep well because: "during the night I fear that somebody will knock at my door and take our furniture away." I asked more about this: Was it a dream?

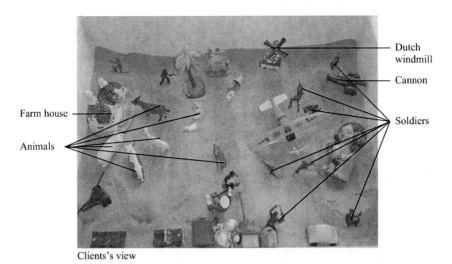

FIGURE 13.4. The fourth sandplay scene: *Difficulties*.

Could she see someone? Did she know of other people who had left the Center? I also associated her fear with other situations in the past, when she had to move. "During the time of the war we did not know that we would have to move, so we were not stressed about it before but it was all very sudden", she told me.

At that time Sara had a dream about going to another clinic for treatment, but she could not talk there. She wanted to talk to me, but she could not because she was in another place.

We spoke about her fear of discontinuing the treatment with me now that she would be moving to another city, and I was able to explain that even if she had other treatment for herself, she could continue our treatment with Denis for a while. We also spoke about the changes earlier in her life, such as when she left her house and moved to live with Andre. She said that her parents did not know that she was going to leave. After she moved, Andre's sister, who lived in the same village, went to talk to Sara's parents but her father said that he did not want anyone from Andre's family to have any contact with them. Sara's father was very angry and threatened Andre's sister. Sara explained me that this behavior of her father is common in their culture, and Sara and Andre were very afraid that her family would find and harm them.

When Sara was talking about this difficult subject Denis hit his head in a shelf and started to cry. He asked for his father as it was difficult for him at that moment to accept that his mother would console him with my help. It was also impossible for Sara to do it by herself. I picked Denis up, spoke to him, put him on Sara's lap, and helped Sara to hold him close and to caress his head. After a few minutes, when Denis was fine and started to play again, Sara continued to talk about her family but Denis got upset again. I could understand and interpret that he could feel his mother's sadness and tension about this subject and that he reacted to it. I explained to Sara this fine example of "psychological mutuality". Dennis came close to me and I told him that we would continue this talk another time.

The changes in the family's life were very positive for Dennis. He showed his happiness during the sessions. He played simple symbolic games, frequently including small dolls representing a "father", a "mother" and a little boy. The "father" was the coordinator who took care of both mother and child, as it was in real life.

Slowly Sara started to talk to me about Denis's good behavior. They liked to watch television together and he also played in the living room while she was there. Sara liked to watch cartoons. She was less depressed and she also smiled more often. She was able to talk to me about her fear that Denis would be taken away from her, when he was at the créche. These fears revealed Sara's ambivalent feelings towards Denis, but also showed her increasing attachment to him and her fear of them being separated.

In another session Sara was looking at Dennis playing and she was able to describe it very well, showing her cognitive capabilities, but at the same time showing that she was not interested in the meaning of his play. She also said that Denis had been sick during the night and he vomited. She had not known how to handle the situation. She remained paralyzed. She was afraid of losing him; she was afraid that he could die. She also started to talk about having had the same feeling before, when she was pregnant and she was also afraid that her baby would die.

While we were talking, Denis came to his mother with a book. This time he could stay sitting on his mother's lap for longer while I played with a figure from the book and he enjoyed and imitated me. Both, mother and child were smiling. It was very good to see this very active and smart boy with his mother, very close to each other, enjoying it.

Sara started to speak again about her family. She told me that she had nobody from her or Andre's family in the Netherlands. She has an uncle, (her mother's brother) who lives in London, and once Andre spoke with him by telephone, asking if he could act as an intermediary between Sara and her family, but it was in vain. The uncle was afraid of revenge, because her father and other uncles in Kosovo were very strict and refused to talk about her.

While speaking about this subject Sara cried, saying that she missed her parents. She would like to have contact with them, especially with her mother, but she explained to me that in her culture, women had to accept and to do what the men said. We spoke about cultural differences: how it was for Andre (who came from a city) and how it was for her, to live in the Netherlands.

Sara explained to me how she wanted to talk to her father, because in her childhood she used to be very attached to him. He was a good father who loved her and was never aggressive to her. We spoke about her blocked feelings, her wishes to contact her parents and the importance of her attempts to build a bridge between them. Sara was able to show more about her grief and her fear to be rejected again by her parents. I understood this and I spoke with her about this conflict which contributed to her passive and blocked behavior.

The Interaction Assessment Procedure

When Denis was two and a half and Sara was twenty years old, we again proposed to record their interaction on video, this time following the Interaction Assessment Procedure – IAP (Wiese, 2006; Batista Pinto, 2007)

The *Interaction Assessment Procedure* – IAP, which can be used in a clinical setting and in research, was developed by the Infant Psychiatry of our clinic (Wiese, 2006; Batista Pinto, 2006), in order to assess the parent/infant interaction. The IAP is an assessment method based on the attachment theory, which proposes holistic clinical judgment, in which the observer uses contextual aspects to infer the appropriate behavior of the interaction partners. The IAP uses a script inspired by the *KIA-Profile* (Stern et al., 1989), for the sequence of the interactive activities to be registered on video. It proposes a global qualitative analysis of the interaction exchanges, based on clinical aspects and on the criteria presented in the *Emotional Availability Scales* (Biringer, Robinson, & Emde, 2000).

In the *Interaction Assessment Procedure* (which takes about twenty minutes), the parent/infant interaction is recorded in video, in the following sequence: to play without toy, to play with toys, to teach, to ignore, to separate, to meet. The analysis must consider the behavior and the affective interaction of the dyads, with special emphasis on the qualitative analysis of the mother/child and father/child interaction. The parents' sensitivity, structure of the play, non-intrusive and non-hostile behavior, as well as the infant's responsivity and involvement are taken into account.

Although Sara understood what she was meant to do during the IAP video recording of her interaction with Denis, she was not able to play with him without toys. Denis waited patiently for his mother, sometimes looking at the toys which were behind him.

In the activity with toys he took the initiative and showed them to his mother, who held them, but was unable to actively play. She interacted with the child in a passive way. Denis explored the toys structuring his play.

In the video-interaction we clearly see that there was still a gap between the expectations of the child and the behavior of the mother. The child seems to know his mother's behavior and her reactions to intrusiveness quite well and he keeps himself physically close, but not directly touching her. When the mother withdrew her attention, Denis noticed it, but he continued to play, accepting the situation. He also searched for support in his surroundings and accepted it.

There were only a few verbal exchanges in Albanian between the two of them during the video recording, but they communicated mostly in a non-verbal way, being able to establish a certain rhythm in their interaction.

Analyzing the IAP video interaction, after a period of one year of mother/child psychotherapy, I saw that Sara showed weak sensitivity, inconsistent structure in the play, partial intrusiveness and covert hostility towards her child. Dennis showed moderate responsivity and moderate involvement in the interaction with his mother.

Nevertheless, this second video-recording of their interaction, when compared with the first one (about one year earlier), showed great qualitative improvement in the mother/child interaction, with both partners in the dyad showing better adjustment to each other's patterns of functioning.

The Last Sandplay

A few weeks after Sara and her family had moved to a new house, she made her fifth Sandplay scenario, which she called "Begging them".

In this scenario we can distinguish several scenes which seem to be connected in a time line to the past, present and future. The first scene closed in a fence that has no entrance, represents the past: Sara's parents' farm, with a house, animals, trucks, trees. Here she placed a couple, symbolizing her parents, facing each other in conversation. She added

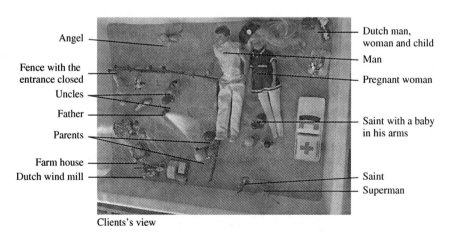

FIGURE 13.5. The fifth sandplay scene: *Begging them.*

three human figures which represent her uncles talking to her father (a soldier figure with a gun). A windmill, which is the most famous symbol of the Netherlands, stands next to the house. Although a part of the scene is bucolic, the addition of the soldier figure, representing her father, placed in a group of male relatives, projects Sara's fear of the aggressive behavior of her father, supported by the other men in the family. The fact that she is living in the Netherlands now is also clearly represented by the windmill.

In the scene, the big dolls of a man and a pregnant woman represent Andre and Sara, and one of the reasons she was rejected by her family: the pregnancy. Between these two figures she placed a saint with a child in his arms, showing the need for protection for the couple, but also for the unborn child. Close to the girl (big female pregnant doll) there is an ambulance, representing the treatment she needs to deal with the situation, and the telephone to communicate from a distance with her parents.

The four figures in front of the couple represent Sara and Andre begging her parents' forgiveness. In this scene, Sara's mother is represented by a saint and her father by a superman. Sara added three Dutch human figures in the corner of the scene, close to the telephone, representing Andre, herself and Denis. The last figure Sara added, again showing her need for protection and her wish to protect her family in Kosovo, was an angel.

In this scenario Sara could express her inner psychological conflict: her grief caused by having left her parents and not having any contact with them since then, her fear for the aggressive reaction of her father and uncles, and her wish to communicate with them and to have their acceptance of her choices in life.

After two years of psychotherapy, in this Sandplay scenario, Sara expressed, in an organized way, a major conflict which was not directly related to the war and the trauma, but which referred to her individual history as a woman in her culture and her family. This projection also shows that Sara was able to move forward in her psychological development. Nevertheless, the mother/child psychotherapy with Sara and Denis is still in progress.

When I was finishing writing this chapter the family received a permanent resident permit to stay in the Netherlands.

Final Remarks

The case of Sara and Denis clearly illustrates the implications of a woman's traumatic experiences since childhood in establishing a severe Posttraumatic Stress Disorder, with depressive and psychotic symptoms. It also exposes the consequences of the mother's mental disorder for her interaction with her baby, and later her infant, putting the emotional development of the child at risk.

The case shows how the individual psychotherapy treatment was important to access the mother, and to help her to express and to elaborate on elements of her traumatic experiences related to the child and how the mother/child psychotherapy succeeded in helping them to develop both individually and in their interaction.

The mother/child *psychological mutuality* (Cramer, 1974) during pregnancy and in early childhood, determines the real and the imaginary mental representations that the mother has of the child and this affects the psychological organization of the child.

Parentalization is a complex process in which the experience modifies the symbolic and vice-versa. This process includes the recognition of the child as the bearer of a psychic heritage, which holds the parent's culture, conscious dilemmas and unconscious conflicts that can exist in the family line: the transgenerational mandate (Lebovici, 1998)

It has as metaphorical paradigm – *The Tree of Life* – *a* transgenerational transmission which tends to be a family myth that defines the axe of the life mandate imposed on the descendent. This heritage is transmitted to the child through the care and the real and phantasmal parent/child exchanges and complex and reciprocal identifications, constituting the inter-subjectivity (Lebovici, 1996, 1998).

The fact that Denis was a healthy child and had a positive interaction with his father was a good basis for the mother/child psychotherapy, during which we could focus on the mother's representation of the child, helping her to diminish her massive projections that were related to the very traumatic experiences she had during his pregnancy on to him.

Moro (2002) and Moro, De la Noë, & Mouchenik (2004) pointed out that the migrant child has to develop in a transcultural situation and, as a consequence, must build a cultural structure in the separation between the two worlds with different natures – one related to the family's culture, the world of affection, and another, to the outside world, the world of rationality and pragmatism – frequently resulting in many conflicts in his/her interaction.

Even though we still see important sequels of the traumas in Sara's personality and behavior, the individual psychotherapy, followed by the mother/child psychotherapy, helped to instill in her the motherhood process as Denis' mother, as well the process of becoming a son of his own mother in the child.

Thus, the mother/child psychotherapy, combined with the Sandplay method, opened an important psychological space for the detection and treatment of the client's maternal conflicts, favoring the development of a better attachment in the dyad, contributing to the emotional development of both mother and child, as well as preventing the development of psychopathology in the child.

As we saw in Sara's case, the transcultural clinical work with clients with PTSD, is very complex and demands sensitivity, strength and emotional stability from the psychotherapist. Several authors have written guidelines (Nader, 1994; National Center for PTSD, 2006) with suggestions for the therapist's attitude to the client. Inspired by these authors, as well as based on my clinical experience with clients such as Sara and Denis, I suggest the following basic guidelines for the psychotherapists who work with traumatized children, adolescents and young adults:

1. be able to talk about the traumatic events;
2. provide means to express the experiences and feelings related to the trauma;
3. support the client in positive strategies to cope with anxiety, anger and other stress reactions/symptoms;
4. be consistent and predictable in your relationship with the client in view of his/her vulnerability;

5. be affectionate and take into account the context and the culture of the client;
6. discuss what is expected in the client's behavior in different situations and contexts;
7. answer the questions and explain what is needed;
8. look for signs of re-enactment, dissociation, avoidance, and reactivity;
9. empower the client to avoid re-traumatization;
10. talk to the client about choices giving him/her some sense of control of his/her own life;
11. ask for help and supervision if necessary.

Most of all, as psychotherapists, we must be aware that traumatized clients need to re-establish their connection with the world and with other persons, and that we are an important element in helping them in their healing process.

References

American Psychiatric Association. (1995). *Diagnostic and Statistical Manual of Mental Disorders. International Version.* Washington D.C.: American Psychiatric Association.

Batista Pinto, E. (2000). Psicoterapia breve mãe/bebê. In C. F. Rohenkohl (Ed.). *A clínica com o bebê* (pp. 125–130). São Paulo: Casa do Psicólogo.

Batista Pinto, E. (2001). L'alchimiste des interactions. *Journal des Psychologues. La passion des bébés: Serge Lebovici. Hors-série.* 72–73.

Batista Pinto, E. (2004). Os sintomas psicofuncionais do bebê. *Estudos de Psicologia,* 3, 451–457.

Batista Pinto, E. (2007). A análise das interações pais/bebê em abordagem psicodinâmica: clínica e pesquisa. In C. Piccinini & M. L. S. Moura (Eds.), *Observando as Interações Pais-Bebê-Criança: diferentes abordagens teóricas e metodológicas.* São Paulo: Casa do Psicólogo. (In Press).

Batista Pinto, E., & Franco, A. (2003). O Jogo de Areia na pesquisa. *Psicologia (USP). Instituto de Psicologia. Universidade de São Paulo,* 2, 91–114.

Biringer, Z., Robinson, J. L., & Emde, R. N. (2000). Appendix B: The emotional availability scales (3rd ed.; and abridged infancy/early childhood version). *Attachment & Human Development,* 2, 256–270.

Cramer, B. (1974). Interaction réelle et interaction fantasmatique. Réflexion au sujet des thérapies et des observations du nourisson. *Psychothérapies,* 1, 39–47.

Fitamant, D.S. (1999). Assessment report on sexual violence in Kosovo. The United Nations Population Fund – UNFPA. In United Nations Development Fund for Women (2006). *Gender profile of the conflict in Kosovo.* Retrieved August 25, 2006 from http://www.womenwarpeace.org/kosovo/kosovo.htm

Franco, A. (2003). *O Jogo de Areia: uma intervenção clínica.* Dissertação de Mestrado. Instituto de Psicologia da Universidade de São Paulo, São Paulo.

Freud, S. (1992). As paraneuroses. In S. Freud. *Obras Completas. Psicanálise II.* (pp. 291–300). São Paulo: Martins Fontes. Original work published in 1917.

Golse, B. (2004). Entre mére et bébé: éduquer les sentiments ou co-construire les affects? *L'Autre,* 2, 215–226.

Grubbs (1995). A comparative analysis of Sandplay process of sexually abused and non-clinical children. *The Arts in Psychotherapy,* 5, 429–446.

International Helsinki Federation for Human Rights, Women 2000. (2000). An investigation into the status of women's rights in Central and South-Eastern and newly independent states. Federal Republic of Yugoslavia: Kosovo and Serbia. In United Nations Development Fund for Women (2006). *Gender profile of the conflict in Kosovo.* Retrieved August 25, 2006 from http://www.womenwarpeace.org/kosovo/kosovo.htm

Jung, C. G. (1991). *A Prática da Psicoterapia.* Petrópolis, RJ: Vozes. Original work published in 1935.

Kalff (1980). *Sandplay: a psychotherapeutic approach to the psyche.* Santa Monica: Sigo.

Lebovici, S. (1989). Le bébé vulnerable: évaluation des risques. In S. Lebovici & F. Wei-Halpern (Eds.), *Psychopathologie du bébé* (pp. 561–566). Paris: Puf.

Lebovici, S. (1996). La transmission intergénérationnelle ou quelques considérations sur l'utilité de l'étude de l'arbre de vie dans les consultations thérapeutiques parents/bébé. In M. Dugnat (Ed.). *Troubles relationnels pére-mére/bébé: quels soins?* (pp. 19–28). Ramonville St Agne: Érés.

Lebovici, S. (1998). L'arbre de vie. *Journal de psychanalyse de l'enfant. Les psychothérapies psychanalytiques.* 22, 98–127.

Mestre, C. (2003). *Mettre au monde loin de sa mére. Vulnérabilité des femmes migrantes au moment de l'accouchement de leur premier enfant.* Mémoire du Diplme Universitaire de Psychopathologie du bébé: Université Paris XIII. Paris.

Mitchell, R. R., & Friedman, H. S. (1994). *Sandplay – Past, present and future.* London / New Youk: Routledge.

Mitchell, R. R., & Friedman, H. S. (1998). *References for the scenario analysis in Sandplay.* Unpublished manuscript.

Moro, M. R. (2002). *Enfants d'ici venus d'ailleurs: naître et grandir en France.* Barcelone: Hachette.

Moro, M. R., De la Noë, Q., & Mouchenik, Y. (Eds.). (2004). *Manuel de psychiatrie transculturelle: travail clinique, travail social.* Grenoble: La pensée sauvage.

Moro, M. R. (2005).Les bébé et les jeunes enfants aussi: pour une clinique transculturelle du trauma de la premiére enfance. In T. Baubet, C. Lachal, & M. R. Moro (Eds.). *Bébés et traumas.* Grenoble: La pensée sauvage.

Nader, K. O. (1994). Countertransference in the treatment of acutely traumatized children. In J. P. Wilson & J. D. Lindy (Eds.). *Countertransference in the treatment of PTSD* (pp. 179–205). New York: Guilford.

National Center for Post-Traumatic Stress Disorder (2006). *Rape in a war zone. National Center for Post-Traumatic Stress Disorder Fact Sheet.* Retrieved September 8, 2006 from www.ncptsd.va.gov/facts/specific/fskosovo.html.

Piccinini, C. A., Moura, M. L. S., Ribas, A. F., Bosa, C. A., Oliveira, E. A., Batista Pinto, E., L., et al. (2001). Diferentes perspectivas na análise da interação pais-bebê/criança. *Psicologia: Reflexão e Crítica,* 2, 469–485.

Rabain-Jamin, J., & Wornham, W. L. (1990). Transformations des conduits de maternage et des pratiques de soin chez les femmes migrantes originaires d'Afrique de l'Oest. *Psychiatrie de l'enfant,* 1, 287–319.

Sayad, A. (1999). *La double absence, des illusions de l'émigré aux souffrances de l'immigré.* Paris: Seuil.

Schwimmer, B. (2006). *Module I: Introduction. The Culture Concept.* Retrieved September 11, 2006 from http://www.umanitoba.ca/faculties/arts/anthropology/ courses/122/module1/culture.html

Stern, D. N., Robert-Tissot, C., Besson, G., Rusconi-Serpa, S., Muralt, M. de, Cramer, B., et al. (1989). L'entretien "R": une méthode d'évaluation des representations maternelles.

In S. Lebovici, P. Mazet, & J.-P. Visier (Eds.), *L'évaluation des interactions précoces entre le bébé et ses partenaires* (pp. 151–160). Paris: Eshel.

United Nations Development Fund for Women War Peace (2006). *Gender profile of the conflict in Kosovo*. Retrieved August 25, 2006 from http://www.womenwarpeace.org/kosovo/kosovo.htm

United Nations Interim Administration Mission in Kosovo – UNMIK (2004) In United Nations Development Fund for Women. *Gender profile of the conflict in Kosovo*. Retrieved August 25, 2006 from http://www.womenwarpeace.org/kosovo/kosovo.htm

United Nations Population Fund – UNFPA. (2006). In United Nations Development Fund for Women. *Gender profile of the conflict in Kosovo*. Retrieved August 25, 2006 from http://www.womenwarpeace.org/kosovo/kosovo.htm

Wiese, E. B. P. (2004). Parents/Baby Psychotherapy with Asylum Seekers in the Netherlands. 9th *World Association for Infant Mental Congress* (p. 20. No. 205). Retrieved September 10, 2006 from http://www.waimh.org/CONGRESS2004/ Abstracts_129–242.pdf

Wiese, E. B. P. (2006). Interaction Assessment Procedure – IAP: a qualitative approach to parent/infant interaction. 10th *World Association for Infant Mental Congress* (p. 3. No. 569). Retrieved September 10, 2006 from http://www.waimh.org/ABSTRACTS%202006/ Abstracts%20561–688.pdf.

Wiese, E. B. P., & Burhorst, I. (2004). Asielzoekerkinderen en-adolescenten in behandeling bij Herlaarhof, centrum voor kinder-en jeugdpsychiatrie. *De Ark*, 3, 34–40.

Wiese, E. B. P., & Burhorst, I. (2007). Transcultural Psychiatry: a mental health program for asylum-seeking and refugee children and adolescents in the Netherlands. *Transcultural Psychiatry*, (In press).

Wilson, J. P. (2004). The broken spirit: posttraumatic damage to the self. In J. P. Wilson & B. Drožđek (Eds.), *Broken spirits: The treatment of traumatized Asylum seekers, refugees, war and torture victims* (pp. 109–157). New York: Brunner-Routledge.

14
Lost in Limbo: Cultural Dimensions in Psychotherapy and Supervision with a Temporary Protection Visa Holder from Afghanistan

Robin Bowles & Nooria Mehraby

Introduction

Many people in refugee work have the view that it is important to match up therapist and client so that they are not from groups which are persecuting or fighting each other. The idea is that it is very difficult to build trust with a person from a group, which has abused you and/or your family and friends. While we would be in agreement with this view, sometimes clients can be matched with a therapist and/or an interpreter, who speak their language and are from the same country, but may be from an opposing ethnic, political or religious group. This case study is of current interest because the therapist and client are from opposing sides in the war in Afghanistan, and the therapist and the supervisor are from opposing sides in the 'War on Terror'. ('War on Terror' is a loose term coined by the US government, which refers to the current international situation where the US and their western allies are trying to prevent terrorist attacks from small groups of people who use Islam to justify their extreme ideas. The term also includes the recent occupation of Iraq and Afghanistan by the US and allies, and the terrorist attacks and fighting in those countries.) From a distance, it would appear that the matching in this case would be a recipe for disaster – yet this has not been our experience so far.

In this chapter we are examining some psychosocial and psychotherapy work with a young male client from Afghanistan, living on a Temporary Protection Visa in Sydney, Australia. His extensive trauma history and emotional and physical issues are introduced in the first section of the chapter. The second section will focus on a number of cultural and political factors in the environment; the third section introduces some thoughts about politics and culture which were relevant for understanding the young man's mental state and aspects of the work with him, including transcultural issues in the therapeutic relationships.

This case study includes two different cross-cultural relationships – both the relationship between the therapist and the client, and the relationship between the therapist and her supervisor. Dimensions of more overt cultural differences in these relationships include ethnicity, religion, class, education, language and gender. Less overt dimensions include ways of thinking, identity, 'flavours' and nuances in feelings, ways of understanding experience, unconscious ideas, internal relationships and images, which also are informed by culture and language.

The therapist and supervisor are both working at STARTTS (Service for the Treatment and Rehabilitation of Torture and Trauma Survivors) in Sydney. STARTTS is perhaps a unique service because it has always employed a majority of workers from refugee and non-English speaking backgrounds, so that it could form strong links with refugee communities. It has developed using a combination of community development and clinical models for interventions with refugees at multiple levels of the system. (Cunningham & Silove, 1993; Aroche & Coello, 1994, 2004). Working in this multicultural staff group has provided a rich environment for ongoing discussions about culture, politics and psychotherapy 'at the coalface'. There has been close contact with the crises and events affecting the local refugee communities, and there has been experimentation working with local healers and religious people. Some of this early work has been documented. (Becker et al, 1990; Silove, Tarn, Bowles & Reid, 1991; Bowles, 1993, 1998, 2005, 2006; Nguyen, 1993; Morris et al, 1993; Bowles & Haidary, 1994; Bowles, Haidary & Becker, 1995; Nguyen & Bowles, 1998; Becker & Bowles, 2001a, 2001b, 2001c, 2004; Aroche & Coello, 1994, 2004; Bowels, Salem & Preston-Thomas, 2004; Haidary, 2000; Mehraby, 1999a, 1999b, 2001a, 2001b, 2002a, 2002b, 2002c, 2003a, 2003b, 2003c, 2004, 2005a, 2005b, 2007a, 2007b; Mehraby & Coello, 2005)

The traumatising nature of the work tends to push the staff together for support. A feature of STARTTS has been the implementation of support structures, for example regular clinical supervision and encouragement to attend personal psychotherapy or other forms of self-development and anti-burnout strategies. We would like to acknowledge the clinical supervision, which both authors have received from Rise Becker, which has informed much of our thinking.

Some Thoughts About Culture and Psychotherapy with Refugees

Ravalico's discussion of culture and psychotherapy (Ravalico, 2007) describes culture as encompassing 'the ineluctable modalities of being', including class, gender and race, with the mother tongue assumed to have important effects on the formation of thought. Ravalico uses postmodernist ideas to describe a complex interplay of different cultures in the therapy room being co-created. Each client and therapist have within them histories and identities, which include ways of thinking. There can be many cultures at the same time within the therapy room.

Bruck, as cited in Ravalico (2007), explores notions about multilingual identities. People who speak more than one language are usually situated in more than one cultural context, and so are exposed to differing notions of identity, the self, subjectivity, values and attitudes, (all of which are encoded in language). Foucault's notions (1975) of structures of culture are language, political systems and religion, as cited in Ravalico (2007). He referred to language as the 'building blocks' from which we create our experience.

Lemma and Levy (2005) write how there is dialectic between the inner (and unconscious) world of individuals, and their social, cultural and political environment. People's responses to traumatic events reflect a range of political issues, as well as the personal meanings, which they have for them. Even if a person has resources in the external environment this may not counterbalance the pain and desperation which they may feel inside themselves. In other words, if one cannot feel at home and comfortable inside oneself, it is very hard to feel at home anywhere. (Becker, 1991, 2006).

In summary, underlying our discussion, we are using ideas from psychoanalytic and post-modern theory about psychotherapy and about culture. We are also using the Cultural Formulation of Diagnosis as designed by the editors, Silove's Psychosocial Adaptive Systems Model (1999), and other models developed by practitioners in the field, as frameworks for thinking about transcultural issues in the case material.

The Story of Mr Hussani

How We Met

Mr Reza Hussani had been referred to STARTTS by his solicitor for support and therapy because during his session with the solicitor he was shaking and sweating, and he had great difficulty recounting his history. He was a 40-year-old man of Hazara ethnicity from a remote village in Afghanistan. He had arrived in Australia by boat, and then had been detained in an Australian Immigration Detention Centre for a number of months. He was finally released from Detention and was granted a temporary protection visa (TPV) for three years. He was living in a flat with some other Hazara TPV holders and working full time in a factory. He said that it was beneath his dignity to accept social security as he had been working since he was a young teenager to support his family. He said '*It is better to eat potatoes that you earn yourself rather than having meat given to you by someone else.*'

Mr Hussani further disclosed, '*I belong to the Hazara ethnic group. As far as I remember, I consider myself as a Hazara to be very poor and disadvantaged. I feel even in Australia that we are low class residents who are never welcomed. It is written on our foreheads that Hazaras should suffer.*' As described in Mr Hussani's history below, as a member of the Hazara ethnic group, he and his family had suffered greatly during the Taliban era.

Mr. Hussani's Life

Mr Hussani's memory of his early childhood and family in Afghanistan did not come to his mind very easily. He found it difficult to talk about his family at all, especially in the early phases of the treatment, partly because he felt so guilty about leaving them behind. At the time of referral, he felt a complete failure as the breadwinner of the family, because he was unable to support them. His feelings of failure were intensified because he was living in relative safety while his family may have been killed in Afghanistan already. He could not tolerate talking about his family with anybody at the time of referral.

However, eventually he did tell the therapist that he was only a young teenager when his father and uncle were killed by Russian soldiers. Soon after this, Pashtun people killed his elder brothers and some cousins. Mr Hussani became then the head of the family and he started to provide financial support for his mother, younger brother, sisters, and his brother's wife and children. Mr. Hussani himself was illiterate in his own language, he had never attended school, and the only education he had received was studying the Qur'an in the rural village where he had grown up. He entered an arranged traditional marriage at the age of 19 with his cousin who was only 14 at that time. They had five children: a girl and four boys. The youngest boy was born after Mr.Hussani left Afghanistan. Although the marriage was arranged, they had a loving relationship and as cousins had many good childhood memories.

Mr Hussani was working long hours on a farm, and also polishing shoes in the street in the evenings. During the Taliban era, his younger brother (aged 22) who was working with him on the farm was captured by the Taliban. Pieces of his brother's body were found in a bag in front of their house a month later. Mr Hussani and his family feared for their lives, so they sold the farm and paid a smuggler to help Mr Hussani escape from the country. Mr Hussani had to leave his wife and children behind, planning to bring them out later. A Pasthun smuggler took Mr.Hussani to Pakistan. He said the most traumatic experience of his life was when he had to say goodbye to his mother and his pregnant wife and children. He left the country with a stranger who told him that he would take him to a peaceful country where he could bring his wife and children. He had never heard of Australia before, nor did he have control over the choice of his final destiny. He was terrified and remained silent through the trip, as he could not speak the smuggler's language, Pashtu. The smuggler also advised him to be quiet during the trip so that he would not create a climate of suspicion while travelling.

Eventually after four days of travelling under hazardous circumstances they arrived in Kawitt, Pakistan. He was then taken from Kawitt to the city of Karachi where he was locked in a room for a month waiting for his journey to proceed. The smuggler provided a false document which enabled Mr.Hussani to travel further to Singapore and from there via Indonesia to Australia. His escape to Australia was a prolonged unsafe journey. Mr.Hussani had to share a small boat with another 150 people. Travelling by boat and being at sea for the first time in his life was a frightening experience for him. Mr. Hussani was rescued by an Australian team when their boat was sinking, but he was placed in detention rather than being allowed to live in the community. During the trip refugees ran out of food and water and he was not only terrified by this experience but was also physically sick. There were times when Mr.Hussani thought that he would die, and he was all the time facing the unknown.

His experiences in detention in Australia were so overwhelming and re-traumatizing that he spoke very little about it. However, he said that when he fled the oppressive regime of the Taliban, he had been expecting Australia to be a society of justice. Instead his suffering from injustice and discrimination continued in detention. He reported degrading experiences in detention, such as being called by number instead of name. He had to prove his identity as an Afghan because of his Hazaragi accent. He was also stripped of his personal belongings including a ring that had been given to him by his mother. This was significant for him as it was his last connection with his mother.

At the time of referral Mr Hussani had not had any contact with his family since he had fled from Afghanistan. It was only later that another TPV holder, who had gained permanent residence and had travelled back to Pakistan, found the whereabouts of Mr Hussani's family. His family had left Afghanistan a year after his departure with the help of one of the wife's uncle. They were living in the city of Kawitt under hazardous circumstances.

Mr Hussani then found out that his little son, who had been born after he had fled, had died, and also that Mr Hussani's mother had died. When Mr Hussani heard this news, he said to his therapist: '*I am not a real father. I did not wait for my son to be born. I could not protect him from dying. I am worse than animals because at least they protect their children and I did not. My mother was a holy spirit. I am a failure because I could not go to her funeral or be by her bedside while she was dying.*'

The family tree (Figure 14.1) was gradually outlined by Mr Hussani during his therapy. It shows the level of transgenerational trauma suffered by his family, and himself, described above.

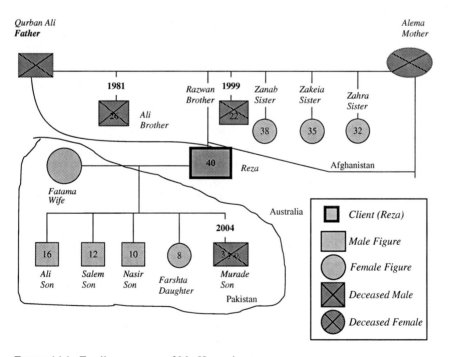

FIGURE 14.1. Family genogram of Mr. Hussani.

Anxieties in Exile

Mr Hussani had never had any psychiatric or psychological treatment before coming to STARTTS. There was neither a history of mental illness in his family, nor had he any history of suicide attempts or emotional problems. He gradually described the following symptoms through his treatment. These symptoms had begun after he had been released from detention in Australia, and they had worsened after his application had been rejected by the Refugee Review Tribunal.

Mr Hussani was worried about his own future and the future of his family in Afghanistan. He was anxious about being separated from his family, and about having temporary visa status. He was certain that if his application was rejected and he was deported to Afghanistan, his life would be in danger again.

His anxiety was exacerbated by the long wait while his application was being processed. His application had already been rejected on two levels in the determination process (both at the Immigration Department level and at the level of the Refugee Review Tribunal). During his treatment, his case was waiting for a Federal Court Hearing.

He was worried that he was going to lose control of himself and harm himself or others. He was also worried that he was going mad. He knew of a TPV holder who had committed suicide in Adelaide, and another who had been involved in a knife stabbing incident and diagnosed with a mental illness.

Most of the time he suffered from headaches, stomach aches and diarrhoea which his therapist believed were somatised aspects of the anxiety, as there were no medical conditions causing these physical problems.

He felt guilty that he had left his family behind in an area still dominated by the Taliban. Mr Hussani felt helpless and ashamed of himself. Many other Hazara TPV holders had gained permanent visas in Australia, and had sponsored their families out already. He said, '*What kind of a man am I, that my suffering cannot be approved of?*' He was ashamed that he was not protecting his family in Afghanistan and felt hopeless about the future. He said he was not worthy of being a husband or a father.

He started to feel powerless and discriminated against as he had been in Afghanistan. He felt angry about the injustice of his situation, both in Afghanistan and in Australia. However, there was a minimum expression of anger both in the sessions and outside. His anger was more a 'frozen rage'.

He would wake up with nightmares about being deported to Afghanistan or being killed by the Taliban. Mr Hussani suffered also from traumatic memories of his family members being killed by the Taliban. Images of war or detention, and other symbolic reminders, were intolerable for him, as they evoked strong feelings of fear and memories of the past.

He avoided situations and activities that reminded him of his past. He avoided any topic related to his past or present trauma. He constantly felt in danger, thinking that something bad might happen to him or to his children. Mr Hussani had lost several kilos in weight over the past few months.

He said that he had trouble falling asleep and staying asleep. He tended to sleep for 3 – 4 hours per night. Usually he awoke at about 3am and could not go back to sleep. Mr Hussani could not concentrate, and at times he would loose his way while driving and drove through red lights. Sometimes, he just had moments of blankness.

During his treatment, he rarely spoke of the past and then would soon try to change the subject of the conversation. Therefore, much of his trauma and early life experiences remain unknown.

Mr Hussani sometimes thought about killing himself, longing for the peace of death, or wishing he had been killed by the Taliban. However, he said that he would never commit suicide because it was forbidden in his religion, and that he cared about his family too much to inflict a suicide on them. Mr Hussani suffered from severe grief because of the multiple losses and separation from his family.

In summary, Mr Hussani eventually described his feelings as a 'deep sharp pain burning in his heart.' Fernandes (2002) cited the phrase 'burning in the fire' as a common description for the feelings of a group of young TPV holders from Afghanistan. This idea of burning is often used by Afghan people to describe extreme psychic pain.

In terms of the DSM IV classification (APA, 1994), he was suffering from symptoms consistent with those of depression and posttraumatic stress disorder (PTSD). These symptoms were of serious concern to him, but were not his primary concern.

Course and Outcome of Mr. Hussani's Psychotherapy

Initially it was difficult to connect with Mr Hussani in psychotherapy because he was quite disconnected from other people and had lost trust in them. He was trying to make some meaning from his experiences and was wondering whether God was punishing him. He began to lose trust in God as well, when his application was rejected twice and when he heard about the death of his son and his mother. He said, '*I stopped praying. Even God is not on our side. Is this fair, the way that I am treated? When we Hazara people were born, I think 'bad luck' was written on our forehead.*'

He stopped going to any social or religious gatherings, even stopped going to the mosque. He just would go to the park and isolate himself there. He was worried that he was going mad and was terrified of being on his own, but he found it shameful to be with others.

In the beginning the therapist focused on establishing safety in the contact (as according to Herman's framework, Herman (1992)), but it was difficult for the client to feel safe when his external situation was insecure. The threat of being returned to Afghanistan was constantly looming with his temporary status. It took several sessions for him to start to engage. The therapy was his only option for ventilating feelings and talking about some of his worries, so he kept attending his sessions on a regular basis.

Practical interventions such as writing a report supporting his visa application and trying to trace his family members through Red Cross were beneficial in developing trust and building safety. Assurances of confidentiality and responding with empathy, and a non-judgemental attitude of the therapist helped to build trust as well.

Communicating a genuine sense of justice helped the client to think that the therapist was with him, rather than against him. The therapist used the word 'we', which helped Mr. Hussani to engage more in therapy and gave him a sense of belonging as an Afghan rather than feeling an outsider as an alienated Hazara. The therapist also said that she used simple concepts and language to fit with Mr Hussani's level of literacy.

In these early sessions Mr Hussani preferred to focus on current issues regarding his visa and his family's current situation. The themes of loss and separation were recurrent, and he discussed losing his son and his mother and his wife's illness. As time went by, he became more depressed and socially isolated as more TPV holders gained permanent residency, and were able to visit their families abroad.

Supported by the therapy, Mr Hussani continued to work long hours, including on the weekends, and was able to send money to his family in Pakistan, so that his children could attend school and buy a computer. He gradually gained in confidence, and started to provide support to other people who had been recently reunited with their families in Australia. For example he established a charity group within the Hazara Community where members of the community would collect money regularly to support the newly arrived families to buy basic necessities. He started to attend community gatherings and go to the mosque again.

Finally Mr Hussani gained his permanent residence in December 2005 and travelled back to Pakistan to see his family. He is currently engaged in sponsoring them to Australia.

Some brief comments on the course of the therapy are that Mr Hussani never explored his trauma history in depth. There was a minimum expression of feelings, particularly at first. The way that the therapist and Mr Hussani, engaged together reflected a collective sense of self (for example using the word 'we'). Religion was a strong theme in the meaning of the trauma and also in the form of recovery. Negative feelings in the relationship were not expressed directly. These issues have interesting cultural/political and therapeutic aspects and will be discussed in the sections below. In addition, the political circumstances as described below influenced the process of the therapy and supervision.

The Political and Cultural Environment

Thinking About the Political Dimensions

Mr Hussani's experiences, and also the experience of the therapy and the supervision, need to be understood in the context of the ongoing war in Afghanistan, the position of the temporary visa holders from Afghanistan in Australia, and the ongoing 'War Against Terror' internationally and in Australia. All these aspects have been contributing to Mr Hussani's ongoing reactions and situation, and have affected the process of psychotherapy and supervision.

The Wars in Afghanistan

Twenty-eight years of war in Afghanistan are still having a profound impact on all aspects of life in this country. The problems began in 1978 when the Soviet-backed regime commenced a systematic political repression, targeting 'enemies of the revolution'. In 1979 the Soviet Union occupied Afghanistan and its army remained in the country until 1989. During this period, tens of thousands of Afghans, mostly from the educated middle class, were imprisoned, tortured and killed. Disappearances were commonplace. Between 1989–1992 fierce fights took place between the communist regime and the opposition groups

After this (1992–1996), a bloody civil war amongst the rival political and ethnic groups took place. From 1996 to 2001 the Taliban led Afghanistan, imposing severe restrictions on the rights and freedoms of the general population. Women were targeted and suffered enormously. Since October 2001 Afghans have been caught in combat between the 'War Against Terrorism' and the Taliban regime, resulting in a significant number of civilian casualties (Mehraby, 2002a).

All these conflicts have cost the country about two million dead, two million internally displaced and three million disabled. More than five million Afghans sought refuge in other countries. Consequently, Afghans comprise the world's largest refugee population. Many of them were able to flee to neighbouring countries including Pakistan, Iran and India, while some left for Australia, the USA and several European countries. These figures are conservative estimates, since in Pakistan alone; there are an estimated number of three million refugees (Mehraby, 2002a).

Most refugees from Afghanistan could be seen as suffering from transgenerationally transmitted trauma as the war in their country has attacked several generations of their families.

Afghan Refugees in Australia

Afghans constitute the fifth largest group of arrivals to New South Wales (Department of Immigration and Ethnic Affairs, 2001). Most of the estimated 14,000 Afghans who currently live in Australia came via refugee camps. The majority of them are middle-class professionals. Like other refugees, Afghans face a range of settlement difficulties such as unemployment, lack of English language, accommodation, and financial problems. All these difficulties affect their integration into a new culture.

Since the end of 1999, a later group of Afghan asylum seekers have arrived on Australian shores by boat and have been detained in Australian immigration detention centres. Following the determination of their refugee status they were released into the community and granted Temporary Protection Visas (TPVs) for three years only.

TPV holders are entitled to basic financial support and Medicare benefits; however they are not able to apply to bring their immediate family to Australia under the family reunion scheme. They are able to work but do not benefit from free English classes, nor do they have access to settlement services or Job Network

Intensive Employment Assistance. (The Acting Federal Race Discrimination Commissioner, 2001). TPV holders from Afghanistan are predominately Hazara men who arrived in Australia on their own without their families. They mostly live in shared accommodation with 3–4 other men which they have found themselves in the private housing market. They share the cost and have a roster in home chores such as cooking, cleaning and shopping. Their excellent financial management skills enable some of them to save money and start small businesses such as Afghan bakeries, grocery stores, Halal butcheries and take away shops.

According to Centrelink statistics (January 2003) around 4000 Afghans were granted TPVs, and to date, the majority have now been granted permanent residence.

In Australia, the cycle of trauma and discrimination is repeated through their experiences. The attitudes of Australians are increasingly polarized about asylum seekers. Whereas some are sympathetic, racism towards Afghans has increased since the terrorist attacks on New York and Washington in 2001 (Mehraby, 2001b, 2002a, 2002b, 2002c, 2007a)

Impact of International and National Events

The global terrorist crisis resulting in the US bombardment of Afghanistan has had a significant impact on Afghan refugees in Australia. Many have been retraumatised, for example, experiencing symptoms of grief, loss, trauma, anxiety, depression, anger, and survivor guilt. Concern about family members in Afghanistan and neighbouring countries, as well as pressure to provide financial support to them, are additional sources of stress (Mehraby, 2002a).

This has become further complicated through the association of terrorism with the words *Islam* and *Muslim*. It has become common to hear reports of stigmatisation, fear, rejection, harassment and discrimination, which have been shown to them by members of the wider society in Australia. Afghans on temporary visas are far more vulnerable in this situation because of their visa class and lack of security and support (Mehraby, 2001b, 2002a, 2002b, 2002c, 2003a, 2003d, 2007a; Mehraby & Coello, 2005).

Events such as the September 11 attacks on New York and Washington, the war in Afghanistan, the War in Iraq, the War on Terror and terrorist attacks in London all contribute to a sense of lack of safety and belonging for Afghan people. Events closer to Australia have included the Tampa crisis (when a large boat load of Middle Eastern Muslim asylum seekers was sent to a Pacific Island rather than being permitted to anchor in Australia) the Bali bombing terrorist attacks which killed and injured many people including many Australians, and the sinking of boats leaving Indonesia and carrying asylum seekers. More recently, the Cronulla riots in Sydney in December 2005 have continued this feeling of insecurity, when large gangs of non – Muslims and Muslims attacked innocent people belonging to each other's community and vandalized property. All these events affect the psychological health and employment opportunities for refugees from Afghanistan.

Thinking About Afghan and Australian Culture

Australian Culture

The host culture of Australia is a diverse multi-cultural one. However, the dominant culture in the media, government and most institutions is still the one derived
from the Anglo-Saxon/Celtic Australian culture which has been developing over
the last two hundred years since the White settlement of Aboriginal Australia in
the late eighteenth century.

The stereotype of Western culture is that of individualism. People tend to
take an active position and see themselves as being in control of their lives, and
the language reflects this. There is a fair degree of tolerance of differences
(broadly speaking). People are free to choose their own marriage partners, and
divorce and remarriage are common. Some couples live together without being
married. While some extended families are closely knit, others are less so.
There is a high proportion of single parent families and people living on their
own. There tends to be a relatively high level of tolerance for practices of
different religious beliefs within the Christian tradition, and outside of it. There
is, in general, a non-judgemental attitude towards sexual identity, for example
the Sydney Mardi Gras parade (a celebration for freedom for gay people) is
held annually. People tend to make eye contact when they speak to another person, and there aren't generally very strict traditional codes of behaviour, speech
and dress.

The history of the subjugation and near genocide of many tribes of indigenous people in Australia has now become part of the education curriculum and
is more openly discussed by the broader community. Since the introduction of
scholarships and financial assistance for indigenous people, they have had a
higher level of participation in public and professional life, and in the arts. The
image of the large aboriginal elder holding the hand of a small white child in the
opening ceremony of the Olympic Games in Sydney recently (in 2000) is a
kindly way of depicting the length of time of the two races in Australian history.
Unfortunately this symbol white-washes over the shameful aspects of the history. One hopes this could grow to be a more accurate representation of the
relationship for the future.

There has been a tradition dating from the convict settlements around the
country, (many of the convicts were of Irish, Scottish or British working class
origin) to distrust the authorities and to ridicule high achievers ('the tall poppy
syndrome'). There is a strong belief in equality and mateship. In this sense there
is still quite a collective emphasis in the culture.

Most Australian families have a quiet history of migration and struggle,
either in the current generation or in the past. For those whose family members
have been in the country for several generations, there is a pride in the sacrifice of their ancestors in the world wars in the past. The earliest wave of
migrants to arrive from non-English speaking societies was the people of
Chinese ethnicity who started to arrive in the mid nineteenth century during

the gold rushes in Australia. However, it was after World War II that many groups of immigrants arrived, and since then the population has become far more diverse.

The place of women in Australian society has undergone dramatic changes since the Women's Movement in the 1970s. There is now a greater proportion of women in higher education institutions, and in public and professional life in general. Gender roles have become far less prescribed, at least overtly, and there is far more flexibility in families about sharing roles, such as work outside the home, childcare, shopping and housework. Hugh Mackay (2004) recently quoted the average number of children in an Australian family as being between one and two per nuclear family.

The stereotype of Anglo-Australian communication is that of a laconic, humble person whose actions speak louder than words. This is a culture of mainly urban people who are only removed from country life by one or two generations, and who still have the traces of rural community in their style. The hundreds of friendly, down-to-earth volunteers at the 2000 Olympic Games in Sydney are a good example of this image of an Australian. Less palatable aspects of communication include the bitter racist comments on talk-back radio and the violent behaviour of groups of racist youths in the recent riots.

Afghan Culture

Afghanistan (Aryana) is land-locked mountainous country located in the heart of Asia. It has a 5,000-year-old history and culture. The exact population of Afghanistan is unknown but it is estimated to be around 21–26 million (www.afghan.com) The modern boundaries of Afghanistan were determined by the interests of foreign powers. Afghanistan's geographical location is at the cross-roads of the east and west. This country is on the trade link between Europe and Indian Ocean. It has attracted the interest of superpowers such as Aryan nomads, Mede, Persian Empires, Greeks, Arabs, Turks and Mongols.

Waves of migration and invasion have brought different ethnic groups to Afghanistan. Hence, Afghanistan has never been inhabited by only one ethnic group. It is a multi ethnic nation with four major groups, Pasthuns (38%), Tajiks (21%), Hazara (19%) and Uzbeks (6%). Afghanistan is a predominately Islamic country (99%) with 85% Sunni and 15% Shiite Muslim. There are also a small percentage of Sikh, Hindu and Jewish people. There are two official languages in Afghanistan, Pasthu and Dari, although, most Afghans are bilingual. Hazargi, Uzbeki and Turkmeni are minority-spoken languages.

Afghan culture is composed of tradition, religion, tribal relics of war, language, romance and magic (Robson et al. 2003). People's loyalties are first to their local leaders, their tribes and to their ethnic identification. This prevents the structure of one solid Afghan nation from forming. In addition, the tool of 'divide and rule' has been utilised by rulers throughout history resulting in mistrust and conflicts between different factions. Despite differences in culture between ethnic groups, the people share common fundamental values. Some of the remarkable qualities of Afghans are their toughness, resilience, patriotism and hospitality, which have been proven through history.

The core system of Afghan culture is characterised by a hierarchical system of intimate relationships within the extended family. There are certain role expectations, strong family ties, and each individual is expected to obey his/her role. The concept of self is collective. The older children, especially boys, are expected to be the 'walking stick' of their parents and take the primary caregiver role when their parents need them On the other hand parents are responsible to ensure that their children are nourished in soul and body so they can fulfil this role. Even when a child becomes an adult, his/her wellbeing is the responsibility of the parents (Mehraby, 2004).

Contrary to some western ideas that women in the east are passive and subservient, women play an active role in this hierarchical system. Afghans give a high value to their mothers, as reflected in the poetry and literature. Afghans usually follow the saying of the prophet Mohammad that '*Heaven lies under the feet of the mother*'. Women have had an active role in all the wars against the invaders through Afghan history. These cultural values and traditions provide women with security and safety. However, it is difficult for them to depart from this traditional identity and become more independent.

There is an emphasis on keeping the family together, resulting in a low rate of divorce amongst Afghans, although the rate of divorce has increased significantly amongst Afghans resettling in Western countries. As it is forbidden in Islam, defacto relationships and homosexuality are not accepted in Afghan culture. The social classes in Afghanistan are based on level of education, family background, wealth and ethnic groups.

In Afghanistan, older family members mainly conduct the counselling. This usually includes advice and direction giving, emotional and financial support and other types of material assistance to the younger members. The problems are kept within the family and are rarely discussed with non-family members or with 'outsiders' (Mehraby, 2002a).

The Pasthuns comprise the largest ethnic group. They have ruled Afghanistan since 1747. They are believed to be the descendants of Afghana, the grandson of King Saul. The Pasthuns are Sunni Muslims, but their cultural values have influenced their Islamic practices and they have many non-religious cultural traditions. They have a rich oral literature and value poetry. Pasthuns are fierce fighters who have actively participated in the wars against invaders through history. Pasthuns' cultural values are highlighted in a code of ethics called 'Pasthunwalia' by which Pasthuns are required to live (see Robson & Lipson, 2003, for a detailed explanation). Pasthuns are known for their strengths: patriotism, bravery, hospitality, honesty and friendship.

The Tajiks are the second largest ethnic group, believed to be the original Persian population of Afghanistan, Tajikistan and Uzbekistan. They speak Dari and the majority of them are Sunni Muslims but there are also some Tajik Shiite Muslims. Tajiks mostly live in the northern region, and in the capital city of

Afghanistan, Kabul. They often identify themselves by their particular valley. Tajiks are mainly urban people with a heritage of rich literature. They are known for their civility, warmth and politeness. They are generally strong in their faith and are devoted Muslims.

The Hazaras are the Hazaragi speaking group largely located in the central remote area of Afghanistan called Hazaristan, and in the capital city of Afghanistan. There is a general view that Hazaras are the Mongol descendants of Changhis Khan's soldiers. The word Hazara refers to 'a thousand', and refers to when Changhis Khan left a thousand of his troops in Afghanistan after the Mongols had conquered the country. The Mongoli appearance of the Hazaras differentiates them from other Afghans. The Hazaras are proud, hard working people and they are accustomed to hardship and poverty. They are known for their hard work, loyalty and good manners. The Hazaras in Afghanistan have suffered from long-standing discrimination, racism and violation of their human rights by other ethnic groups. Figures from a Human Rights Watch report of August 1998, which described a massacre of 2000–3000 Hazaras in the city of Mazar-I-Sharif and elsewhere, show that they also suffered enormously under the Pashtun dominated Taliban regime (Hazara.net). They come from the working class and the majority of them are illiterate. They were often forced into manual, serving and construction jobs. Their contribution to the construction of Afghanistan is priceless. They were not accepted into the broader Afghan community, and in Australia other Afghan ethnic groups may still reject them (Mehraby, 2002c).

Amongst Afghan people today (and in the past) there have been, and still are, many mixed marriages between people from different ethnic backgrounds. This has led to a mixing of the different cultures and more understanding between them. However, it becomes particularly stressful for people in mixed marriages, when the different ethnic groups are in conflict.

Thinking About Culture and Politics in the Work with Mr Hussani.

Mr Hussani's Identity

Mr Hussani had grown up in an extended family situation, and had taken on the role of head of the family while still a young teenager, following the murder of his father and his elder brother. In Australia, he suffered greatly from feeling that he had let his family down, and failed in his role as head of the family.

He still displayed many characteristics of having a collective self. For example, he had an indirect style of relating to others, and was respectful towards senior people for example his mother and the therapist. His priorities were towards the welfare of his family and fulfilling his duty as the head of the family, rather than his own self-development and personal welfare. He began to recover when he was fulfilling his responsibilities towards his family and began helping others in the community.

Mr. Hussani said that praying helped him a lot. He said that what had happened to him had come from God, and if it was God's will, it would be solved. He said that he felt relieved from praying. Although at one stage he fell into such despair that he lost his faith, he managed to regain it again and this was one of the central pillars which had held him through all the losses and stresses, which he had survived. However, he said that he didn't go to the mosque because he didn't want to be labelled as a terrorist.

His identity as a Hazara on a temporary visa was central to his self concept. He said, '*As a Hazara, I never feel that I am above anybody. I am sick, powerless and helpless . . .*' At the same time he missed the collective activities of being in a family and in the Hazara community . . .'*I miss those moments when I was coming back from work and my wife and children were valuing me. My clothes were washed and my food was cooked. I miss the call to Prayer in the evening and going to the Mosque and praying. I miss the breakfast during the fast month and having dinner with the family.*' (Mr. Hussani was almost in tears while disclosing this.)

Most of his distress was expressed in terms of his relationships with others, and how he was missing them.

Mr Hussani could be defined as having a collective self in transition. When he was referred to STARTTS, he felt completely lost, almost as if a crucial part of him was missing, without having his immediate and extended family close by. His collective sense of self at that time was disintegrating. We are using Marsella's (1985) notion of non-Western people having a self which includes a wide variety of significant others. Roland's work (1988) which uses the idea of the 'expanding self' – for people who are living in a new culture – and the 'spiritual self', is also relevant for understanding the self of Mr Hussani.

Cultural and Religious Ideas About Mr Hussani's Health and Recovery

Mr Hussani frequently used the idiom 'burning' to describe his feelings, which is commonly used in Afghanistan. The only illness category he used was that he was afraid he was going mad ('dawana'). In his culture people who are mentally ill are considered crazy or possessed by Janes (Djinns). There is no concept of psychological problems in Afghan culture; people are either mad or healthy. Sufferers of mental illness are often cared for and looked after at home by their families rather than being sent to mental institutions. Not having his family around him exacerbated his fear of madness and of being left alone in case anything went wrong. He said that he was afraid to tell anyone about how he was feeling because others would think he was mad.

He also expressed psychological distress through somatic complaints such as headaches, backache, stomachache and general body tension. This is an acceptable way of expressing distress in many non-western cultures where psychological problems are stigmatising, and sufferers risk being labeled 'mad' (Mehraby, 2002a, 2001a).

He was a religious person who interpreted life events as being according to the will of God. He wondered whether all the things, which had happened to him, were punishment from or a test from God. He also looked to religion for healing, and had participated in praying in the mosque and reciting the Qur'an with others to sustain himself.

Mr Hussani came from a remote area where access to medical help was extremely limited. He said that if someone was mentally ill in his village, the family would look after him. Treatments were provided by respected religious leaders in the community. *"They will pray for him. They will talk to the Imam or Sheikh to pray for him. The Imam or Sheikh might write verses from the Qur'an with saffron on a piece of paper. They would then soak the paper in water, and give the sick person the water. They might also write verses of the Qur'an on a piece of paper, fold it and cover it with different layers and pin it on the sick person's clothes or give it to him/her to wear around the neck. They might also take the sick person to spiritual people's graves and pray for him/her. They will try to give the person good food, such as almonds and nuts.'*

This traditional religious healing does have some parallels with western therapy as it has elements of a trusting relationship with a healer, and some recognition and holding of suffering and feelings in the rituals. The relationship is nurturing (e.g. giving almonds) and also links the persons with their spirituality and relationship to good internal figures (e.g. holy people who have died).

Mehraby (2002a, 2003a, 2003b, 2005b, 2007a, 2007b) described how Islamic rituals and beliefs are healing for people who practice them. Understanding and exploring those beliefs can be valuable for the treatment of Muslim clients who are experiencing depression, anxiety, stress, loss and grief, and posttraumatic stress symptoms. For example, in accepting grief and loss, the relatives of the deceased are urged to be patient (*sabr*) and accept God's decree. *"Be sure we shall test you with something of fear and hunger, some loss in goods, lives and the fruits of your toil, but give glad tiding to those who patiently persevere. Who say, when afflicted with calamity: To Allah we belong, and to Him is our return"* (Qur'an: 2:155). People who have patience in accepting God's decree will be given a reward from Him. *"[And thus it is with most men-] save those who are patient in adversity and do righteous deeds: it is they whom forgiveness of sins awaits, and a great reward"* (Qur'an 11:11).

The use of religious parables, the life story of the Prophet Mohammad and *Surahs* from the Qur'an and Hadith (sayings and customs of the prophet Mohammad) can all be therapeutic. For instance, some clients benefit from reciting the Qur'an when they are frightened, or from listening to the Qur'an to acquire body relaxation. Prayer is also a time to remember God, thank Him and ask for forgiveness. It also gives some exercise to the whole body and is a source of meditation and a combination of relaxation and physiotherapy. *"He guides to Himself those who turn to Him in penitence, those who believe and whose heart has rest in the remembrance of Allah (Qur'an 13:27–28).*

This enables the person to accept the self and the pain because one is not in isolated existence but part of a total wholeness in relation to God. In life situations when nothing can be done except observing patience, trust in God can reduce feelings of excessive responsibility and lead to the creation of constructive methods to deal with, and perhaps overcome, the situation. According to Islamic beliefs, only God knows the ultimate destiny. The Muslim therefore feels reassured that trust is well placed and that God will not forsake him or her (Mehraby, 2007a, 2005b).

Group prayer, especially Friday congregational prayer, contributes to a sense of identity and belongingness. Both group prayer and fasting have substantial social elements that give Muslims a sense of identification with others as well as social support.

In many Islamic cultures, religion plays a significant role in every day practice. Religious beliefs change over time in an individual, and become more critical at different stages of the life cycle. It is therefore difficult to practice psychotherapy without considering culture and religion.

Thinking About Culture in the Psychotherapy Relationship

Developing Trust Between a Pashtun Sunni Therapist and a Hazara Shiite Client

For the therapist, developing trust with a Hazara client was challenging. She felt moments of intense guilt when Mr Hussani spoke of his suffering and pain at the hands of the Pasthun people, and the murders of his brothers and cousins. As their relationship developed, she encouraged him to express his feelings about having a Pasthun Sunni therapist. He never expressed any negative thoughts about Pasthuns and Sunni people. He said *'We are all Afghans, not all Pasthuns are bad.'* He said that his therapist was the person who most understood him – and otherwise he mostly had help from non-Afghans. He said that *'In our culture we have a saying that only those people will burn who are in the fire* (meaning people only understand each other when they are in the same situation) *– but I don't expect anyone to do anything more for me.'*

The therapist was thinking that his positive feelings towards her could be seen as idealizing her. However, Mr. Hussani's attitude could also be understood as being influenced by cultural attitudes of negative feelings not being expressed to respected people. It could also be a fear of another loss, which could happen if something negative was expressed. However, he genuinely had a positive attachment to the therapist, and had the capacity to be open to a new experience of being cared for by a Pasthun person.

Sense of Self and Merging in the Therapeutic Relationship

As described above, the therapist and Mr Hussani used the term 'we Afghans' to describe common feelings and tended to join together in a collective sense within the therapeutic relationship. This idea of merging between collective selves in a psychotherapy relationship is discussed by Bowles (1993).

Bowles (1993) describes how within the relationship where there is a strong sense of 'togetherness' and collective identity, this identity coexists with the individual one. This is more evident when there is a third party in the therapy group such as an interpreter or a bicultural cotherapist. This sense of closeness has a different, elusive quality: the sense of group identity becomes dominant, and anxiety tends to diminish, as all three people feel they belong to the unit. There is a heightened sense of awareness of others and concern for others as part of the unit which includes yourself.

This kind of relationship is not viewed as pathological, or as inferior to the closeness experienced by more individualistic people, but arises out of a different culture, and different sense of self. The challenge for the parties involved in this kind of therapeutic relationship is to keep an individual thinking space going, and at the same time allowing oneself to feel and think about the developing collective unit. All parties in the group have their own internal meanings about this group identity, and this can be thought about as well.

Expression and working through of negative feelings in this kind of relationship is possible and may occur in some cases on a subtle level, both verbal and non-verbal. An issue which arises here is to what degree does an issue need to be discussed verbally in order for it to be resolved.

Gender Roles and Expression of Feelings

It was difficult for Mr Hussani to talk about his problems and to show any emotion, especially at first. Culturally, in Afghanistan, men are expected to be stoic, and expression of emotion is generally inappropriate for them. Men should be strong enough to tolerate suffering without crying; it is generally considered shameful for men to express emotion in front of a woman. On the other hand, the mother is the dominant caring figure in Afghan society, so identifying the therapist as a maternal figure probably encouraged Mr Hussani to express his feelings.

Mr.Hussani initially kept minimal eye contact with the therapist. This could be related to his low self-esteem or depression. It could also be related to his Islamic beliefs that direct eye contact with the opposite gender is considered sinful, and cultural mores that lower class people should be respectful to those in authority (Mehraby, 2005c). Islam values knowledge and this encourages respect of educated people.

However, as the therapy progressed, Mr. Hussani was gradually able to cry in a number of sessions, expressing feelings about his situation and multiple losses, and he was able to maintain direct eye contact.

In one session, which occurred towards the end of his treatment before he travelled to see his family, he expressed his ideas about seeking help from a woman:

'I am not sure (whether he would prefer male or female). I don't want to go to a female doctor; it's embarrassing to talk about some of the issues. But I think with emotional issues it's better to talk to a female. I feel embarrassed to show my weakness to another man.'

Class and Education Differences

The therapist said that she was very aware of the power difference between herself and Mr Hussani in terms of her education in Afghanistan and in Australia, her financial position and social class background, both in Afghanistan and in Australia compared with his. She said that she sometimes tried to deny – or overcome – the differences by being humble and modest when she was with him.

However, when he was asked about the issue of having to follow advice, Mr Hussani very plainly said that as a Hazara he never felt above anybody, and that he felt that his therapist knew better than he did. He felt he should follow her advice. He quite openly accepted the power difference, although he did not really express his feelings about

Countertransference Issues

The therapist said that she was able to identify with many aspects of her client's story as she herself was from Afghanistan, and had her own refugee experiences. She was also affected by the ongoing national and international events, as was her client. There were moments of traumatic and painful countertransferences, which the therapist discussed in the supervision. This external process helped to maintain the therapist in her role with Mr Hussani despite her own suffering.

Working with Negative Feelings Towards the Therapist and Working with the Trauma

These aspects of the process were difficult to deal with in the treatment of Mr Hussani.

Many therapists who work with refugees document being able to successfully work through trauma and losses, and to allow the patient to work through the issues of persecution and hatred in the therapeutic relationship. Lemma (2004) describes how there is an attempt to avoid psychic pain associated with loss, and to avoid destructive impulses, which become aroused in the self in response to the trauma. In her view it is critical to work with these negative feelings in the therapeutic relationship order for the client to recover. She also describes how there is a tendency in refugee work to act rather than to sit with the pain of the patient.

Mr Hussani was in a precarious external situation, living in poverty and being extremely anxious about life and death issues in reality for himself and his family. His concern was to survive and save his family. He said that he could not bear to think too much about his family, as he became far too distressed and anxious. The therapist did act on his behalf (writing the report for immigration and contacting the Red Cross) – however, as far as possible she tried to think about his feelings and mental state as well. In addition, Mr Hussani was relying on the therapist for survival in a real sense at the time; it was not his priority to process the trauma nor to examine his negative feelings about the therapist.

A thinking space was created in the supervision where the pain of Mr Hussani's experience could be survived and faced, so that a similar space could be created for him in the therapy. (Becker & Bowles, 2001c) While he did not process much of the trauma, he did express some of the agony of the separation from his family and the loss of his son and his mother. This perhaps was something significant, given his situation and also that counselling was such a new concept for him.

Lemma (2004) writes that while we are all wary of idealization, interpreting the defensive aspects of it prematurely may cut off a lifeline to a person whose hope is very precarious. Melanie Klein, as cited in Lemma (2004), pointed out that longing for a good object to love is a condition for life. The need for a good object is universal. The distinction between an idealized and a good object cannot be considered as absolute.

The Cultural Dimension in Internal Relationships

We are now tentatively entering further into the cross-disciplinary world of anthropology and psychoanalysis. While we are aware that there are cultural dimensions in psychoanalytic theories, (as there are in any theory) we have found that many of the psychoanalytical concepts are useful in our clinical work with refugees from non-western cultures (Bowles, 1993).

Lemma and Levy (2004) discuss how traumatic events have personal meanings for survivors, which reflect aspects of how the person engages with the world. These responses tell us something about the nature of people's inner worlds and the quality of their attachments. A trauma is taken inside the mind and processed in a way that makes the experience specific to that individual. People's experience of trauma is idiosyncratic. A trauma is experienced through the person's particular internal object representations. These are felt to be real, but can be understood as maps or images which are formed as the individual develops and interacts with their external world. These internalised configurations become the lenses through which trauma is experienced. (Becker, 2006)

Lemma and Levy (2004) write that there is a dialectical process between the person's inner world, and their social and cultural background. External relationships and other structures, such as family, home, and work, can offer alternative realities to the pain and suffering within the person. Similarly, the nature and quality of a person's internal resources will deeply affect how they perceive and respond to external life events.

Mr Hussani had very few sustaining external structures to support him. However, his internal resources must have been strong enough for him to survive. Although, we know little about Mr Hussani's early childhood, we hypothesise that he had a strong attachment to his mother or major caregiver/s. He was able to bond so positively to the therapist despite major cultural obstacles which could hinder developing trust. He had the capacity, despite his trauma history and current situation, to look beyond stereotypes and see the good in the therapist, and to some extent to hold the good and bad about his situation together in his mind

It is interesting to think about the cultural aspects of our internal relationships and how they affect our external ones (and vice versa). Cultural and political factors affect our early childhoods and the quality of our relationships – for example growing up in an extended family in a village under attack from another ethnic group must influence the quality of internal relationships in people. For example, for many people from close extended families, their internal relationships must have a collective, merging flavour.

The therapist has had close, positive associations with Hazara people during her early childhood, and was struck by their hard work and endurance, and by the injustices which they had suffered. It is generally believed that the Hazaras are known for their loyalty to people who accept and appreciate them. These internalized relationships from the therapist's early life probably infused her attitude to Mr Hussani.

Cultural Issues in the Supervision Relationship

Many of the processes in the therapy were mirrored in the supervisory relationship, as well as many of the cultural issues.

The therapist and supervisor are from different cultures. They differ in ethnicity and religion: the supervisor is anglo-saxon and is from a Christian family background. Both have grown up in very different circumstances.

The supervisor felt ashamed (being from the mainstream society) about racist behaviour and comments towards innocent Muslim people, and about first world countries' imperialism in Asia in general. At the same time, the therapist felt ashamed, through association, about the terrorist attacks on innocent western civilians in the name of Islam. However, as they had been working very closely together for many years prior to this current political situation arising, the trust and respect in their working relationship had already been established and overcame these tensions.

In their own personal experiences the therapist and the supervisor had much in common. The supervisor has had a positive experience of living in a predominantly Asian Muslim country, and the therapist has had positive experiences with many western Christian people. Probably they both have incorporated aspects of eastern and western, collective and individual, senses of self, and both are women. They have also worked at the same agency together for many years, and shared that common culture and commitment to Human Rights.

Concluding Remarks

Cultural dimensions, including religious and political factors, were of primary importance in working with Mr Hussani, both in understanding what was of primary concern to him, and in the therapeutic and advocacy work with him.

Although he had suffered from severe trauma and losses as a teenager, he barely mentioned these. His concern was with immediate survival (gaining a permanent visa) and with trying to rescue his family once he discovered that some of them were still alive.

His symptoms were consistent with symptoms of grief, anxiety (PTSD) and depression, although he described them as 'burning in his heart' and understood them as part of God's will. If it was God's will, he would recover and find his family again.

Most of his distress was expressed in terms of lost relationships with other people and his lost world with his family and his Hazara village. He was in agony because he felt he was a failure as a husband and father and had failed to protect and care for his family. Much of his suffering and 'frozen rage' were due to loss of face with others in his current life because he was still on a temporary visa. He suffered also from anxiety about being returned to a situation where his life was in danger and where all his brothers and some cousins had been murdered. He was becoming more and more isolated when he had been referred to STARTTS, and had lost his hope in God as well.

The way that he was able to attach to the therapist, despite her being from the Pasthun ethnicity, (members of which had murdered his brothers), was of critical importance for his survival. The authors hypothesise that Mr Hussani had strong internal attachment figures and relationships, and a capacity to hold good and bad together, which helped him to bond with and trust his therapist. Gradually, from this relationship, he began to trust others again, to manage to link with his community and survive until he gained his permanent residence and went back to Pakistan to reunite with his family. The therapist also assisted in crucial practical matters, like writing a report supporting his application for permanent residence.

There were interesting cultural dimensions in both the therapeutic and supervisory relationships in this case study. These include differences in ethnicity, gender, class, and religion, and cultural aspects of the internal less conscious worlds of the client, clinician and supervisor. There was an interesting collective experience in the relationship, a sense of merging and orientation to the group. These cultural aspects emerged and developed in the relationships between Mr Hussani, the therapist and the supervisor.

Having three languages (at least) in the minds of the therapist, client and supervisor also added a complex dimension to the process. This meant that there were subtle shifts in meaning in the translations, which would be interesting to examine more closely. The cultural nuances in the languages give a different colour to the feelings, the relationships and the experiences. Although, the therapist and the client both spoke in Dari language, this was not a mother tongue for either of them.

Mr Hussani did not process his past trauma in much detail, nor did he express directly negative feelings towards the therapist; however, he did work through some feelings regarding the losses and separations, and the injustices in his life. This was of note, because of the cultural inhibitions on men expressing 'weak' feelings, especially to women, and because the therapy process in its western construction was a new idea for him. Mr Hussani was so overwhelmed that the therapist felt that pushing him to explore more deeply would traumatize him further, while he was in a situation of ongoing external insecurity.

This psychotherapy was a form of 'reconciliation' for Mr Hussani and the therapist, and in a different sense for the therapist and the supervisor; it was the forming of healing bonds between people whose communities are at war. It was the beginning of a restoring of Mr Hussani's family and social identity, his collective self, as well as the genesis of restoring his spiritual and individual selves.

The authors wish to thank Jorge Aroche, Rise Becker, Marc Chaussivert, Mariano Coello, Peter Davis, Fatana Rahimi and Julie Savage for their comments and proof reading.

We also wish to acknowledge Mr Zalmai Haidary, the first worker from Afghanistan at STARTTS, and from whose article title 'Living in Limbo' we have created our title.

References

Acting Federal Race Discrimination Commissioner. (2001). *Face the Facts: Some Questions and Answers About Immigration, Refugees and Indigenous Affairs*. Sydney: AGPS.

American Psychiatric Association (APA). (1996) *Diagnostic and Statistical Manual of Mental Disorder* (DSM-IV) (4th ed.) (pp. 424–429). Washington DC: American psychiatric Association.

Aroche, J., & Coello, M. J. (1994, December). *Toward a systemic approach for the treatment and rehabilitation of torture and trauma survivors in exile: the experience of STARTTS in Australia*. Paper presented at the fourth International Conference of Centres, Institutions and Individuals Concerned with Victims of Organised Violence, Caring for and Empowering Victims of Human Rights Violations, Dap Tagetay City, Philippines.

Aroche, J., & Coello, M. J. (2004). Ethnocultural considerations in the treatment of refugees and asylum seekers. In J. P. Wilson & B. Drožđek (Eds.), *Broken Spirits: The Treatment of Traumatised Asylum Seekers, Refugees, War and Torture Victims* (pp 53–80). New York: Brunner-Routledge.

Becker, R. N. (1991, August). *Refugees in search of a home*. Paper presented at the Conference Trauma and Its Wake, Sydney.

Becker, R. N. (2006, March). *Phenomenology of trauma*. Seminar given to Clinical Supervisor Training, Service for the Treatment and Rehabilitation of Torture and Trauma Survivors, (STARTTS), Sydney.

Becker, R. N., & Bowles, R. A. (2001a). Interpreters' experience of working in a triadic psychotherapy relationship with survivors of torture and trauma: some thoughts on the impact on psychotherapy. In B. Raphael & A. Malak (Eds.), *Diversity and Mental Health in Challenging Times* (pp. 222–230). Sydney: Transcultural Mental Health Unit.

Becker, R. N., & Bowles, R. A. (2001b, May). *The experience and role of the clinical supervisor in work with torture and trauma survivors: managing deep projections and an unbearable reality*. Paper presented at the international conference, Diversity in Health: Sharing Global Perspectives, Australian Transcultural Mental Health Network, Sydney

Becker, R., & Bowles, R. (2001c, May). *When three's a crowd. Ethical considerations in the practice of psychotherapy with traumatised refugees when working with an interpreter*. Paper presented at the international conference, Diversity in Health: Sharing Global Perspectives, Australian Transcultural Mental Health Network, Sydney.

Becker, R. N., & Bowles, R. A. (2004). Stuck in the middle. Debriefing for interpreters. *Refugee Transitions, 15*, 40–42.

Becker, R., Haidary, Z., Kang, V., Marin, L., Nguyen, T., Phraxayavong, V., et al. (1990). The two-practitioner model – bicultural workers in a service for torture and trauma survivors. In P. Hosking (Ed.), *Hope After Horror* (pp. 138–156). Sydney: UNIYA.

Bowles, R. A. (1993). *Culture, self and the analytic relationship: the relevance of some Kleinian ideas for working with survivors of torture and trauma.* Unpublished Masters Degree thesis. Sydney: UNSW.

Bowles, R. A. (1998, June). *Sexual assault and torture: some thoughts about clinical work with refugees who are sexual assault survivors.* Paper presented at the conference of the NSW Sexual Assault Forum, No More Falling Through the Net, Sydney.

Bowles, R. A. (2005). Social work with refugee survivors of torture and trauma. In M. Alston & J. MacKinnon (Eds.), *Social Work Fields of Practice* (2nd ed.) (pp. 249–267). Melbourne: Oxford University Press.

Bowles, R. A. (2006). Supervising bicultural counsellors in their work with traumatised refugees. *Psychotherapy in Australia, 3*, 17–18.

Bowles, R. A., & Haidary, Z. (1994, December). *Family therapy with survivors of torture and trauma: issues for women in an Afghan case Study.* Paper presented at the fourth International Conference of Centres, Institutions and Individuals concerned with Victims of Organised Violence, Caring for and Empowering Victims of Human Rights Violations, Dap Tageytay City, Philippines.

Bowles, R. A., Haidary, Z., & Becker, R. N. (1995, October). *Family therapy with survivors of torture and trauma: issues for women in an Afghan case study.* Paper presented at the third National Women's Health Conference, ANU, Canberra.

Bowles, R. A., Salem, M., & Preston-Thomas, C. (2004, October). *Working with refugees. A resource developed for social workers.* Paper presented at the International Social Work Conference 2004, Global Social Work Congress, Adelaide.

Cunningham, M., & Silove, D. (1993). Principles of treatment and service development for torture and trauma survivors. In J. P. Wilson & B. Raphael (Eds.), *The International Handbook of Traumatic Stress Syndromes* (pp. 751–762). New York: Plenum Press.

Fernandes, P. (2003) 'Burning in the fire'-the continuing saga: An analysis of group work with Temporary Protection Visa Holders in NSW. In D. Barnes (Ed.), *Asylum Seekers & Refugees in Australia: Issues of mental health and wellbeing* (pp. 55–79). Parramatta: TMHC.

Haidary, Z. (2000). *Living in Limbo.* Mimeographed, Sydney: STARTTS.

Hazara Online, www. hazaraonline.

Hazara.net

Herman, J. L. (1992). *Trauma and Recovery.* New York: Harper Collins.

Lemma, A. (2004). On hope's tightrope: reflections on the capacity for hope. In S. Levy, & A. Lemma (Eds.), *The Perversion of Loss: Psychoanalytic Perspectives on Trauma* (pp. 108–126). London: Brunner-Routledge.

Lemma, A., & Levy, S. (2004). The impact of trauma on the psyche: internal and external processes. In S. Levy & A. Lemma (Eds.), The *Perversion of Loss: Psychoanalytic Perspectives on Trauma* (pp. 1–20). London: Brunner-Routledge.

Mackay, H. (2004, May). *Keynote Address.* Paper presented at Social Justice Expo, Uniting Church of Australia, Sydney, Australia.

Marsella, A., Devos, G., & Hsu, F. (Eds.). (1985). *Culture and Self: Asian and Western Perspectives.* New York and London: Tavistock Publications.

Mehraby, N. (1999a). *Re-visiting a harsh place in transitions* (pp. 13–14). Sydney: STARTTS.

Mehraby, N. (1999b). *Therapy with refugee children. The Child Psychoanalytic Gazette, 1999,* 45–66.

Mehraby, N. (2001a). Refugee women: the authentic heroines. *Transitions, 9*, 18–22.

Mehraby, N. (2001b, December). *The forgotten voice of Afghan refugees.* Paper presented at the International Conference of The Refugee Convention – where to from here?" 50th Anniversary of UN Convention, Sydney.

Mehraby, N. (2002a). Counselling Afghan torture and trauma survivors. *Psychotherapy in Australia, 3*, 12–18.

Mehraby, N. (2002b). Healing the Body, healing the soul. In W. Dal Bosco (Ed.), *Tales from a suitcase: the Afghan experience,* Thomas C. Lothian, South Melbourne, (pp. 148–166). Melbourne: Psychoz.

Mehraby, N. (2002c). Unaccompanied child refugees: a group experience. *Psychotherapy in Australia, 4*, 30–36.

Mehraby, N. (2003a). Psychotherapy with Islamic clients facing loss and grief. *Psychotherapy in Australia, 2*, 30–34.

Mehraby, N. (2003b, June). *Suicide in Islam.* Paper presented at 10th Annual National Conference on Suicide Prevention, Brisbane, Australia.

Mehraby, N. (2003c, October). *Islamic Beliefs in Healing of Loss and Grief.* Paper presented at the Diversity in Health National Conference, Sydney, Australia.

Mehraby, N. (2003d). September 11 and Re-traumatisation. *Psychotherapy in Australia, 1*, 65.

Mehraby, N. (2004). The concept of self in different cultures. *Psychotherapy in Australia, 24*, 47.

Mehraby, N. (2005a, February) *The effect of 11th of September 2001 and its aftermath on the traumatized refugees from the Middle East: Re-traumatisation of a vulnerable group of clients.* Paper presented at 7th International conference on Human Rights and Health, Vadodara, India.

Mehraby, N. (2005b). Suicide its pathway, perception and prevention amongst Muslims. *Psychotherapy in Australia, 2*, 60–65.

Mehraby, N. (2005c). Body language in different cultures. *Psychotherapy in Australia, 24*, 27–28.

Mehraby, N. (2007a). Isolation versus integration: the impact of 'war on terror' on Muslim refugees resettling in western societies. *Transitions, 18*, 14–17.

Mehraby, N. (2007b). Loss and death in Islam. In G. Bozan, McMahon & Wilcox (Eds.), Spirited Practice. Sydney: Allen & Unwin.

Mehraby, N., & Coello, M. (2005, February) *A Systemic framework for working with Muslim Refugee Communities Re-settling in Western Countries.* Pre-conference training presented at 7th International conference on Human Rights and Health, Vadodara, India.

Morris, P., Silove, D., Manicavasagar, V., Bowles, R. A., Cunningham, M., & Tarn, R. (1993). Variations in therapeutic interventions for Cambodian and Chilean refugee survivors of torture and trauma: A pilot study'. *Australian and New Zealand Journal of Psychiatry, 21*, 429–435.

Nguyen, T. (1993). Parents and naughty children: two Vietnamese perspectives on conduct disorders and their implications for intervention. *Australian Social Work, 2*, 50–53.

Nguyen, T., & Bowles, R. A.(1998). Counselling Vietnamese refugee survivors of trauma: points of entry. *Australian Social Work, 2*, 41–47.

Ravalico, P. (2007). Working with other cultures.' In J. Crawley & E. Shaw (Eds.), *Couple Therapy in Australia: Issues Emerging in Practice.* Melbourne: PsychOz Publications.

Robson, B., Lipson, J., Younos, F., & Mehdi, M. (2003). *Afghans: Their History and culture.* Washington DC: Centre for Applied Linguistic and Cultural Resources http://www.culturalorientation.net/afghan/index.html.

Roland, A. (1988). *In Search of Self in India and Japan. Toward a Cross-Cultural Psychology*. Princeton: Princeton University Press.

Silove, D. (1999). The psychosocial effects of torture, mass human rights violations, and refugee trauma. Toward an integrated conceptual framework. *The Journal of Nervous and Mental Disease, 4*, 200–207.

Silove, D., Tarn, R., Bowles, R., & Reid, J. (1991). Psychosocial needs of torture survivors. *Australian and New Zealand Journal of Psychiatry, 25*, 481–490.

15
Latino New Yorkers and the Crash of Flight 587: Effects of Trauma on the Bicultural Self

David C. Lindy, Rebecca Morales & Jacob D. Lindy

Introduction

An Argentinean therapist working in a clinic in the United States meets with a new client from the Dominican Republic. Sharing Spanish as their native language, the therapist is confident that he will understand this woman. In reviewing her family history he asks about the gender of her two children. She replies that one child is *el niño*, male, and the other *la hembra*. The therapist becomes deeply disturbed because *la hembra* describes a female animal, and he presumes this reflects the client's pejorative, self-hating view of females. Only later does he learn from a Dominican colleague that, in the Dominican Republic, *la hembra* is a commonly used expression for girls and women which has no negative connotations. This vignette is an example of the "myth of sameness," the assumption that one person understands another because of ways in which they are the same (Young, 2004). It is a myth because these shared characteristics may or may not create shared understanding. Indeed, the assumption of understanding when in fact it does *not* exist creates misunderstanding. The myth of sameness is a fantasy, unexamined and unexpressed until it comes to light as a result of the confusion and misunderstanding it creates. For the Argentinean therapist, this occurred in the peaceful, everyday setting of his clinic. For mental health workers in the disaster situation, the myth of sameness can greatly complicate an experience which is already overwhelming, traumatizing, and extraordinary.

In this chapter, we will tell the tragic story of American Airlines flight 587, which crashed after take-off in New York on its way to the Dominican Republic. This was a disaster in which mental health workers and the victims they cared for shared *some* cultural characteristics, but, importantly, not others. We will examine ways in which the myth of sameness affects the establishment of empathy in the disaster situation, but also how it bears on the experience of the self. Since many of the workers and victims involved were Hispanic, or Latino, the flight 587 disaster provides an opportunity to explore what might be called the cultural self. The cultural self represents that complicated aspect of identity comprised of our experience of ourselves in relation to our race, ethnicity, culture-driven effects on perspective and behavior, and our sense of our relation to other cultures. Language is a basic constituent of the cultural self. In a paper on the psychiatric evaluation of the Hispanic patient, Marcos notes that "bilingual patients often report the experience of a language-specific sense of self; that is, they feel and perceive themselves as two different persons according to the language that they speak" (Marcos, 1980). For the bilingual person, this "language-specific sense of self" will manifest itself in ways that will be characteristic of both a particular culture and a particular, bilingual individual.

Bicultural people will experience traumatizing disaster situations through their particular bicultural lens, and this will affect their response and behavior. Their cultural selves will affect their relationship to the group and its role in disaster response. The trauma membrane (Lindy, 1993) is constructed by the survivor community at these times to protect itself in relation to an outside world which has shown itself to be dangerous. The trauma membrane determines who is allowed in and who is kept out, and is an important variable for helping professionals in their efforts to be effective with these groups. The bicultural self will also determine the nature of the trauma membrane with certain communities, and how it operates.

Let us see how the myth of sameness, bicultural self, and trauma membrane interacted and influenced the experiences of the people of flight 587 as they coped with this disaster.

The Story of Flight 587

For many years, American Airline's flight 587 was a popular staple of the Dominican community of Washington Heights, a neighborhood in northern Manhattan with a large Dominican population (Michaels, 2001). Leaving John F. Kennedy International Airport first thing in the morning, Dominican New Yorkers could get home by lunchtime to see family, do business, purchase essentials for their Dominican way of life. On November 12, 2001, two months and one day following the 9–11 attack on the World Trade Center, the vertical stabilizer and rudder of the Airbus A-300 that took off that morning separated shortly after take-off and the plane broke apart in mid-air. Some witnesses claimed to see a mid-air explosion. At 9:16 am the plane crashed into Belle Harbor, a quiet, middle-class neighborhood in Far Rockaway, Queens. JFK is so close to Belle Harbor that its control tower can easily be seen from across Jamaica Bay. Parts of the plane were found in the bay within one mile of the crash site, close to the Far Rockaway High School. All people on board were killed, 251 passengers, including five unticketed infants in laps, and nine crew members. Five people on the ground in Belle Harbor were also killed.

A look down the list of flight 587's passengers shows that the vast majority of passengers were Dominicans (American Airlines, 2001). The list shows numerous collections of similar names—12 de la Cruz, 5 Diaz, 6 Martinez, 6 Sanchez. Juana and Manuel Abreu are at the top; her passport is from the Dominican Republic, his from the US. This reflects a fact of life for many Dominicans in

Washington Heights: members of the same family, living in the same home, in the same country, hold passports from different countries. The passport, a kind of identity card reflecting a basic aspect of one's place in the world, assumes a less concrete meaning in their lives. This accompanies a parallel phenomenon: the family, cornerstone of Dominican and Latino culture, is not the same creature as the family of mainstream, white America. Even though the classical version of the American nuclear family is undergoing profound change, many Dominican families have a more fluid, complex structure that, like their passports, reflects differences in their relationship to the world. These differences became very important in the aftermath of flight 587's crash.

Forty passengers on the plane were from Washington Heights, re-traumatizing a neighborhood that already had been hard hit by 9–11. Many residents had worked in the Twin Towers as waiters, cooks, janitors, and clerical workers. Others were New York City firemen and police officers who participated in the relief effort. Many were lost that day. The reported explosion seen with the 587 crash prompted rumors of terrorist activity. (The National Transportation Safety Board determined that the crash was caused by pilot over-reaction to turbulence (National Transportation Safety Board, 2001), although on-line websites argue that the NTSB was hiding the truth of a terrorist attack (Vialls, 2001)). Washington Heights was plunged into new mourning at a time that the rest of New York was still reeling from 9–11 and the on-going threat of Anthrax bioterrorism.

Dynamics of Minorities

The crash of flight 587 reflects several dimensions of the dynamics of a disaster that primarily affects a minority population within a dominant culture. First, the subordinate status of the ethnic minority bears on how the disaster is experienced and metabolized. Second, the bilingual nature of many of the mourners reflects the bicultural nature of their life in the U.S., their on-going connection to the Dominican Republic as home, and the effects that this bi-national existence has on their identity and experience of grief. Finally, Latino mental health workers dealing with this particular disaster found that their identification with its victims and their loved ones made the experience very difficult, not least because it high-lighted their own ambivalent relationship to the minority culture of their birth and the dominant culture with which they have become professionally identified.

Dynamics of Latino Culture

Earlier in 2001, Lynn DeLisi, a research psychiatrist who usually studies schizo-phrenia, volunteered for several weeks to help victims of a massive mudslide caused by an earthquake in El Salvador, decimating the Las Colinas neighbor-hood of San Salvador. She describes her first approach to one of the relief camps set up for victims.

Santa Tecla, by far the biggest tented community, had been established by the government for all those inhabitants of San Salvador who had lost their homes. Santa Tecla was an awesome sight. It could be approached from high above with a view of 1,000 pointed, white tents neatly lined up in the distance. It appeared quiet and peaceful.

(DeLisi, 2004)

Not surprisingly, DeLisi's experience of life *in* the camp was very different. Indeed, outsiders approaching the world of Hispanic culture might at first observe a monolithic, homogeneous "camp" where everyone appears to share most things, as they share a common language. This could describe the approach of non-Hispanic disaster workers wanting to help the Dominicans affected by flight 587. One step inside, however, reveals a very different, more complicated reality. For instance, there is controversy over the term "Hispanic" itself. A product of the Nixon administration's need to categorize peoples of Central and South American origin, no such cultural category had previously existed. While it denotes the countries that have a historical connection to the Spanish empire (from the Latin *Hispania*), many people object to its use for the same reason, namely, that "Hispanic" implies the subjugated, inferior status of colonized peoples to colonizer. The term "Latino," reflecting cultural and ethnic origins in Latin America, is often considered preferable (Moreno & Guido, 2005). Whatever we call members of this culture, it is clearly a richly heterogeneous group. Particular cultural legacies and experiences will bear on the individual's experience of identity and self, and these will bear on the nature of the connection points available for empathic bonds in the disaster situation.

Focus Group

Although there is a growing literature on cultural dimensions of disaster relief work, much of it is related to developing cultural sensitivity and competence in mental health workers and systems of care (United States Department of Health and Human Services Substance Abuse and Mental Health Services Administration's National Mental Health Information Center, 2004). We wanted to examine the impact of cultural identity and sense of self on the experience of the flight 587 crash, focusing on the Dominicans who lost loved ones and the mental health workers involved with them. We convened a focus group comprised of mental health clinicians and administrators who had been involved with the disaster relief work of the 587 crash and who volunteered to look at this with us. They were all American, and fell into two cultural sub-groups: (a) non-Spanish speaking white, (b) bilingual, Puerto Rican American with some familiarity with Dominican culture.

Mr. A

Mr. A is a clinical social worker, and former administrator with the New York City Department of Mental Health's mobile crisis and disaster relief services. Culturally, he is a bilingual, first generation American of Puerto Rican descent.

Despite extensive previous experience with disaster work, nothing could have prepared me for September 11th. I was deeply involved from the beginning, and worked 20 hour days to establish a family reception area and oversee coordination efforts with other mental health and relief operations. This had been my life when flight 587 crashed on November 12, creating a new trauma for New York. I immediately knew that, given the Latino population affected by this new disaster, my services as a bilingual, Latino mental health administrator would be badly needed.

When the Mayor's office went about setting up the initial family reception center in the Ramada Hotel at JFK, they used the blueprint developed at earlier crashes, such as Swiss Air 111 (September 2, 1998) and TWA 800 (July 17, 1996). For these disasters families had gathered at individual tables in the hotel's ballroom. They had traveled great distances and waited long hours for news which was reluctantly released by airline and government officials, anxious not to let out information that might be inaccurate. These families—largely affluent, European and American whites—expected to be treated well by the airlines, as indeed they were. Nonetheless, the families had been critical of this withholding of information that they had wanted as soon as it was available. They were part of the "Anglo" culture of grief in which tragic news should be directly imparted and then handled stoically.

But the flight 587 group was different. Local yet foreign at the same time, these Dominican families were all from areas inside the five boroughs of New York City. As immigrants and minority people of color, they anticipated the second class treatment they usually received from the authorities, especially compared to the white families of the earlier disasters. In addition, I knew that this group would express its grief in the extreme, dramatic, but normative style of its culture, and I was very concerned about how this should be handled administratively. The reactions of this tightly-knit Latino community would not be characterized by single families grieving their respective loses. The grief of one would quickly become the grief of all and I worried about the development of mass hysteria.

I recommended to the Mayor's office that, in contrast to the ballroom procedure we'd used before, the Dominican families would need smaller, more private spaces where they could display emotion physically without harming others or creating a dangerous contagion. Unfortunately my recommendations were ignored, and because it had worked before, the families were gathered in the ballroom once again. As the first confirmation of death came in, screaming broke out and then quickly careened from one table to the next. People fainted, fell off their chairs and began writhing on the floor. Others threw ash trays and vases, whatever was closest. One man grabbed the lit light bulb in a wall sconce and crushed it with his bare hand.

Finally my advice was heard. For this group to grieve, they needed a safe, personal space, and the presence of understanding representatives of the larger society (mental health, Red Cross, government and airline officials). Once we established a more orderly process, I was able to identify selected mourners, who, according to family members and available clinicians, appeared to need medication. Some were willing to accept it, especially from a Latino doctor.

While ultimately successful in restructuring the family reception procedure for the flight 587 families, I felt very badly that I had not been able to prevent the traumatic hysteria that caused more damage and pain. I had been intensely involved in other disaster situations, but they had not gotten to me in the same way. Although I thought of myself as a fully acculturated American, I was surprised to feel such a profound identification with this immigrant community. That put me in a very different relationship to this disaster. I understood their culture and while that helped, it also made the experience hard, maybe too hard. I saw politics everywhere and felt that city officials and leaders from the Dominican community were motivated by their desire for power, not to help their constituents in need. I felt cynical and bitter. These disadvantaged immigrants were not getting the treatment they deserved—of course. I remembered from childhood the sound of my mother screaming in grief when someone had died. Later I wondered why I had had such an angry, negative reaction to this experience, and realized that I was burnt out. I left this job shortly after that, and now, I don't do disasters anymore.

Ms. B

Ms B is a clinical social worker and program director of a community-based agency which provides mental health services to Latino youth in a disadvantaged area of New York City. Many of her program's clients are Dominican. Like Mr. A, she is first generation, bilingual, and of Puerto Rican heritage.

When I heard about flight 587, I volunteered to do grief counseling for some of the families who had lost loved ones. Although I thought I was familiar with the cultural orientation of the Dominican families, I encountered one particularly inconsolable young woman who surprised me. The mother of a small child, she was four months pregnant when her husband, father of both children, died in the crash. She kept saying that he lived with her and that she had the right to bury him. She emphatically reiterated details that would establish her legitimate claim to him. She held up the comb from the bathroom that she claimed had his DNA on it.

Gradually, the situation became clear to me. Like many Dominican men in Washington Heights, the victim had two families: a legal family in the Dominican Republic, and a second family in New York where he actually spent most of his time. Although they were married as far as she was concerned, my client knew that she could not produce the official documentation required to prove this legally. She might therefore be denied the entitlements, emotional and financial, that would then go to the other family. Just as importantly for her and her children, she would have no legitimacy as the grieving widow and thus no respect, values of immense importance in the Dominican community. While she desperately hoped that proof of domesticity could help her make her claim, she was frantic because she knew it was impossible. She was trapped.

I empathized deeply with her, maybe too deeply. This was a family with many complicated social, emotional, financial, and immigration problems. This case felt personally stressful to me, and I realized that I felt more than just compassion for this woman. I was angry at her man. How could he leave this poor woman and her children in this predicament? My pity for his tragic death gave way to anger at Latino men and their *machismo* values. But my anger made me feel guilty: how could I feel this way about a young man who'd lost his life, and even more, couldn't I understand why he had lived his two lives? The immigrant experience, with its extraordinary circumstances, demands, and hopes, was still close enough to my own experience to leave me with this conflicted, uncomfortable mix of compassion, pity, and anger.

Ms. C

Like Ms. B, Ms. C is a clinical social worker who works as a director of a community-based mental health agency which serves many Latino clients. In addition, she is psychoanalytically trained and has a private practice. She is first generation, bilingual, and her family is from Puerto Rico.

I was raised with strong Latino values which shape who I am, even as they sometimes conflict with my professional values. Values from my two worlds are often in opposition to each other. For example, basic Latino values include: *collectivism*, the group is more important than the individual; *familialism*, strong identification with the nuclear and extended family, personal needs are secondary to family needs; *fatalism*, belief in higher power or fate; *machismo*, traditional gender roles place authority and power in male figures, and *simpatia*, avoid confrontation, hide negative feelings (Moreno & Guido, 2005). While I was growing up, my grandmother, aunt, and godmother lived in one building and my cousins lived next door. This felt like the way the world was supposed to be, and, in many ways, still does. However, when I studied at a psychoanalytic institute, *familialism* was viewed as resistance to separation and *fatalismo* was unheard of. I was told that my own personal needs should never be sacrificed for my family. Family meant nuclear family, not extended, and optimal mental health was viewed as the capacity to move away from one's family of origin. I was the only Latina in this institute and these concepts were foreign to me.

I liked living close to my family and putting my needs in front of theirs seemed selfish, no matter how many classes I took. Although I considered my analytic training important for my professional development, I worried about being perceived by the Latino community as a Latina who had sold out to the larger system, a Latina who had accepted the values, customs, and beliefs of the "American" culture. I also worried the American culture did not understand or respect my Latino values.

When flight 587 crashed, the New York City Department of Health and Mental Hygiene contacted the mobile crisis teams with city contracts, requesting that all Spanish speaking clinicians with disaster training report immediately to Alianza Dominicana. This is an agency, based in Washington Heights, which provides social and mental health services to New York's Dominican community. Many of the clinicians volunteering to help were of Puerto Rican descent. While the Dominican Republic is only about 30 miles away from Puerto Rico, in New York there has often been tension between the two groups. This may relate to the power struggles that often develop between older, more established immigrant groups and newcomers of related, but different backgrounds. These struggles can involve the sibling rivalries of groups that see themselves as competing for the good graces of the host country while still feeling basically insecure in their respective relationships to this important "object." Puerto Rican communities have worked since the 1950s to establish themselves in New York, and they sometimes see the more recent influx of Dominican immigrants as threatening to their economic, professional, and political gains, which they still experience as tenuous. While they are acutely aware of the differences between the two cultures, they worry that these differences will be lost on the host country, which sees no differences between one Hispanic immigrant and the next. This was seen, for example, at the turn of the last century with the ambivalent reactions of German Jews in the United States to the arrival of the poorer, Eastern European Jews (Akhtar, 1999).

Alianza needed Latino clinicians to attend a memorial service and visit the Belle Harbor crash site with family members. I thought I was well prepared for this event since I had recently worked at the 9–11 memorial service at Ground Zero and I am extremely familiar with Latino culture. I told one of the Alianza administrators we needed a psychiatrist at the memorial service as a precaution. I felt that we might need medical intervention for possible *ataque de nervios*, a distinctively Latino form of hysteria expressed as screaming, crying, trembling, fainting, shouting, or even becoming physically aggressive. Alianza Dominicana was very clear that they wanted Spanish speaking, bicultural clinicians. Not surprisingly, there were no Spanish speaking, bicultural psychiatrists available. I explained to the administrator that I had experience providing mental health intervention through translation. I offered to bring Dr. D, a Jewish, non-Spanish speaking psychiatrist with whom I'd worked, and helped them to understand that medication through translation was better than nothing.

On the buses we were issued "family badges." Alianza wanted the clinicians to be designated as "family members" at the memorial. They hoped that this would reduce the stigma attached to mental health services and make it easier for family members to utilize the help available. Distinguishing mental health workers from families also increased the risk that we'd be separated at the memorial services. We were part of the Alianza Dominicana family. We would be sitting next to our families at the service, walking with them at the crash site, assisting them in whatever way needed, feeling their grief. I took a deep breath and tried to prepare myself and Dr. D for what was to come. I felt responsible for her since I was the one who insisted she be there. But they welcomed her with open arms, saying, "Today she's part of our family."

Besides Dr. D and me, there were two other support personnel on the bus, both volunteers from the Red Cross. Neither spoke Spanish. One was a rabbi who had just flown in from Denver and the other was a nurse. I was the only one who spoke Spanish. As we began our journey I introduced myself to everyone on the bus. More than half the passengers were members from one family. I met a man I had known as a child who told me that the owner of my own neighborhood *bodega* had been on the plane. Another passenger who stood out was Luz, a 30 year old female who had lost her cousin in the crash. She cried most of the way there.

We arrived and walked towards the tent where the memorial service would take place. Red Cross workers glanced empathically at me, offered me water, or cookies and potato chips. At first I didn't understand these gestures but then I remembered I was wearing a "family badge." They thought I had lost somebody in the crash. I felt vulnerable and wished there was a way I could explain that I was staff, I was not one of *them*. I didn't like the way it felt to be identified as family member. I also sensed how they were using their empathy to put a distance between me and them. My mind flashed back to a Puerto Rican family I had met with on 9–11. They were waiting to identify their son's hand, his only remaining body part, and realized I had probably done the same thing.

New York's Governor George Pataki, Senator Hillary Clinton, and Mayor Rudi Giuliani attended the memorial service along with various other officials. Prayers were said in English, Hebrew, and Spanish. There was lots of crying, fainting, vomiting, and hyperventilating. I helped people walk to the triage room where mental health services were supposed to be provided, but the clinicians had already been moved to the crash site. The outpouring of grief in the tent was contagious, like at the Ramada ballroom. I knew it was going to be awful and decided I had to focus my energy on those people assigned to me. Although I felt extremely guilty leaving the room, I knew I had to protect myself emotionally. Dr. D and I gathered the people from our bus and slowly made it back to the parking area. I used my family badge and gathered whatever water and snacks I could find. I felt angry that there were no bathrooms on the buses and prayed that no one would get sick. I was also angry that they had moved the clinicians assigned to the triage room. There should have been psychiatrists at both sites. I was grateful we had our own psychiatrist. I knew someone would need medical attention and I felt supported by Dr. D and safe with her. I later learned Dr. D also felt supported by me because she didn't know the language, culture, or what to expect, having never personally experienced the Latino grief reaction. I realized how much I identified with these people and how much harder this was for me than the World Trade Center disaster. On the other hand, my familiarity with this culture made me feel better prepared to deal with their needs.

The buses were very delayed in leaving the memorial service to go to the crash site. We had to sit on the bus for two hours with hungry, thirsty, hot, angry, overwhelmed, grieving family members. There were no bathroom facilities on the bus. Since the passengers had to leave the bus to go to the bathroom there was always the fear that the buses would leave without them. Tensions were running high. It was dark by the time we got to the crash site. We were given instructions to walk through with our family members as quickly as we could and return to the buses. Luz was nearly hyperventilating by then. The memorial service had been very difficult for her and I knew seeing the crash site would be devastating. We had to walk past the large hole in the ground made by the plane, now papered with flowers, stuffed animals, and notes written to the victims. Dr. D and I tried to help Luz, but with each step she got heavier until she ultimately collapsed.

Dr. D shouted she needed water and a brown paper bag. Everything was happening so fast. I could still smell the smoke and ashes and I envisioned those last moments for my neighborhood grocery man. Had he suffered? Was he burned? Did he die instantly? I'd never have answers to these questions but then it wasn't about me. Yet in some way it was. These family members were suffering with similar reactions. Who thought putting them through this was a good idea? I was so angry at whoever had arranged this. It felt like torture and yet somehow with all of those feelings racing through my mind, I managed just to act and get my job done. We walked Luz back to the buses and sat her on a nearby stoop where emergency personnel evaluated her. They wondered if she should be hospitalized. I didn't know if she'd be able to withstand the ride home, but I worried about leaving her in a strange hospital so far from home. We decided to try and get her back to more familiar surroundings. She got on the bus and slept for a while.

We were stuck in traffic on the hot buses for more than an hour trying to get out of Belle Harbor. By then Luz was inconsolable and 911 had to be called to transport her to the hospital. As we waited for the ambulance, passengers started getting off the buses. We were in a residential area and there were no public bathrooms. People started to ring door bells asking to use the bathroom. Several homeowners opened their doors and let them in. Finally the police opened up the traffic jam and insisted we move the buses immediately. I had already lost one family member and I couldn't leave anymore behind. An officer yelled to leave immediately but we managed to get everyone accounted for before we headed home. We got back to Alianza Dominicana's offices after midnight. I hugged some of the people on the bus as they exited. I never saw any of them again.

Dr. D

Dr. D works as a psychiatrist with a community-based agency. She is also an experienced emergency and disaster psychiatrist who has been involved in numerous events, large and small, in New York City. She is white, Jewish, and English-speaking only. Since a considerable amount of her work involves members of the Latino community, she often relies on a translator.

I volunteered to be the psychiatrist to treat distraught family members at the memorial service and visit to the Belle Harbor crash site. I was concerned about the visit to the site, but deferred to the better judgment of the officials planning the day. While smaller than Ground Zero, this site had many of the same compelling psychological links. It had acquired almost sacred dimensions as the place where loved ones had died. An organized, communal visit would hopefully help with mourning, and thereby, with healing. The Dominican family members hoped for a solemn visit at the final site where their loved ones had taken their final breaths. They wished to say the required number of rosaries at the site in order to carry out their familial and religious duty. Many also believed that this ritual would speed up the time their loved ones would need to spend in purgatory before they could ascend into heaven.

But as the day unfolded, I had the feeling that this event was not going to turn out well. The buses were held in traffic so that by the time we arrived at the scene, the mourners had been traveling for over two hours. There were no lavatory facilities on the bus. The local Belle Harbor community showed no signs of welcoming them. Indeed, we had the impression that, as far as Belle Harbor residents were concerned, the Dominican "foreigners" should pay their respects, then leave as soon as possible so that the unsightly hole in the ground could be repaired and their community could restore its quiet, out-of-the-way existence. For them, precious little attention seemed to be going to the local families who had also experienced death from the crashing plane. They experienced their own version of being "second class citizens." The plane had crashed in *their* neighborhood, it had killed *their* residents, yet all the attention and concern seemed to be going to these foreign immigrants. As working class, white Americans, they had their own sense of alienation from the mainstream, and had created their own, remote community within which they could feel at home in a world which often seemed not to care. The plane which dumped itself in the middle of their world brought with it the reminders of their own marginality.

As family members surveyed the burnt hole in the ground, reactions were horrific. I had never seen anything like it. There was a build up of dread, anxiety and grief, then hyperventilation, retching and vomiting from the people at the site. This spread as if by contagion to the people inside the bus. Individual mourners fainted, fell and remained unconscious, with others hovering frantically around them. One collapsed mourner, Luz, had a panic attack and was sent back to the bus, where she had a second attack. Everyone was frightened. For a moment I couldn't find my translator, Ms. C, and I began to feel the panic that was all around me. I was supposed to function as a physician, but there were no clear parameters for me to define my appropriate professional responsibilities in this setting. Alianza Dominica expected the doctors to distribute medication as needed, and Luz's family certainly wanted me to treat her immediately. Yet I knew nothing about her medical or psychiatric condition and I had not even been able to evaluate her. In addition, the nurse on the bus opposed my providing any medication at all, which is indeed in line with Red Cross policy. This made me worry about getting sued. In the midst of this grief and chaos, I was acutely aware that I did not belong. I am Anglo, I do not speak Spanish, and the hysterical grief all around me felt frightening and strange. It was so different from my background. I was able to sense how the white residents of Belle Harbor were frightened by these reactions, and felt intruded upon by these darker skinned "foreigners" and their foreign ways. It was somehow vaguely and irrationally connected to the dark terrorists who had crashed into the Twin Towers, and now there were new victims of what may have been yet another act of sabotage. I absorbed the neighbors' paranoid anxiety connected with the crash site ceremony. For them the hole at the crash site was a scar in their neighborhood, not a sacred space. They felt an urgent need to end the ceremonies quickly, get the bus out of there, and bull-doze the scar. I felt ashamed that I could identify with these angry, intolerant feelings.

Even though I could identify with the people of Belle Harbor, I could also feel for the pain and grief of my Dominican "family." I could draw on my relationship with my translator, Ms. C, who, more importantly, is also my friend and colleague. This bond gave us the strength to span the cultural divide, for example, to knock on doors to gain access to neighbors' bathrooms, expanding the empathic connection between the two communities. It also helped us to make common decisions about the need to medicate, when to evacuate a traumatized survivor, and when to insist that all move on.

Cultural Style and the Bilingual Self

The story of the crash of flight 587 is not only about a disaster and its tragic impact on the lives of those involved; it is also a bicultural story of people living in and between two worlds, and of their struggle to connect across this cultural space at a time of trauma. The people in this story live on both sides and within this divide, and perhaps we have learned some things about what happened to them when they were thrown—some by choice, some by trauma— into this space. According to SAMSHA, "culture refers to the shared attributes of a group of people. It is broadly defined as a common heritage or learned set of beliefs, norms, and values" (United States Department of Health and Human Services Substance Abuse and Mental Health Services Administration's National Mental Health Information Center, 2004). Lionel Trilling, the great literary critic, took this a little farther. He suggested that culture can be "thought of as having a certain organic quality, an autonomous character and personality which it expresses in everything it does . . . a *style*, which is manifest not only in its conscious, intentional activities, . . . but also in its unconscious activities, in its unexpressed assumptions . . ." (Trilling, 1955, p. 34).

This organic, autonomous cultural style, conscious and unconscious, affects how we organize our experience of the world, including our encounters with different cultures. For Latino New Yorkers, we have seen that cultural identity varies widely depending on multiple factors, such as Latin country of origin, length of time in the U.S., education and social class, bilinguality. (Polls have shown that by the third generation, 78% of Hispanic Americans do not speak Spanish. Pew Hispanic Center, cited in Newsbatch.com [News Batch, 2006].) But perhaps more importantly for our exploration of the dynamics of culture in the traumatic situation, we must examine these unconscious, "unexpressed assumptions" of cultural identity. Often preconscious, known and not known, these assumptions will tend to *get* expressed in trauma, an issue which becomes critical as we try to connect empathically across an untranslatable, cultural divide. The bilingual Latino American of course knows that she can speak both Spanish and English, but she is probably not typically focused on how this influences her sense of self. She will have similar relationships to other aspects of her bicultural identity, such as her degree of assimilation, her ambivalence in relation to her culture of heritage vs. her new culture, and, for bicultural mental health clinicians, her points of countertransferential vulnerability. Working on the disaster scene with survivors representing the part of the bilingual self that accesses childhood memories, and especially exposure to adult grief in childhood, accentuates these tendencies. The bilingual mental health professional may feel suddenly de-skilled and regressed as the culture of childhood is accessed. Yet, as Ms. C points out, this state can also offer her immediate access to the grief of the traumatized community and acceptance by them. The Latino mental health workers who have told us their 587 stories illustrate these points.

The Culture of the Ataque

Mr. A confidently predicted the "mass hysteria" that he knew would develop as the Dominican families learned of their awful losses. He based his prediction on multiple levels of cultural knowledge: his awareness of Latino culture in general, Dominican culture more specifically, and most particularly, his knowledge of the Dominican community of Washington Heights. He also had intimate, personal knowledge of loss in his own Puerto Rican family, different yet ethnically connected to Dominican culture, with painful memories of his mother's grief. This pain came to the fore as he related to the pain of his Dominican clients, who now felt like "his people." This occurred despite the tradition of tension and mistrust between New York's Puerto Rican and Dominican communities noted by Ms. C.

In this context these conflicts disappeared. Puerto Rican American Mr. A expressed his view of a bitter reality, perhaps an "unexpressed assumption" unconsidered by outsiders though basic to all insiders, namely, the "second class" status of Latinos in the United States. All Latinos involved with 587, loved ones and helpers alike, shared the conviction that these people would not receive the same respect and consideration as the affluent whites of earlier crashes. Whether true or not (New York's top politicians all turned out for the memorial service), Mr. A felt this deeply and none of the other Latinos in our focus group disagreed. An on-line search of items related to flight 587 reveals articles like "Death of the Invisibles" (Cruz, 2001), suggesting that others share this feeling as well. Mr. A clearly felt unheard and invisible as he struggled to get his non-Latino superiors to listen to his advice regarding the propagation of "mass hysteria," strengthening his connection to the Dominicans' feeling of invisibility. Ms. C, dealing with the *ataques* at the memorial service and crash site visit, also angrily wondered who had thought that this was a good idea? Certainly not anyone who was culturally sensitive to Latino ways of grieving.

Mr. A, Ms. B, and Ms. C are all first generation Puerto Rican, bilingual, mental health professionals. They are among the most highly educated, "successful" (as defined by mainstream, American values) members of their families. All of them were highly ambivalent about *ataques* and "mass hysteria" as a mode of grieving typical of Latino cultures. On the one hand, this was as familiar as every other aspect of the life of Puerto Rican children of immigrant parents growing up, at least mostly, in the United States. Their absorption of traditional Puerto Rican and Latino values was militated by exposure to the values of American education and culture. As such they live somewhere in between. Ms. C told a story of traveling to Puerto Rico with Dr. D when *their* flight encountered mechanical problems. Both were understandably concerned, and anxiously awaiting information from the flight crew. The message in Spanish was long and reassuring, full of details and lengthy explanations (perhaps the mellifluous nature of Spanish promotes a more comforting response to anxiety provoking situations). The message in English was, "We have experienced mechanical difficulties. We're turning back now." That was apparently all that English speakers needed to hear.

These two approaches to the threat of trauma perhaps speak to aspects of the cultural nature of grief. The more dramatic mode of expression goes with a more dramatic mode of grief, which on the up side allows for the therapeutic expression of despair but on the down side might not provide as much control against overwhelming affect. A study of how elderly Hispanics deal with end of life issues showed that many would rather not be told a fatal diagnosis but would prefer to have the information given to a family member (McLean & Grahm, 2003). This is consistent with a story Ms. C told about a daughter who wanted to view her sister's body so that her distraught mother would not have to. An unexpressed assumption seems to be that someone not as directly affected must function as the "strong one," an idea that was not appreciated by the people who planned the ballroom gathering and crash site visit. Mr.A assumed the "strong" role for the grieving Dominican families that day, taking on their disenfranchised status and burden of grief. He understood and empathized, wondering in the end if he had understood *too* well. At the same time, they all also felt discomfort, if not a guilty, Anglicized disdain for the *ataques*. They were just too much.

The Culture of Machismo

Ms. B encountered an aspect of Latino culture that evoked an unexpectedly strong reaction in her. Her countertransference to the plight of the second wife, the other woman, left her enraged at the irresponsibility of the man who died on the flight. We can speculate that this was a multileveled reaction for Ms. B, although she made nothing explicit and it could probably apply generically to many Latina women (indeed, women of many cultures). Her reaction reflects the angry helplessness of the woman bound by the sexist *machismo* values of Latino culture, and by the poverty which forces her to be the other woman. She also feels guilty that she does not willingly accept the traditional place of the Latina woman she was raised to be (Moreno & Guido, 2005), and that she is not more understanding of the plight of the Latino man, caught between two worlds, now dead. But Ms. B is also the partially emancipated American woman who has at least been *told* that she is the equal of any man. This is a frightening posture to assume in the face of her internalized *machismo* father/lover who will brook no rebellion, at the same time that it is liberating and energizing. Ms. B, who has been able to lift herself to some degree out of the *machismo* bind, found herself empathically helpless and constrained as she struggled to find ways to help her suddenly widowed client, disenfranchised not only as an immigrant in New York, but now even within her own community as the other woman and so entitled to nothing. This is an example of the trauma membrane operating within different parts of the same community, here to extrude one member who is seen as more morally culpable than another.

Identification with the Victim

Ms. C, like Mr. A and Ms. B, identified deeply and painfully with the Dominicans' grief in reaction to the crash of 587. She saw their *ataques* as reflections of "the straw that broke the camel's back," a displaced outpouring of emotion related to a life of poverty, dislocation, and constant hardship. It can be seen in other cultures as well (e.g., Egyptian, Sicilian), often expressed by others who share similar socioeconomic conditions. Like Mr. A and Ms. B, her story shows her ambivalent relationship to bicultural identity, here within the specific context of psychoanalytic training and conflicts between her analytic and Latino values. It also shows the conflicts her training created with her family, who told her that she should "leave that white shit at work." The achievements of the children, the realized aspirations of immigrant parents, are sources of great pride but are also grave threats to the old ways. It is in many ways the story of all immigrants struggling to assimilate yet retain their connection to their heritage. We see it in "Fiddler on the Roof," "West Side Story," and countless other stories.

While she focuses very much on the points of Latino contact between her and her clients, Ms. C's story is also universal for us: we see the anxiety every disaster worker feels confronting the encounter with victims of trauma, the sense of helplessness, the fear that we will have nothing to offer in the face of such tragedy and need. This was striking in relation to her story of the "family member" badge she wore to the memorial service at the request of Alianza Dominicana. Her reaction to the sympathetic glances of other workers who thought that *she* was a family member evoked a feeling of, "*I'm* not one of *them!*" This could be seen as an example of identification with the victim, the defensive rejection of empathy with the victim's experience of trauma, an empathic experience which is traumatizing itself (Lindy, 2004). Here the myth of sameness functioned to create a connection that Ms. C needed to reject because it felt too painful to bear.

The Trauma Membrane

Dr. D experienced the trauma of flight 587 from the other side of the cultural divide. She is white, non-Spanish speaking, a member of the majority culture as seen by Latinos. Her own cultural identity is probably somewhat different, in that she may see herself as belonging to another minority given her status as a

Jewish American. This may create a sense of connection and identification with minorities for her which is not apparent to Latinos unfamiliar with Jewish culture. This is the opposite of the myth of sameness: connection exists where it does not appear to. But there were powerful connections for Dr. D that she did not expect in her identification with the white residents of Belle Harbor. This was created in part by her anxious reactions to the *ataques*, alienating in their power and strangeness. She could relate to the Belle Harbor residents who were reluctant to let Latinos into their homes to use their bathrooms. They wanted the Dominicans to leave, and Dr. D wanted to get home where it was safe, comfortable, and familiar. Despite her experience with other disasters, she felt more vulnerable this time, almost as if she was succumbing to the contagion of mass hysteria. There was less of the usual professional, protective distance with this group. This suggests that the trauma membrane of the Dominicans was porous enough to let her in—she was embraced as "family member"—but once inside, it did not feel safe, but dangerous and difficult to get out. Yet she was also feeling a second trauma membrane, that of the Belle Harbor community. She was excluded by its paranoid rejection of the foreign outsiders, even as she identified with that feeling. Clearly, the collective trauma story of each community reflected aspects of their respective cultural styles, and influenced the ways in which the mental health workers were kept outside, or invited in.

The Myth of Sameness

The myth of sameness suggests that appearances of sameness do not necessarily mean that sameness actually exists. We have seen that the Latino world is highly complex and variegated, with many particular variations related to being Latino American. For the Puerto Rican American clinicians working with the Dominican families of flight 587, differences in country of origin, education, and degree of assimilation mattered less than their identification with the pain of people who felt like family in the crucible of disaster. The bicultural self was highlighted in their ambivalent reaction to the extreme form of grief displayed, but this was also related to their clinical understanding of the pathological aspects of these reactions. The Anglo psychiatrist just wanted to escape. But these feelings did not keep them from performing, sometimes courageously, in appropriately caring and helpful ways. All of the Latino clinicians felt that perhaps they had identified *too* much, and each discovered roots of those connections in their own backgrounds. The trauma membrane of flight 587 surrounded them and made them part of the disaster community, perhaps to the point of discomfort for the non-Latina clinician. The bicultural self, trauma membrane, and myth of sameness all influenced the process of connecting on that day, but perhaps, in the end, the culture of trauma creates a unifying force to bring people together in the wake of disaster. Trauma makes us all members of a disadvantaged minority. In that culture, the differences do not mean so much.

Acknowledgements.   The authors wish to thank Leila Laitman, Lori Rodriquez, Isaac Monserratte, Oscar Serrano, Katherine Levine; and Joanne Lindy for reference to the "myth of sameness."

References

Akhtar, S. (1999). *Immigration and Identity: Turmoil, Treatment, and Transformation.* Northvale, NJ: Jason Aronson Inc.

American Airlines. (2001). Updated Partial Passenger List for AA Flight 586. PR Newswire. Fort Worth, TX. Retrieved from http://www.prnewswire.com/cgi-bin/stories.pl?ACCT=104&STORY=/www/story/11-13-2001/0001615180&EDATE=

Cruz, A. (2001, November 18). *Death of the Invisibles.* Long Island, NY: New York Newsday. Retrieved from http://www.commondreams.org/views01/1118-06.htm

DeLisi, L. (2004). The Acute Aftermath of an Earthquake in El Salvador. In A. Pandya & C. Katz (Eds.), *Disaster Psychiatry: Intervening When Nightmares Come True* (p. 136). Livingston, NJ: The Analytic Press.

Lindy, D. (2004). Upheaval of the Stars: From Happy Land to the World Trade Center. In A. Pandya & C. Katz (Eds.), *Disaster Psychiatry: Intervening When Nightmares Come True* (pp. 229–247). Livingston, NJ: The Analytic Press.

Lindy, J. (1993). Focal Psychoanalytic Psychotherapy of Posttraumatic Stress Disorder. In J. Wilson & B. Raphael (Eds.), *International Handbook of Traumatic Stress Syndromes*, (pp. 803–809). New York, NY: Kluwer Academic Publishers.

Marcos, L. (1980, April). The psychiatric evaluation and psychotherapy of the Hispanic bilingual patient. *Research Bulletin.* New York, NY: Hispanic Research Center of Fordham University, *2*, 1–7.

McLean, M., & Grahm, M. (2003, Winter). Reluctant Realism. *Issues in Ethics 14*(1). Santa Clara, CA: Santa Clara University Markkula Center for Applied Ethics. Retrieved from http://www.scu.edu/ethics/publications/iie/v14n1/elipse.html

Michaels, S. (2001). *The Most Popular Flight in Washington Heights. In Two Months and One Day Later: The Tragedy of Flight 587.* New York: Columbia University Graduate School of Journalism. Retrieved from http://www.jrn.columbia.edu/studentwork/flight587/dominican.asp

Moreno, C., & Guido, M. (2005). Social Work Practice with Latino Americans. In D. Lum (Ed.), *Cultural Competence, Practice Stages, and Client Systems: A Case Study Approach* (pp. 88–111). Thomson Brooks/Cole.

National Transportation Safety Board. (2001). *News and Events.* Retrieved from http://www.ntsb.gov/events/2001/AA587/default.htm

News Batch. (2006, August). *Immigration Policy Issues.* Retrieved from http://www.newsbatch.com/immigration.htm

Trilling, L. (1955). *Freud and the Crisis of Our Culture* (p. 34). Boston, MA: The Beacon Press.

United States Department of Health and Human Services Substance Abuse and Mental Health Services Administration's National Mental Health Information Center (2004). *Developing Cultural Competence in Disaster Mental Health Programs: Guiding Principles and Recommendations.* Retrieved from http://mentalhealth.samhsa.gov/publications/allpubs/SMA03-3828/default.asp

Vialls, J. (2001, November 14). *The Crash of American Airlines Flight 587 in Queens. Hard Scientific Evidence Proves United States Government Trying to Mislead the American Public.* Retrieved from http://www.geocities.com/mknemesis/airbus.html

Young, R. (2004). Cross-cultural supervision. *Clinical Social Work Journal, 1*, 39–49.

16
Clinical Supervision and Culture: a Challenge in the Treatment of Persons Traumatized by Persecution and Violence

Ton Haans, Johan Lansen & Han ten Brummelhuis

What is Clinical Supervision?

Supervision has become a familiar element in teaching and training of future mental health professionals all over the world. Psychiatrists, psychotherapists, social workers, counsellors and other professionals know supervision as a regular part of their education. Besides this professionals often realize that, even after many years of practice, it can be helpful to go through some supervision again. Learning a profession does not end with certification and registration.

But what do we mean when we talk about 'supervision'? In this article we prefer to talk about 'clinical supervision', which differs significantly from administrative supervision. Administrative supervision is a form of quality control, an evaluation by a senior professional who incorporates the right way of doing things; it is an administrative control within a hierarchic organization. But clinical supervision is something else. Here the relation is based on shared reflection by the supervisor and supervisee and not on instructions within a professional hierarchy. Educational supervision incorporates both elements; on one hand it is a quality control of the senior professional supervisor who trains the junior supervisee in the do's and don'ts of the profession. On the other hand the supervisor warrants an increasing capacity of self-reflection and independence in the supervisee.

The shared reflection in clinical supervision is between an expert, preferably an outsider, and another professional, the supervisee, and it is focused on the supervisee's work. Its aim is to help the supervisee to acquire more cognitive, emotional and methodical depth and skill. Supervision should lead to a more independent position of the supervisee, based on his competence – and we assume that the supervisee's clients will benefit from this increase in competence as well (W. Lammers, personal communication; see also Lansen & Haans 2004, p. 330).

We can describe clinical supervision as a form of hands-on learning, learning from concrete practical experience by the combined reflection of supervisee and supervisor. They reconstruct what has occurred in a treatment. They examine together the meaning of what has happened, what they did themselves, what interpretations they gave and they also assess their own feelings – a process that is highly based on their intuition and on a whole domain of common assumptions and understandings, in other words on the culture they share.

The challenging question of this article is indeed what will happen – or what has to be done – when the element of cultural difference is introduced in clinical supervision, when the life experiences of the patient are located in another culture or when patient plus supervisee come from a different culture? Will this result in a lack of common understanding and mislead the interpretative work? Theoretically this may sound as an unsolvable problem, but in practice therapists are confronted with it everyday. They are forced to find immediate solutions when they meet refugees who fled terror and violence in their own country or when they participate in international relief organizations that attempt to reduce the suffering caused by international conflicts or disasters.

Let us first explain why the problem is challenging for theoretical reasons. Culture and supervision are closely connected in at least two ways. First, clinical supervision can be seen as something that has its origin in western cultural values. But does this mean that its validity is limited to the West? Supervision is based on autonomy of thought, critical reflection and thinking beyond or even against our self-interest. In this sense it is part of an achievement of western humanistic culture. Other cultures may have similar traditions of radical reflection, but they are not institutionalized in the medical and social professions. Clinical supervision is part of an approach which is defined as scientific and it contributes to a professional identity. This does not mean that it is widely used and acknowledged; in fact it is marginal and sometimes disputed. Although we may argue that clinical supervision is 'western-bound', it does not imply that individual autonomy of thought and critical reflection only work in a western environment. In this article we hope to demonstrate its wider and general value.

Second, clinical supervision necessarily works with material that is formed by, in the first place, a patient's culture, but also by a supervisee's and a supervisor's culture. Despite differences in, among others, religion, education, class, generation, gender and so on, understanding the life events and experiences of their clients is something that is within the reach of most therapists who treat patients from their own culture. Psychiatrists and therapists in Western Europe, the USA, and Canada (and their western-educated counterparts in many other countries) have a common corpus of more or less accepted ideas that excludes many other interpretations held by other groups or in other societies, e.g. explanations in terms of astrology, karma or the influence of spirits.

When we state that supervision works with cultural material, 'culture' has an ambiguous sense. To avoid confusion we have to distinguish between culture as a universal human characteristic that enables – and not constricts – human behaviour, and the specific or concrete culture in which a person is socialized. Supervision works always within a certain common framework of culture and it assumes the existence of common structures, categories and mechanisms. In this article we address however the specific problems related to the different concrete cultures in which the individual patients or supervisors are socialized. We may compare this with language. Languages have a certain grammar in common and when people do not know each other's language, this does not mean that it is totally impossible to communicate. As there are individuals who have a gift to pick up a completely foreign language, so it is expected from a supervisor to be open to the world of a patient or supervisee of another culture and to understand what at first sight seems not understandable. Apart from this, openness and reflection are general characteristics of all clinical supervision; they are also required when working in the own culture.

How clinical supervision can work in a non-western environment will be elaborated in this article. We will do this by describing and commenting on a number of selected cases. These cases reflect two quite different situations. The first situation occurs when supervision is given to a therapist who is in charge of treating a patient from abroad, for instance a refugee from Afghanistan living in Holland. The therapist can be a professional who is new in the treatment of refugees, or he can be an experienced therapist who has run into some difficulties with this particular case. In these cases the supervisor is mostly a Dutchman. Within this supervision system, the main cultural split is between the Dutch therapist and his patient, although there also may exist some minor 'sub-cultural' differences between supervisor and supervisee.

The second situation occurs when a supervisor goes abroad as a team member of a training project. This can happen at several places in the world where the violence of civil wars and tribal conflicts has made many victims. Often elementary help is given by the Red Cross or other charity organizations. When they have left, people may need other help, including psychological assistance. Western organizations may assist in the form of training projects, which can include a training of trauma counsellors. Here the major cultural split in the training system is between a western trainer and his trainees. The trainees are confronted with a new, western method of helping patients, while they are familiar with their patient's culture and often belong to it. When the trainees are medical doctors, teachers or social workers who are trained in western concepts, the cultural difference with the trainer will be smaller, but there might be some cultural split between them and their patients. In most cases however they know their patient's culture and have working experience within their culture. They have thus learned how to handle new input from the West.[1]

---

[1] This situation can be even more complex if supervision is a part of the training method. In most cases an expat staff member of the international NGO will supervise the local workers. He (or she) introduces supervision as a western concept like we described above. But his long stay in the region may lead to a fruitful interchange of cultural elements in the supervision. It also happens that local, senior counselors are appointed as supervisor of junior colleagues. The seniors are often trained by a western trainer-supervisor. He comes for a restricted period of some weeks to give some form of supervision training. In these fleeting encounters the intercultural components are even more difficult to handle, even if the same trainer-supervisor returns at regular intervals when the supervision trainings are continued during a certain period of time.

Western Therapists and Foreign Refugees

Let us start with an example of the first situation, supervision of therapists who are treating patients from abroad, thus also a case of group supervision.[2]

Case I

Supervised is the therapeutic work done by Peter, a 70-year old retired psychotherapist, who is giving support to a refugee family of the Middle East. The central person in this family is a refugee woman of 41 years old. Her name is Aisha. Peter started his work with Aisha by doing supportive sessions. She has recently been admitted to the psychiatry department of a general hospital, as she was considered suicidal. Doctors at the hospital have treated her well, to his opinion. After two weeks she has been discharged and now she is at home again.

Peter, who knows this family for several years now, has changed his approach in the course of time from supportive sessions with the mother to 'accompanying the family', as he calls his work now. The family has taken refuge from a country in the Middle East, where they as members of an ethnic minority people were subject to severe restrictions, and even threatened to be persecuted on a local level. The husband, whom we shall call the father, was a member of a forbidden political organization that sought independence from their country. Police raids resulted in arrests of family members (father and his two eldest sons), who after some routine ill-treatment at the police station were interrogated and kept in prison for some days. A few days later and after some further ill-treatment they were released with a serious warning. They had to refrain from any political activity. But they did not; they went on with secret meetings with political friends. The result was another police raid, ill-treatment, arrest and release after a few days, and another grave warning. They went on, however, meeting political friends in secret. Apparently police was able to trace their activities and a third police raid followed, accompanied by a military squad. The soldiers have beaten the family members up and took the four-year old youngest boy in a separate room, battered him too and flung him against the wall. The boy cried terribly but suddenly it became quiet. In the meantime the handcuffed father and his sons were carried off to the police station. Later it came out that the boy was heavily injured, and after a short period in hospital the child died from his injuries. Furthermore the soldiers troubled the mother and the eldest daughter in a way that could not be spoken of until today.

The prisoners, the father and his two eldest sons, were told that they would be transferred to a faraway prison under a strict regime. During their absence Aisha and her eldest daughter had to report to the police station every day. It was obvious what threats were imminent for them. If they wanted to prevent this,

---

[2] Names and locations in this article have been changed in so far as they can give any information about the identity of patients or therapists.

they had to be law-abiding and loyal to the authorities. This implied that they had to report about all activities of persons from their political party. Only on this condition they would be released instead of being transferred. The father, seeing no other way out, decided to accept these conditions, and after that they were soon discharged. The father had no intention to obey the authorities and on the first occasion the family fled the country. They applied for asylum in a German speaking country where they arrived in 1999 (father's brother was living there). At that time the family consisted of father (then 37), mother (35), a son of 17 years, a son of 16 years and three daughters of 12, 9 and 6 years old. They were six years older now.

In the story that follows the matter of obtaining a permission to stay in the country of asylum plays a very important role. As regulations became more and more strict appeals for a residence permit were rejected time and again. A local committee of church members took care over the family. Procedures were protracted when they moved to other districts; and psychological support was organized. When the mother got into problems, the psychologist Peter, member of this committee, offered to help. He had regular talks of a supportive nature with her. As no official interpreter was available the eldest daughter, who had acquired a reasonable knowledge of the language, acted as interpreter.

Peter's Efforts

The continuous insecurity about a residence permit made the mother desperate. Authorities considered the situation in the home country as much improved and saw no reason to let them stay. For this family going back was however unacceptable. Neither the father could cope with the situation. He let off steam against wife and children. Outwardly things went better for the children: they learned the local version of German, they did odd jobs, and they managed to go to school. There was some contact with other refugee families from their country. But Aisha became more and more unbalanced. She did not sleep well and she often cried. She felt neglected by her husband and she thought that he was deficient in caring for his family. Her eldest daughter supported her by doing household chores. But Aisha's situation worsened. She collapsed at times, she had fits of screaming, and she got anxious and threatened with suicide.

Then Peter decided to help the family. He had talks with the father, he spoke with the children separately, he learned to know all of them and he even held a few family sessions. As no regular social worker could be obtained – again, this country leaves the case of not yet recognized refugees to charity, which means that regular services are not available in most parts of the country – Peter acted as such, assisted at times by other citizen volunteers. The family held Peter in high esteem. He carefully kept some distance when they tried to become closer to him.

About one year and a half ago (early 2005) a turn for the better seemed to come for this family. New rules determined that refugees had the right to stay for treatment reasons in the country where they had applied for asylum, as long as the same treatment was not available in the country of origin. Mother's mental condition was recognized for treatment. The need to be treated gave her and her family the right to stay temporarily, as long as the treatment required, and as long as treatment would not be available in the country of origin. Together with a psychiatrist Peter had written a medical report for this purpose, which was recognized by the court. His conclusion: Aisha was suffering from chronic PTSD with depression as co-morbidity.

The family got a house. The father as well as one of the sons found a simple job. Peter kept in touch with the family. Mother made regular visits to the local psychiatric clinic on an outpatient basis. With the help of medication she found some rest. Her condition improved for some time. The girls went to school. But after half a year the mother's condition started to decline again. When she complained of suicidal thoughts, she was admitted to the psychiatric department of the local hospital, as mentioned before. After her discharge her condition went up and down without showing real progress for the better. The hospital's outpatient department followed her with supportive contacts and anti-depressive medication.

As Aisha had psychiatric treatment now, Peter could give his attention again to the family. He had the impression that mother was the carrier of the stress of the whole family. Every once a while he had a session with the father, and he had also sessions with the eldest daughter. At times he had a session with the whole family about their stressful situation. This situation can be summarized as follows. The mother cannot become better; her disorder allows the whole family to stay. This also means that domestic care for the family, and care for mother, is in the hands of the eldest daughter, now 18 years old. She does her best to keep the family going. She has almost no contact with peers from outside the family. But she got an eating disorder (frequent vomiting) which makes Peter think of anorexia nervosa. Father is worried about his wife and daughter, who are very ill he thinks. He insists on a thorough physical examination, but no physical disease was found after it took place.

'Accompanying' this family became a bit too heavy for Peter. He saw the family sliding down, since now also the 15-year-old daughter showed up with symptoms. She had complaints of anxiety when walking in the streets and started to stay at home from school. A school social worker showed up, who worried about the girl. He tried to help her overcome her anxiety, and when this did not succeed, he wanted her to see a psychiatrist.

The Supervision

Peter brings this case in the supervision group. All members of this small group of seven people are therapists of traumatized refugees. The group meets on a regular basis every month and they have agreed to follow a certain sequence in their sessions for group supervision as proposed by their supervisor.

After Peter has finished his story about the family, there is room for some clarifying questions. Then Peter states his question for supervision: "What more could be done for this mother, as she seems to be the center of the problem?" He has an additional question: "Could something else be done for the eldest daughter?" Before starting the supervision *with* the group, two special rounds are made according to the 'structured group supervision': one from the perspective of identification with the *patient* and one from the perspective of identification with the *position of the therapist*.[3] After a minute of silence in order to concentrate on the reality and life of the patient everybody, except the supervisee and supervisor, is asked to tell how he or she feels as the patient (Aisha). This round of identification allows the supervisees to come closer to the difficult and sometimes impossible and stressful situations a refugee family is living in.

All participants reveal how they feel in the role of Aisha, the mother of this refugee family. They worry about the children, since they do not receive support from the husband. They feel the oppression through the traditional role of men and women in the family and have no idea what more misery the future may bring. Furthermore they feel alone, because now Peter, the psychologist with whom Aisha could talk so well is letting her down. He is a nice man and she sees him as a sort of grandfather for the family, but evidently he does not know anymore what to do. And neither she nor her daughters are able to speak about what happened when the soldiers had carried off her husband and sons. One of the group members feels as if she ought to have been killed. As a mother she was absent when her child was so badly beaten up and smashed against the wall so that it died shortly after.

Peter is asked to give feedback now. He has recognized everything that has been said. Aisha had expressed herself in fact like this: "I have earned death, but I can't leave my children now alone". Peter does indeed not know what to do with this family and he thinks that the family needs psychological assistance. The best thing to do now is to find another social worker who works intensively with the whole family, besides the psychiatrist for the mother, a psychiatrist for the eldest daughter and the social worker for the younger daughter. Where however to find another expert to work with refugees from another culture?

The supervisor asks the participants now to make a round of identification, in which they identify with the task and position of the psychologist (not with the psychologist Peter himself, as a person). They have to imagine that they really work with the family in Peter's place. After a minute of identification the supervisor asks again how they feel – and not what they should do now. This should avoid that they

---

[3] It is important to emphasize that the supervisor works *with* the group of supervisees (Proctor (2000:38). He follows the lines of a 'structured group supervision' (Lansen & Haans 2004:340–3), where the group executes several rounds during the supervision process: (1) presentation of the case; (2) questions for clarification; (3) identification with the patient; (4) identification with the task and position of the therapist; (5) supervision *with* the group; and (6) a final round. After the case has been presented (1 and 2) and before the discussion with the group starts (5), two rounds of identification are held in which explicitly the feelings of the participants are discussed. The purpose of these rounds is to attune the participants to a climate of reflection instead of giving comments and advice from a distant observer position.

speak from the perspective of an audience in an easy advice-giving position. Participants express now feelings like: "I feel insecure, confused, helpless and desperate; I cannot work with my regular 'instruments' and that makes me feel miserable; I feel the desire to offer 'holding' to the family; I feel that I have to work very carefully". But also: "I feel irritated, furious with those soldiers, shocked by the ill-treatments".

Peter is asked to give his reaction. He says that he feels helpless himself. As a man he cannot imagine, he says, the things that happened to the women. It must have been awful. He himself is furious with the father, who is relatively indifferent to the difficulties and sufferings of his wife. Peter tells now how furious he becomes any time he thinks about the helplessness of these women when their little son and brother was so deadly ill-treated. His words are followed by an impressive silence.

The supervisor then proposes to make a normal round of supervision *with* the group. He opens the joint reflection with the question "What more could one do here with this family?" and "What suggestions are living in this group?" A profound exchange of ideas takes place, out of which several are taken to the foreground here. It is clear that individual therapy for the mother may be indicated, but at the same time it is impossible that she will heal completely. She cannot, as long as she has the unpronounced duty to remain ill. The secondary gain for the family is huge, as family members can stay in this country as long as treatment is necessary. Going back is impossible for the time being, even if the political situation and the behavior of police and military would improve. The members of this family have not yet come to terms with their traumatization and for several reasons it does not look like this will soon be possible in their place of origin. Politically they still run the risk of persecution by local authorities; psychologically they fear to be seen as cowards by their former comrades for their flight to the West; and also culturally because everybody in their village will have a misgiving about what happened to the women by the police (which means that the girls cannot marry in their region of origin).

A treatment concept for this woman should imply a compromise: she may get a supportive therapy, which would enable her to cope with mourning and also would make her 'self' grow. As for symptoms, medication could take care of that. If the psychiatrist is satisfied with a limited objective, the mother will be able to function much better, while a number of complaints will remain.

Peter's role is also discussed. He has a role as a sort of 'adopted grandfather' (as he calls it himself), a wise old man, who gives advice and help and who is seen as a personal helper. This role is very important for this family, but also for himself. Instead of loosing courage and leaving things completely to others, he should reflect about his role and accept this role in a sensible way. Peter has a role in reality for this family. He is respected and all are very grateful for what he has done so far. He has the uneasy feeling that this family puts him too high on a platform, whilst he should like to be on more familiar and equal terms with them. They decline to call him by his first name and to consider his rather egalitarian wish (during this supervision we might have explored the issue whether this wish is coming forth from his training as a western therapist or from a personal need of Peter). They call him 'Herr Peter' which sounds a bit absurd but evidently they do not feel the freedom to call him by his first name, as they see their contact more in terms of doctor and patient in their own culture, notwithstanding all sympathy and even friendship. In fact Peter would like to be one of their people or tribe. But on the other hand, is it wise to be in the 'grandfather' position? Why not take some distance while going on being sympathetic to them and declaring his solidarity by his deeds? He might have a role as adviser but also as somebody who confronts them with unwise behavior. He is a sort of 'elder', but a bit different from elders in their Muslim village community; he is allowed to be different, because he has his own identity as a citizen of his own country. Why isn't he satisfied with this role? Why does he want to be part of them? In fact, as an outside 'elder' he can do a lot. He can take the father apart and show him in a quiet, respectful conversation that he has some shortcomings and might be more considerate to his wife. He may tell the sons that they may help a bit in the household. He can also support the children. He may watch the treatment of mother and eldest daughter from a distance and if necessary act as a consultant to the psychiatrists. Maybe he can do something for the girl with the school phobia. If mother and eldest daughter will experience less stress, the overall level of stress in the family might decrease. Most probably it will not be necessary at all to add a new caregiver, a social worker, to this family as he has proposed. That would make things more confusing.

Peter reacts to this with a broad smile. He feels that he can do something with this. It is as if he has got something like a permission to do what he wanted himself but did not dare to accept. The role as 'elder' is a nice compromise between his wish to be close with the family but to take some distance too.

What about the other participants? For some of them, what happened in this supervision is an eye-opener. Others have to get used to the idea that a psychologist leaves his usual position in treatment (that had happened already a long time ago in this case) and gets a supportive role for this family. For one member it is unsatisfactory that the mother will not get a thorough, effective treatment. This member sympathizes very much with the mother; she fears that her suffering will not be adequately tackled. Another member points out that a social group has just been established for adolescent refugee-girls from the same minority in their country. It might be good to invite the eldest daughter to this group. Finally it is agreed that Peter will bring in this case for some follow-up in future sessions of this group again. It might be useful to give him more support in his role.

Evidently Peter has a role problem that is often seen in therapists working on a voluntary basis with refugees from other cultures. He is part of a group of volunteer citizens. For volunteers it can be difficult to draw a line to their assistance. Peter acts as a volunteer but on the other hand he also tries to act as a professional, because he continues to give psychological assistance. No doubt, it is tempting and laudable to help people in distress when there is no regular assistance available from the mental health system during the crucial time of entry in the country of asylum. It is also tempting to underestimate the problems that may arise. From his wish to assist he was a bit blind for the complications that might arise. Gradually these complications became too heavy. He liked to withdraw by calling in more professional help, but he did not really believe that this family would make any progress this way. He has a sense of reality, but also feelings of guilt. At one hand he liked to withdraw, at the other hand this was not acceptable to him.

Saving this refugee family by trying to arrange a provisional residence permit and hoping that in some magical way a definite permit would be given has been an important motive for his actions. Did it give him a feeling of power to fight against authorities without knowing what the outcome of the war would be? Was it naivety? Was it the battle against injustice? Has he unconsciously been motivated by unfinished conflicts with his parents or teachers? He has saved the family for the time being, but things are not going well. He is committed to the family and feels stuck. He is looking for supervision in order to prevent worse.

Looking Back at Supervision

Peter hardly expresses himself on his motives in supervision. Yet the supervision group knows what is going on. Problems like these often arise, maybe not as hectic, in working with traumatized refugees who fight for a residence permit. Almost all members of the supervision group have experienced how their role as a therapist can interfere in their work. They don't have to explain this to Peter. He knows that he has rushed into helping this family with the best of intentions. He is familiar with the pattern of a passionate caregiver, who is hampered by the impossible context of the people he tries to assist and by the disappointing outcomes. He knows how often a man or woman resigns from this work in frustration or ends up with forms of burnout or 'traumatoid states' (Wilson & Thomas, 2004). He also knows the temptation of a savior's role.

These topics were hardly discussed in this supervision; they were seen as a matter of course and as a well-known theme. The supervisees, amongst whom some experienced therapists, shed some light on other possibilities. Peter does not have to withdraw, but he can better style his role than he has done up till now. This family is open to his role as 'elder'. He has to give up his role as a 'beloved grandfather' belonging to this family, and he should rather accept the role of respected wise man from this European country. An 'elder' at some distance can have more influence than a close pseudo-family member. Why not being a wise and humane western psychologist with empathy, but also distance? Wherefrom this tendency to over-identification? Why such a need to be recognized by the family as 'one of them?'

Looking back at this question an answer might be found in the special situation of giving care and assistance to refugees in Peter's country. At first sight there are a lot of differences between those refugees and their helpers. The people being assisted come from another culture, the culture of a minority people within their home country, whose culture is rather different from the culture in this German speaking country where they have sought asylum. They come from a technically primitive, rural area, whereas their assistants in the new country do often belong to an academic or semi-academic milieu. But there is an important matter that these groups have in common: both groups, these refugees as well as their assistants, are in a certain sense people living in the margin of the society in which they live now.

The group of refugees is not welcomed and the other group's work for refugees is hardly well received. Assistants can seldom show off with their efforts as their neighbors and friends are scarcely interested in this kind of work, or worse even, have a negative opinion about it. Working for traumatized refugees has got a negative note in their country. It is not recognized as a regular part of the work in the mental health system. This means that in practice idealists are engaged in doing this work. Politically they are rather actively engaged against the prevailing opinions in their country about refugees. When refugees do not get a residence permit, lawyers ask them to write a report about the traumatization of their clients. That means another source of unpaid or badly paid work, a source that often takes more than one half of their time. This situation brings along a whole series of particularities in the psychological sense. We see them in this case especially in Peter, the therapist, who asks for supervision in the first case. He is over-involved with this family and finally he phantasizes to be part of it.

Such identification with the victim role can lead to errors and mistakes. It can make an assistant blind to important elements in a case or in a patient system. In this case Peter lost his distance. The case of this family had a strong emotional impact on him. He is in trouble with his role – is he a volunteer like any citizen, a professional or some sort of family member? – and he has problems with the case concept.[4] He has also made an error in assessing the role of men and women in this family. He seems to consider the fact that it is self-evident in this family, that women are more burdened with tasks of internal family life than men, as a personal deficit of the father. He has not seen that this might be a structural given in their culture. Probably it did not occur to him how in countries in the Middle East women behave in regard to emotions.

Females are encouraged to express emotions that elicit support and reflect weakness, such as fear, unhappiness and helplessness. Men are encouraged to express emotions and encourage actions, such as anger, anxiety and revenge. Second, emotional distress is caused by conflicting value demands on women in a society that is both collectivist and paternalistic. The general feeling is that society is a threatening entity that pursues women and prevents them from fulfilling themselves. Very often men are not conscious of the intrapsychic and social pressures on their wives and are not aware of their distress. Third, the notion of suffering in silence is glorified. There is a term for a woman who suffers in silence without complaining: the 'Mastoura' woman. Abu-Baker (2005) describes this as the wife and mother who is to the outside world the sick woman, pleading for help. To the inner family she has to be strong. Se has to fulfill her domestic duty. The husband and father does not know better, to him it is self-evident. He thinks that she does not need support; she is a strong woman, even if she is sick. Anyway she should

---

[4] For a more detailed explanation of 'case concept' see the next section.

be. Two of the daughters are on the way to fulfill the same role. The psychologist Peter in his role as 'elder' has to give a nice package of psycho-education in order to clarify that father has to adjust his expectations and behavior, also in his own interest.

Preliminary Remarks

In this case we have shown that clinical supervision can play an important role in the support of traumatized refugees by western therapists. The open and free-floating reflection of the group helped to find new ways in dealing with a difficult case. The reflection on the role of the supervisee Peter exemplifies the main reasons why supervisors ask for supervision that we have distinguished elsewhere[5].

The first reason why Peter asked for supervision was the emotionally overwhelming impact of his involvement with the family. In a more generalizing manner, we distinguished such reasons as *problems of personal impact*. We can specify them as problems in counter-transference reactions and emerging problems of burnout, heavy emotional impact or even 'traumatoid states' (Wilson & Thomas, 2005).

The second reason for supervision was Peter's lack of a proper assessment of the case and therefore his error of judgment in understanding the case. We took these reasons together under the heading of *problems with the case concept*. They can consist in using unproductive working models, a lack of knowledge about trauma and culture and as a result application of inappropriate therapeutic methods; a concept of the case exclusively formulated in clinical terms, discounting the social, economic and political processes. In the case of Peter the personal impact and the problems with the case concept have led to an unclear conception of his role. Role confusion is often seen; we have put it in a rest group of dissimilar problems, together with problems like aggression in patients, treatment of perpetrators, conflicts with interpreters, unstable work situations or lack of experience in certain therapies.

What clarifies this case however in terms of culture? We like to spell out three points:

(1) The most outspoken cultural difference we noticed were related to the characteristics of gender in the Middle East. The notions about the tasks of men and women held by this Middle Eastern refugee family were initially hard to understand for the psychologist Peter. Instead of acknowledging its cultural meaning, father's dominance made him angry. The case shows how a lack of familiarity with a patient's culture can disturb an adequate perception of the family relations of the patient. Cultural difference was outspoken here, but in principle not dissimilar to

---

[5] The authors have elsewhere made an inventory from their own work in supervising therapists treating traumatized patients, amongst whom the majority consisted of refugees; they selected notes from 100 cases (Lansen & Haans 2004).

what is encountered in the treatment of more common patients. In practice, however, it can be much more difficult to get sufficient cultural knowledge. Sometimes interpreters can give it or there are staff members from other cultures, colleagues with a long experience or a supervisor's expertise.

(2) Cultural differences are not only more outspoken but also more intense. The story is dramatic; it involves persecution and homicide in the country of origin, and the threat of deportation to their asylum country. At the same time we are forced to look beyond culture and to take into account the political context, not only the story behind their flight but also the refugee situation in the asylum country, as no regular psychotherapeutic help exists for refugees who have not yet got a residence permit. All psychological and most social support has to be organized in an impromptu manner and a regular and solid financial base and organizational structure are lacking. An appeal is done on the therapist for more than therapeutical activities (help with money, transportation, making a phone call to authorities about non-therapeutical affairs, involving friends or the church community for accommodation or other support). In such cases supervision is essential.[6]

(3) Of particular interest is the intense cooperation between persons from two different cultures, here the psychologist Peter and the Middle Eastern family. For such interactions no clear-cut models are available and it is more difficult to develop professional neutrality than in common treatments. There are risks like victimization, exotization or identification. Peter's over-identification, which became clear to him in the supervision session, is perhaps understandable given the massive indifference and political harshness towards refugees in his country. This cultural interaction, which is a cooperation and confrontation at the same time, is an eminent theme to be subjected to clinical supervision.

Expatriate Experts

In this part we will discuss several cases that represent what we have called 'the second situation', when western supervisors go abroad and present their method to therapists, professionals, and social workers from non-western cultures. What are the effects, possibilities and limitations when the 'western-bound' method of clinical supervision is applied to counseling and clinical work in, for example, Cambodia, Uganda or Sri Lanka? We limit our description to supervision in areas that have been hit by natural disaster or organized violence. Here we may be confronted with huge numbers of survivors who have lost almost everything: family members, limbs, house and dwelling-place, facilities for practicing their

---

[6] Practical experience has learned that supervision can also be important in countries where care for refugees is part of the regular health care. In such cases the main issue is not the definition of the professional role, but dealing with the emotional impact the agonizing lot of these people can have even on experienced team members.

profession, and so on. They are forced to live in bad conditions, are poor, often hungry and sad, and suffer from disease or mental health problems.

After the first emergency help, a process of rehabilitation starts. When the first-aid NGO's, often helped by the Red Cross, have dealt with the most urgent problems, new NGO's enter the field, by their own initiative or invited by governments or local organizations. These "second wave helpers" often focus on mental health conditions and psychosocial interventions of a more permanent kind. During this period local counselors have to be trained in helping methods, they can use as community worker or mental health counselor. Students in these trainings are often local volunteers, grass root workers with little education or other professionals like nurses, teachers, clergy, leaders etc. The methods taught are often forms of fundamental counseling based on their local helping practices (Van der Veer, 2003).

To support them in their work *clinical* supervision is provided. Most ideal will be to have this supervision applied by supervisors from the local helping organizations and to give more experienced senior team members the formal role and position of supervisor. In reality this option is not always possible. Often outsider experts from the West will be brought in, to provide the capacity and expertise for adequate supervision. If local senior counselors are available to execute clinical supervision, the western expert can limit his task to provide more or less regular trainings as a trainer-supervisor.[7]

In this section we will look at the interaction of cultural differences in a setting where western expatriate experts cooperate with local counselors as long term supervisor or brief trainer-supervisor. The expat supervisor has a western background, but acts within a local – and for him 'strange' – environment. The following examples, where supervisor and supervisees are Tamil, and the trainer-supervisor is Dutch and male, illustrate situations which are quite usual.[8] Most of the following examples occurred in 'structured group supervision' sessions, as described above.

---

[7] We are using the following terms: 'supervisees' are counselors and local staff members from non western helping organizations, and the 'supervisor' is also a person with the same cultural back ground. The 'expat supervisor' or 'western supervisor' is a non local expat who works for a longer period with the local staff. The 'trainer-supervisor' refers to the western trainer who provides the supervision training, often in short blocks of one or two weeks.

[8] During the years 2004 and 2006 one of the authors (Haans) executed a supervision training as a trainer-supervisor with local NGO's in the Tamil region in Sri Lanka and the southern part of India. These organisations had started as a branch of Doctors without Borders and had become independent institutions in due course. The trainer-supervisor offered trainings in individual, group and team supervision. The intended local supervisors were senior counsellors and community workers. They executed supervision within their own organisation and for external organisations like secondary schools and local staff from other NGO's.

Case II

In case II we describe a phenomenon that often occurs when a western supervisor tries to attune to local circumstances.

The local supervisor asked one supervisee to describe her problems. The supervisor listened attentively and empathically, and so did the other group members. There was a warm, supportive climate and at a certain point the supervisor and group members interfered by asking questions. These questions clarified the actual situation and the client's problems. And then, quite unexpected for the western trainer-supervisor, the group members started to give advice and to advance solutions in a quite directive manner. The supervisee who contributed the case listened attentively, nodded and after a few minutes she expressed her acceptance of the solution.

The trainer-supervisor had the feeling that the case presented was a complicated one that, according to his experience, requested a meticulous elaboration of the motivations behind the supervisee's helping strategies. The solution was – to his view only – a variation of other solutions that had failed, but everybody was happy with this outcome and this result of the discussion. "This is like we always do, so what is your problem Mr. Trainer-supervisor?"

Emergency work is often done within the framework of a kind of casualty department. This case is a clear illustration of such an attitude. Significant is that the urgency of the immediate problem, the need to find concrete solutions, convinces all participants of the adequacy of quick answers. For the trainer-supervisor it was like watching the American television series "ER", an emergency ward where problem presentation and solution agreement are reached in a very high speed and within a subordinate frame of relationships. One could wonder if in distress all humans act like this, or whether this American export product had such a strong impact on the local community. The latter is quite implausible and a tendency towards hierarchic quick solutions in catastrophic circumstances seems a likely general human response. Such a response can be consolidated by the influence of expats in the emergency aid and supervision of the local staff. Often supervision is provided by one of the expats in the organization, mostly a doctor or skilled nurse, who is familiar with a medical emergency way of supervision and induces this in the local staff with good results; the effectiveness of the emergency and rehabilitation work often improves considerably.

Apart from the urgency of a problem, this local culture (like most Asian cultures) may support such an attitude when a strong tendency exists to await and to follow the advice of authorities, an attitude that hinders reflection and which is also a pattern that is particularly common in the medical profession. In our case it seems that the local supervisors and supervisees responded from this mixture of general and cultural common behavior.

When the trainer-supervisor questioned this response, the local supervisors and supervisees were quite astonished about the nature of this question, they did not see a problem. The trainer-supervisor explained that this emergency attitude is less required during the rehabilitation and even less during the following reconstruction period, in which the team was now. It can be effectively replaced by a more clinical way of supervision. The supervisees agreed to give a try to this joint reflection. Despite the common occurrence of this submissive supervision attitude, it has struck the trainer-supervisor again and again how easily it is abandoned by both supervisees and supervisors and replaced by a more mutual cooperative attitude in later phases.

Case III

The next example shows the contrary. Here we have a group of counselors who are well-trained during four years of counseling; they have much experience and knowledge regarding the psychological consequences of man made disaster for refugees and displaced persons. They are well-equipped to deal with complex psychological and relational problems. This was a dynamic, non-structured supervision group.

A supervisee presented a case of a woman who had to take care of her mentally disabled son in a refugee camp. She explained to the supervisor and the group how she became more and more demoralized by the incapacity of the mother to care for her son. There was no housing equipment, no food, and the neighbors were mocking her son and herself. The supervisor interrogated especially on these feelings of helplessness of the supervisee. The group members revealed that they had the same experiences in the shelters. They shared their feelings and after a supervision session of 45 minutes all ended in despair.

The trainer-supervisor expressed his concern about the emotional morass they were all in. They confirmed his observations and got stuck again! No alternatives came to their mind, no allies turned up and the local supervisor and the supervisees took the same emotional and professional positions.

This case illustrates the effects of the shared blind-alley job experiences many counselors find themselves in. Shared feelings of powerlessness and despair are quite common among supervisees and supervisors working in the same area and having the same background as their clients. Here the work of the local supervisor becomes very complex. Not only must she (or he) release herself from these feelings of misery and hopelessness, she has also to stimulate the group to a constructive and professional attitude and at the same time she has to do justice to this emotional layer. Irrespective of their cultural background, trauma relief workers and counselors all over the world tend to respond with these feelings of futility and humbleness. Of course, these feelings are colored by the cultural environment, but they reflect shared worldwide experiences. Being a western supervisor can bring an advantage here. He (or she) is more distant, can easily take a 'helicopter view'. Supervisor and supervisee can engage in a dialogue about more unusual local resources, and about the strength and coping capacities of clients, counselors and supervisors. This can help to get out of the blind alley. We will elaborate this in more general terms in a later section.

Case IV

Male-female relationships are a common feature of all supervision relationships, but often they play a more outspoken role in non-western countries.

This group started to work along our structured group supervision framework. From the preceding dynamic supervisions the members were accustomed to the supervisor's question: "Who encounters what problems in his work?" Mostly all supervisees presented a case and the supervisor quite naturally selected the case the supervision group would deal with, irrespective of the supervisor being male or female. The following pattern emerged when within the structured framework, the trainer-supervisor asked the supervisor to encourage the group to decide themselves to select one of these cases for supervision. In this group (and many other supervision groups) the females form the majority; the males are always counselors, the females are either counselors or less-trained community workers. When the group engages into a selection process, nearly always the problems of the male members are chosen. Women's topics only are dealt with if a male group member has the same supervision question.When the trainer-supervisor noticed this pattern, the group and the supervisor responded with surprise, as if they were made aware of something obvious that did not require special attention. When this was brought to their notice by a stranger, they were able to question this automatic pattern and change it. Male group members normally show no discomfort in restraining themselves, female group members have however much more difficulty to convince the others that their problem is an important one. Here the intervention of the trainer-supervisor made them aware of a questionable relation pattern in their cooperation.

Culturally internalized relation patterns are present in the group sessions as well. It takes the 'eye of a stranger' to question this 'natural' daily routine. Case IV points to a common feature in both western and non-western supervisions, the inferior position of women in society. In western societies the supervisees themselves take the initiative to balance male-female relations, but it is also a point of continuous concern for the supervisor. In non-western countries this balancing is less self-evident. The 'natural' characteristics of these relationships are used as a rationalization of the maintenance of existing power structures. When an expat trainer-supervisor mentions this uneven balance within the supervision training, it is often recognized as something that can be changed. Most counselors working in mixed teams, are willing to cooperate on an even gender balance.

Case V

Within supervision the realities of the outside world can not be excluded from the sessions. The social relations and power structures within a community are often mirrored in the supervision session. This happens in this example, where a supervisee, a young female counselor in a secondary school, discussed the difficulties she had with a pupil.

The pupil had lived for a long time in a shelter nearby the school town in the Tamil region of Sri Lanka and had moved with her family to a new house in a new neighborhood. The girl (14–15 years old) caused great problems at school. She often skipped school, was irregular in performing her duties and misbehaved in various ways. She had been expelled from school for some weeks and returned much later than was arranged. The counselor was ordered by the principal to discuss this case with him, and he summoned her more or less to make sure that this girl would stop her deviant behavior. The normal procedure of returning was that the girl talked to her mentor and the school principal and that engagements were made to control and reduce the disturbing behavior. Neither of these happened. The girl was attending school, but officially she was not there, nobody knew about the guidelines she had to keep; she just roamed around and her behavior was even worse than before.

In the supervision the female local supervisor was talking to the supervisee only in terms of her relationship with the girl: "How could the supervisee-counselor improve her working alliance with this unstable young woman?" In the following training exercise, the Dutch trainer-supervisor stimulated the supervisor however to inquire about the mentor and the principal. After some reluctance of the supervisee, it turned out that they had not properly fulfilled their duties and had seriously dropped a clanger by not inviting the girl into their offices. Both were men, the mentor was of the same, the principal of a higher caste than the counselor. This caste issue became only addressed when the trainer-supervisor explicitly asked about it. Both women (supervisor and supervisee) avoided the power relationships involved in it. In their social perception men were naturally more dominant; and at an informal level, the caste shudder towards the principal was still very powerful in these lower caste women. During this supervision they agreed that the counselor should have confronted these men with their negligence, although both were men and one was of a higher caste, which made it very difficult to call them to account. There were two hurdles to be cleared, which proved to be too heavy for the supervisee and the supervisor. Therefore they avoided the issue and concentrated on the client-counselor relationship.

In the outside world there are many socially constructed gender hindrances. The female supervisee, the group members and supervisor were all dissatisfied with the treatment by both male officials, but their behavior was considered proper and natural to a certain extent. Women had to subordinate and show respect, so was the general, culturally accepted agreement. The interventions of the "stranger", the expat trainer-supervisor, brought their neglected feelings of personal and professional injustice to light, made them aware of their avoidance and opened new tracks to grasp the situation. In this way the counselor-supervisee could protect her client, continue the counseling in a responsible way, as well towards her client as to her superior.

In Case V we could observe the basic ingredients of the supervisor's fecundity as an outsider. Often the difficulties that result from the cultural differences between supervisor and (western) trainer-supervisor are stressed, but the position of a stranger can also be very helpful. If the supervisor and supervisee have the same cultural background, many contextual and social boundaries are taken for granted. This also happened in this situation. Both supervisor and supervisee got together in an unconscious collusion and avoided the influence of the misbehavior of both men towards the girl, and towards the supervisee-counselor. They took these socially prescribed male–female power relations for granted and thus avoided a clear analysis of the professional role.

Case VI

Counseling in the area of natural and man-made disaster is often very complex. Decisive cultural influences emerge not only in the assessment of symptoms of distress, they also show up in the counseling relationship and the evaluation of human relationships between family members, community members and counselors, as this case shows.

In a structured supervision session, the supervisee presented a case that was going on for more than half a year now. The father of a family had been very demoralized by the tsunami disaster. His boat was destroyed; he had lost his reason of existence and had become mentally ill. He withdrew himself more and more from friends and family members, he roamed the other villages, slept in the woods and became more and more dependent on charity by the church. He had no longer contact with the other family members. Both his wife and the two adult daughters also drifted apart. One daughter got married to a fisherman and moved to his nearby village; the other one went to the neighboring city, leaving her mother alone with the counselor. The mother became more and more dependent on the counselor, who together with the son-in-law tried to find the father and to reunify the family. The supervisee told about his feelings of exhaustion, entanglement and confusion. These feelings reached a climax after a rare meeting with the father, who mistrusted him, yelled and called him all sorts of names. He was so shaken up that, after this session, he escaped to a Hindu temple, although he was a Christian. In this quiet atmosphere he was able to calm himself down and resume work. The supervisee also reported that there were few team members available to support him.

In this organization the "doll method", described by Diekmann-Schoemaker and Van der Veer (2003) was frequently used by counselors and clients. It is a visualization method in which the counselor uses small dolls, puppets and other objects to visualize the inner and outer world of the client. Together they signify on the table all the relevant relationships. They can "represent the whole family, their neighbors, or anybody else who plays an important part in the client's life. Even a dead person may be depicted: by laying a doll on its back". It makes the problem of a client visual and "helps both the counselor and the client to get an accurate overview; not only of the people involved, but also of the way the client feels that they interact." (Diekmann-Schoemaker & Van der Veer, 2003, p. 38).

The local supervisor and supervisees also used this method in the group supervision. During the exposition round the dolls were frequently used as a tool to visualize the problems of the supervisee.

In this case the supervisee depicted the father fifty centimeters away from the rest of the family, behind a barrier. The mother and the two daughters were close to each other, the married daughter was close to her husband. This son-in-law was replacing the husband for his mother-in-law, he visited her often, took care of her misery during long talks and supported her financially. He became closer to his mother-in-law than to his own wife. The counselor put himself nearly in the centre of this family. He was close to all the remaining family members and much closer to the mother than the youngest daughter, a rebellious teenager, who lived in a sheltered house because of psychological and behavioral problems. He vividly described his warm relations to the mother, the oldest daughter, his compassion for the youngest and his feelings of despair and anger towards the father who had left them all alone.

The supervisees responded empathically to him, and had great difficulties in making critical remarks about his emotional over-involvement. This had to be done by the supervisor who did so in an indirect way by questioning the position of these dolls. The father was put accurately in a very remote position, but the supervisee put the other dolls much too close to the mother. The youngest daughter saw her mother only at rare occasions; the elder one visited her one or two times a month. The only regular visitors of the mother were the son-in-law and the counselor, who were in a kind of rivalry. Both neglected the father and were rejected by him. The supervisor discussed the more appropriate distances of the dolls towards the mother, they were rearranged much more remote from each other. So it became clear that the supervisee idealized the interconnectedness of the family members.

To the trainer-supervisor it was clear that this was a very unproductive family situation. The group agreed, it also considered this family structure as very unacceptable, but the rejection of the father and the stepfather position of the-son-in law were not questioned, neither by the other supervisees nor by the supervisor. The supervisor also questioned the unproductive counseling position of the counselor. Not only was he very alone within the family system, also his rivalry with the son-in-law hampered his helping capacities towards the mother. When the supervisee told more about the recent history of this helping relationship, it became clear that his original client was the father. He was referred to him by a community worker because of his increasing signs of distress. The father had lost his boat and his dignity as a fisherman; and he was afraid of going to the sea again. He was unable to support his wife anymore. He also was a bad father to his younger daughter.

The counselor was supportive to him, gave educational and practical advice, which the father half-heartedly tried to put in practice. The counselor got dissatisfied with it; the client became angry and came no longer to the meetings. He then increased his wandering life style. Then the mother showed up as a client, she could no longer cope with the youngest daughter; her son-in-law was a great help, but he could not deal with the increasing problems. Therefore the counselor supported the mother, found a temporary shelter for the daughter and became a "second son-in-law". This seemed quite acceptable for the supervisor and the group members.

Here the trainer-supervisor intervened, questioning this shift in clients, the professional isolation of the supervisee-counselor and his inability to get in contact with the father. How could he find allies to make contact with this man, who was his original client? It seemed that a catholic priest still had irregular charity contacts wit this man. So the trainer-supervisor asked if he could approach this priest for help. This suggestion was met with great reluctance. Feelings of animosity dominated the discussion and the trainer-supervisor did not understand from where they originated. At a certain point the local supervisor insisted on the autonomy of the counselor and warned him that his role could not to be taken over by the priest. "Counselors work along their own methods and within their own dignity". On this condition the supervisee could approach the clergyman and ask him to help in establishing contact.

In this example several important elements come together; it is a quite thorough description of the post-traumatic cases counselors have to deal with. It is a complex case where the traumatic events have severely affected the client-fisherman and his family. The supervision group members, inclusive the supervisor, look at this family as a pitiable group of people. The behavior of this family is not considered as extraordinary in comparison to other severely affected members.

The description of the family relations is idealized by the counselor and the other supervisees. The position of the counselor as a second son-in-law neither causes much amazement in the group. On the contrary, when the supervisor asks how adequate the distance in his interventions was, he is at first met by suspicious disbelief. If he interrogates further on the actual signs of this strong relationship, it gradually becomes clear that the family members are much more distanced from each other than he originally presented. The dolls' positions are adjusted to this new awareness and then the loneliness and despair of the counselor fully come to the surface.

The complexity of the family and the emotional distress of the counselor is increased by the delicate issues that are mentioned when the seeking of allies becomes a subject of supervision. These issues are dealt with in a nearly secret language. It becomes clear to the trainer-supervisor that there are a lot of religious differences in the area that are not openly discussed. The translator has a lot of problems in finding the correct English words for the phrases that are used. She tries to avoid the joking and sometimes bitching expressions of the counselors.

At first this priest is unacceptable as an ally in supporting the fishermen. The priests are seen as competitors, who do not accept the counselors from the outside, although they are from the same region. If the counselors are accepted in their village, the priests will try to dominate and modify the counseling relationships into a Christian direction.

When discussing other opportunities to establish contact with the father the result is nil, so the counselor has to fall back on this clergyman. Reluctantly he admits he has no choice, but then the supervisor warns him and nearly prescribes him strong boundaries he has to take into account between himself as a counselor and the priesthood. During this part of the supervision the trainer-supervisor estimates that many cultural and possibly even ethnic issues are touched upon, but not openly. It apparently has to do with religious differences, with authority and power struggles in the villages, with generation conflicts between the elder clergy and younger counselors. But it becomes not clear to the trainer-supervisor, the conversation takes place in a scornful atmosphere. It is as if a taboo field is explored in a mystifying way, where the trainer-supervisor is a real outsider and is effectively kept outside. And he simply has to accept these boundaries.

What the trainer-supervisor did not mention, since he had too little evidence, is the problematic psychological situation of the father. Although the whole population had suffered enormously from this flood, the material losses of this actual family were relative petty. It looked like a strong post trauma psychological reaction and according to western nosology one could suspect a psychotic decompensation or a schizoid regression of this man. Neither the counselor nor the supervisor mentioned any clear-cut symptoms pointing in this direction. On the contrary, they considered these reactions as an appropriate, though vehement response to the tsunami. And maybe they were just simply right in their cultural context.

Reflection on the Cases

All the preceding five cases (II–VI) have in common that there is a search for a productive relationship between local counselors and supervisees at one hand and a western trainer-supervisor at the other hand. The difficulties in the development of these interactions were clarified in close connection with the examples. We will now deal with some more general characteristics of this cultural interaction. There are three important strategies that an expat supervisor or trainer-supervisor can use to realize an intercultural dialogue in his or her work in non western countries. The first strategy is an attitude of benign contest, an empathic approach to the people he or she encounters in the other culture. The second strategy is the installment of adequate reference power; and a third strategy is the use of a specific methodology. The combination of these three approaches enables the supervisor to vouch for the viability of exchange in a meaningful social context. In the following paragraphs we will work out these strategies.

Supervision as a Benign Contest

A supervisor must create a climate in which a supervisee feels himself safe; a supportive atmosphere that allows to make mistakes regarding the technique, as long as they are no mistakes of the heart. Especially community workers and counselors feel often vulnerable and doubt about their own possibilities. A good atmosphere should make them receptive for positive feedback. (Van der Veer, De Jong & Lansen, 2004).

Here we approach the middle of cultural tension. Supervision is in non-western countries usually seen as a strict control of work. It mostly takes local supervisors and even more the supervisees a long time and a great effort to find autonomous ways of interaction and reflection. In the follow-up of a humanitarian crisis the help questions become more complicated, and so become the answers. Although there are in the aftermath of a disaster problems that still need such a practical approach through e.g. psycho-educational advice and guidance, in this phase more serious cases of suffering from complex psychological consequences become immanent. Then more community work and trauma counseling is needed.

Many community members cannot cope with their losses and mourning, notwithstanding good advice and good practical support from their environment. The relationship between client and helper will become more intensive, with a deeper emotional impact. She or he must learn to recognize the emotional interaction between clients and herself. Clinical supervision helps the counselor-trainee to become aware of this emotional interaction and stimulates her to evaluate her own feelings and behavior.

One may question whether the original orientation towards effective solutions is not been replaced by the strong emotional tendencies of western counseling methods. Trauma counseling is in western societies very much associated with and even identified with "emotional discharge" or "catharsis". Also the more behaviorist trauma methods concentrate on a "central or core trauma" that has to be dealt with (Foa, Keane, & Friedman, 2000). It is our impression that many untrained counselors focus on immediate solutions for practical problems, but that the more classically trained counselors are more directed at emotional expression. Western trauma counseling methods are therefore pretty culturally insensitive and it requires a lot of reframing to adapt western counseling trainers to local perspectives (Kos, 2005). The same applies to western trainer-supervisors. They tend to follow the "emotional discharge" approach and should take more care of the other supervision tasks. In this complex dialogue the expat-supervisor or trainer-supervisor does not have to give up his own cultural notions and orientations, but he has to be prepared to put them into a benign battle field, where they will enter into a confrontation and conflict with those of the local supervisees and supervisors.

Expat Power in Supervision

We like to present a wider perspective on intercultural supervision by expat or trainer-supervisors. We remind, that they are both outsiders and experts and this capacity gives them a certain amount of power and prestige. Often the interests of international NGO's differ from those of the local people. Although their aim is to give help, they are also committed to their donors, who expect results according to their western criteria. Not always can results be achieved within these terms of reference. Many NGO's have short-term interests; once the emergency phase is over, they leave the country and abandon their local staff. Sometimes their interests may even be selfish, the writing of a PhD thesis or the opportunity to publish articles (Sri Lankan psychologist, 2006). It needs no further comment that when interests are so different, clinical supervision is inapplicable. The basic condition of clinical supervision is a shared mutual understanding of expat and local staff, a strong cognitive and emotional congruence between both parties. Even in that case the expat trainer-supervisor is seen as an expert. He has great guiding power in the selection of the topics that will be reflected upon and he can be quite manipulative. In order to control this selective power as much as possible, the selections and interpretations of the external expert are only "viable if [they are] granted coherence within a significant interactive context". (Krause, 1998, p. 148).

In the supervision process itself expert power is only one of the powers that are influential. Holloway gives a description of several power relations affecting supervision. "Types of power inherent to the role of the supervisor are evaluative (i.e., reward and coercive), expert and legitimate power." These powers are more or less socially given. Referent power on the contrary is immanent to the supervision process itself. It "results from the personal and interpersonal attributes of the supervisor. Referent power can emerge only as a relationship develops" (Holloway, 1995, p. 32).

The notion of referent power is a kind of safety valve in the actual intercultural dialogue. Expats are from the very beginning invested with expert power. Often, especially when they have academic qualifications or are high ranking officials of an internationally respected NGO, also a lot of legitimate power is attributed to them in the host country. In supervision they therefore can wield many 'reward' and 'coercive' power. These powers are easily asserted, all the more by a short term visit of a trainer-supervisor who comes only for some weeks.

The building of adequate reference power requires more personal investment from all parties involved. Supervisors and supervisees together "come to know each other's values, attitudes, beliefs and actions". Although both participants share their commitment to the development of the supervision relationship, it is the supervisor who is responsible to "create an effective learning environment for the trainee". (Holloway, 1995, p. 32) Especially the trainer-supervisor must be aware that he has to build a significant interactive context, in which he has to bring about reference power and promote its constructive effects. In that sense he has to accept the supervisees as equal contributors in this intercultural dialogue and to stimulate their independent thinking and acting.

The Limits of the Outsider

In the preceding examples we mentioned several times that the expat supervisor or trainer-supervisor can have an inducing effect on questioning the casualness of the professional and personal experiences of the local supervisees and supervisor. In an empathic exchange he (or she) might question the naturalness of professional and social relations. These behaviors are often pre- or unconscious, they are "written into behavior, practices and interactions without the participants being immediately aware of this or aware of it at all" (Krause, 1998, p. 144). Often we can observe that these relations are performed as an unconscious, second nature. Although learned in preceding developmental stages (childhood, youth or professional training) they became part of the immediate psychological make-up, they are internalized in the common behavior of people within their cultural environment. Krause, inspired by Bourdieu (1990), refers to this as a "doxic experience"[9].

Such doxic experiences can be exemplified by what occurred in many supervision groups. The participants sat, for instance, on the floor and the supervisor and the supervisees at the same level, but mostly the men and women sat in subgroups next to each other, leaving an open place between them for the local supervisor. Whenever a dispute arose, it often took the form of a "battle" between men and women, the supervisor sitting in-between as a mediator. When the western trainer-supervisor asked not to sit in separate subgroups but to mix in a one-woman-next-to-one-man shape, they immediately found this quite awkward. They could not explain why, but in the arguments that followed, it was much more difficult to distinguish the two "battle camps". The group members were more talking for themselves and from their own opinion. But in the first exercises most group members showed some discomfort, which later was explained as "being alone". Later on they appreciated the more personal exchanges that were made possible by simply changing the sitting order.

These are doxic experiences; people perform this sitting "rules" without noticing them and without even being aware of these rules. They are natural and provide "the illusion of immediate understanding". Its naturalness has two major consequences. It is unquestioned; it is a "characteristic of practical experience of the familiar universe". And "at the same time excludes from that experience any inquiry as to its own conditions of possibility". (Krause, 1988, p. 144).

The expat as an outsider, within the framework of his (or her) benign questioning, has the opportunity to enable this enquiry and stimulate new perspectives. He (or she) must connect to the feelings of doubt that exist in the supervision group and help people to develop new strategies and insights. It is not needless to say however that in these cases his own social concepts are subjected to discussion too. But this procedure, in which multiple and often contradictory meanings are questioned, is not an endless procedure. Cultural relativism has its boundaries. The doxic experiences seem natural and to a certain extent they are perceived as unchangeable. Especially in power relationships this unchangeable naturalness is used as a powerful tool to maintain the power position. This means that the external supervisor or trainer-supervisor must not only search for alternative strategies together with the supervisees, she or he must do so in a way that the "attacked" party can change without losing face. And she or he must realize that some doxic

---

[9] 'Doxic' can be recognized in the words 'heterodox' and 'orthodox' that refer to manifold or single meanings. Doxic experience can be understood as 'meaningful experience'.

experiences cannot be changed, cannot be questioned in the actual cultural circumstances, neither by the local supervisor, nor by the local supervisee.

The long stay western expat working as a supervisor or the passing western trainer-supervisor working in non western countries also has his or her own doxic experiences. From his own original culture he also embodies subconsciously "natural" ways of behaving professionally, socially and culturally. The joint reflection of supervisor and supervisee under guidance of the external supervisor is therefore always a mix of complex doxic experiences, cultural and quasi-natural values. In case IV, for example, the trainer-supervisor could easily connect to the hidden expressions of polite discomfort of the women supervisees in the group. When he raised the issue of the gender steered decision making his remarks fell in a fertile ground, both with the women and men of the group.

In the preceding example (Case III) the participants could rearrange their behavior in the group according to a new value system they were already familiar with from their training. During these trainings they had appreciated and internalized the equality of men and women, but they had difficulties to put it into practice. With the help of the trainer-supervisor this was a relatively easy job.

In case V the resistance of the female supervisor and supervisees was much greater and the social structures were much more robust. To appeal to these high official men, did not only require a sense of self-esteem from the counselors and supervisors, who were "just learning" their job; it also called for a strategy to approach these men about their "mistakes" without "losing face". Here the social and cultural constraints were much more powerful and limited the modes of action substantially. For the trainer-supervisor it was quite a thrill to observe and participate in this strategic thinking within the boundaries of the Sri Lankan culture; it taught him a great deal of the ways in which in western and in particularly Dutch society status constraints are immanent in these kind of conflicts.

Formal Structure as a Warranty

In the third strategy the methodological framework that is used, is closely connected to Holloway's system of supervisory tasks and functions. It is a formal scheme which she developed by investigating what clinical supervisors actually do and how they do this (Holloway, 1995; Lansen & Haans, 2004). It serves as a general, maybe universal, frame of reference of the themes a supervisor has to address and how he has to go about with the supervisee or supervision group. This formal framework offers a maximum opportunity to be filled by all parties involved. It is a kind of umbrella for the cross cultural dialogue.

According to Holloway (1995), the supervisor performs several tasks during a supervision session. She/he observes the skills of the supervisee, her (or his) case concept, the professional role, emotional awareness and the capacities of self evaluation. If the supervisee has a supervision question, this question can be categorized under one of these tasks. The supervisor monitors to which tasks the supervision question applies, and also searches for the more complicated interconnectedness of these tasks and a, sometimes hidden, theme that the supervisee in unaware of. (Hawkins & Shohet, 2000)

What the supervisor is actually doing during supervision, his actions, are called the functions of supervision by Holloway (1995). The supervisor monitors and evaluates the professional activities of the supervisee; and he can provide instruction and advice if required. The supervisor is also a model, both explicitly and implicitly. He can give advice to the supervisee, support him and share his own professional or, if necessary, personal experiences with him.

A similar formal procedure for warranting an optimal socially valid and viable exchange in group supervision is the one developed by Lansen and Haans (2004), briefly described above (note 3). Here several supervision rounds are used: case presentation and questions, identification with the patient as a person, identification with the position of the therapist and supervision with the group. We see these rounds as a formal structure that allows an optimal exchange of meaning, viewpoints and perspectives. During this exchange a vast complexity of multiple meanings (heterodoxy) can emerge. Local culturally accepted and non-accepted behaviors and attitudes can become more conscious. But it brings also a great benefit to move and mix cultures. When people from the same cultural or ethnic background meet, it becomes obvious to them that their culture is not a static, monolithic entity. Within such a formal structure, group members become aware of the individual ways the group members construct and build, internalize and externalize the culture they share. At the same time they produce their culture and are a product of their culture.

Concluding Remarks

Although clinical supervision can be seen as a "western" expression of professionalism it is more than that. We consider it as a general human and professional tool that is effective in helping people to increase their professional skills. Clinical supervision as we describe it offers a formal structure that is evocative and inviting all participants to engage in a joint reflection on the helping activities within the actual social and cultural environment.

In a situation in western countries, where intercultural supervision is exceptional, the supervisor should be aware of his tasks and study, together with the supervisee, the failings and potencies of the supervisee. He must do so with respect to the professional standards of supervision and execute his work within the boundaries of the supervisory functions. Within this framework he must be able to promote a good cooperative relationship based on growing reference power. In these situations the culturally mixed supervision group offers good opportunities to become aware of the cultural and ethnic opportunities and constraints.

In non-western countries another requirement emerges next to the preceding ones. In this intercultural setting clinical supervision offers an effective tool for increasing awareness of cultural and ethnic influences on the helping relationships. In this way, well applied clinical supervision offers many opportunities for indigenous helpers to increase their professional expertise within the framework of their current local, cultural and societal circumstances.

References

Abu-Baker, K. (2005). The impact of social values on the psychology of gender among Arab Couples: A view from psychotherapy. *Israel journal of Psychiatry and Related Sciences, 2*,106–15.

Bourdieu, P. (1990). *The Logic of Practice.* Cambridge: Polity

Diekmann-Schoemaker, M., & van der Veer, G. (2003). An extra language in counselling and training, *Intervention, 2,* 36–9.

Foa, E., Keane, T., & Friedman, M. (Eds.). (2000). *Effective Treatments for PTSD: Practice Guidelines from the International Society for Traumatic Stress Studies.* New York: Guilford Press.

Hawkins, P, & Shohet, R, (2000). *Supervision in the helping professions.* Buckingham – Philadelphia: Open University Press.

Holloway, E.L. (1995). *Clinical supervision. A systems approach.* Thousand Oaks, CA: Sage.

Kos, A. M. (2005). Training teachers in areas of armed conflict. *Intervention supplement, 2,* 1–64.

Krause, I. B. (1998). *Therapy Across Culture.* London: Sage

Lansen, J., & Haans, A. H. M. (2004). Clinical Supervision. In J. P. Wilson & B. Drožđek (Eds.), *Broken Spirits* (pp. 317–353). New York: Bruner/Mazel.

Proctor, B. (2000). *Group Supervision. A Guide to Creative Practice.* London: Sage.

Sri Lankan psychologist (2006). INGO's and international trainers in Sri Lanka, *Intervention, 2,* 169–170.

Veer van der, G. (2003). *Training Counselors in areas of armed conflict within a community approach.* Utrecht: Pharos.

Veer van der, G., de Jong, K., & Lansen, J. (2004). Clinical supervision for counsellors in areas of armed conflict. *Intervention, 2,* 118–28.

Wilson, J. P., & Thomas, R. B. (2004). *Empathy in the Treatment of Trauma and PTSD.* New York: Brunner-Routledge.

17
Are We Lost in Translations?: Unanswered Questions on Trauma, Culture and Posttraumatic Syndromes and Recommendations for Future Research

John P. Wilson & Boris Drožđek

Introduction

As discussed throughout this publication, the relation of trauma and culture is an important one because traumatic experiences are part of the life cycle, universal in manifestation and occurrence, and typically demand a response from culture in terms of healing and care. To understand the relationship between trauma and culture requires a "big picture" overview of both concepts (Marsella & White, 1989). However, because of the complexity of both, reactions to trauma and cultural phenomena, a "big picture" raises also many questions.

What are the dimensions of psychological trauma and what are the dimensions of cultural systems as they govern patterns of daily living? How does culture influence an individual's reaction to trauma? How do victims across the world make sense of their experiences in situations of extreme stress? In this regard, Smith, Lin and Mendoza (1993, p.38) state: "Humans in general have an inherent need to make sense out of and explain their experiences. This is especially true when they are experiencing suffering and illness. In the process of this quest for meaning, culturally shaped beliefs play a vital role in determining whether a particular explanation and associated treatment plan will make sense to the patient . . . Numerous studies in medical anthropology have documented that indigenous systems of health beliefs and practices persist and may even flourish in all societies after exposure to modern Western medicine . . . These beliefs and practices exert profound influences in patients' attitudes and behavior . . ."

How do cultures create social-psychological mechanisms to assist its members who have suffered significant traumatic events? In terms of mental health care, cultures provide many alternative pathways to healing and integration of extreme stress experiences which can be provided by shamans, medicine men and women, traditional healers, culture-specific rituals, conventional medical practices and community-based practices that offer forms of social and emotional support for the person suffering the adverse, maladaptive aspects of a trauma (Moodley & West, 2005). As shown throughout this publication, these different approaches can and sometimes must be combined with each other in order to diminish the suffering of trauma victims. Intercultural trauma treatment can be based on the combination of various "cultural wisdoms" and not on their exclusion from the healing process.

In this chapter, we will discuss the issues of convergence and divergence between healing principles across cultures, raise some fundamental questions on relationships among trauma, culture and posttraumatic syndromes, and propose some directions for future research. In this trajectory, not only the knowledge on psychology and anthropology, but also mythology has been a valuable source of inspiration.

What can we Learn From the Myths?:The Mythology of the Hero, Traumatic Encounters and Personal Transformation

The discovery of how cultures deal with trauma can be found in the great mythologies of the world (Campbell, 1949, 1992). Mythology contains themes which converge across cultures, literary forms (e.g., epochs) and style. Their analysis is a rich source of inquiry as to the interplay between culture, traumatic events and their transformation by facing challenges to existence itself.

The mythologist Joseph Campbell (1949, 1992) researched the universality of myths in many of the worlds' literature, including the myth of "the Hero" who journeyed into "zones of danger" only to emerge transformed in mind, body and spirit. Figure 17.1 presents an illustration of this important myth which includes personal encounters of trauma, disaster and war. In brief, the core elements of the Hero and trauma survivors' journey include:

- A life journey that can begin at any point in life-cycle development
- The encounter within trauma, loss, bereavement and disaster
- The entry and exit from a zone of danger with powerful or supernatural forces
- The four tests of the human spirit
- Trauma and the great cycle of living and dying
- The return of the Hero and the task of transformation upon re-entry

As discussed by Campbell (1992), the mythology of the Hero concerns the travails of ordinary people through extraordinary experiences. In some cases, the myths characterize the life journey, beginning with youthful innocence and naiveté and the eventual encounter with powerful forces of seemingly insurmountable proportions. There are many variations on the themes of this myth and how the individual is transformed by the nature of their experience. For example, young men become war-hardened combat veterans; the apprentice shaman enters the "underworld" of spiritual entities; the knight of the king's realm challenges dragon beasts and the search for sacred, lost objects that have secret powers.

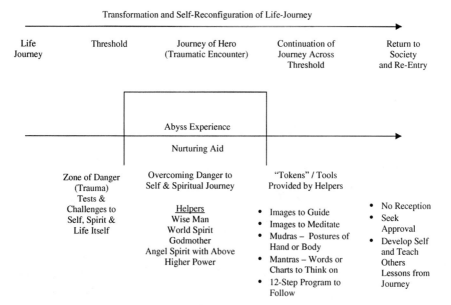

FIGURE 17.1. Mythology and the journey of the hero: The abyss experience and transformation of psychic trauma©.
Source: John P. Wilson, 2005©

The mythological journey of the Hero is also the journey and psychological sequel of the trauma survivor. They both encounter dark, sinister, life-threatening forces and then cross a threshold to re-enter normal life and society. The power of life-threatening dark forces constitutes the nature of the Abyss Experience (Wilson, 2005). During the Abyss Experience the individual confronts the specter of death, extreme threats and overwhelming immersion into traumatic stressors. There are five dimensions of the Abyss Experience which include: (1) the confrontation with evil and death; (2) the experience of soul death with non-being; (3) a sense of abandonment by humanity; (4) ultimate aloneness and despairing; and (5) cosmic challenge of meaning. For each of these five dimensions there are corresponding posttraumatic phenomena: (i) the trauma experience: (ii) self/identity; (iii) loss of connection; (iv) separation and isolation; and (v) spirituality and sense of the numinous. Upon re-entry into society after the Abyss Experience, the survivor faces the task of transformation and the psychic metabolism of these experiences. As part of this process, the mythical Hero is assisted by "helper guides" who take the form of wise old men, a spirit guide, a deceased elder relative, an angelic person or another person who has had a similar experience (e.g., a recovering addict, war veteran, etc.).

After the Abyss Experience, the trauma survivor (Hero) faces the arduous and painful task of re-entry where he or she is met with additional stressors and psychic burdens. Contrary to expectation, the hero or survivor does not receive a warm welcome from those left behind. Campbell (1992) notes that there are three prototypical patterns of reentering the society: (1) no reception; (2) the search for approval, validation and confirmation of one's journey, travails and suffering; and (3) the need to share their story of survival and teach others in generative ways.

Upon re-entry into the culture of origin, the trauma survivor, like mythical Hero, encounters some or all of the following reactions to their journey and life-transforming experiences:

- The absence of recognition of the true nature of suffering, sacrifice and survival
- The absence of recognition of the perils endured
- The absence of appreciation for personal injuries and changes
- The absence of treatments, health care, or opportunities to engage in traditional healing rituals
- The emergent realization that meaning must be created out of the trauma experience

The above mentioned can also be observed in "modern" trauma survivors entering a different society and culture of their own after being forced to migrate.

According to Campbell (1992), mythology suggests that the heroic survivor seeks to find pathways to healing. Thus, we can identify six consequences of healing pathways within the diversity of culture: (1) to restore harmony in mind, body and spirit; (2) restore vital physical and mental energy; (3) promote well-being through mindfulness and psychic integration; (4) empower personal energy for life-course development; (5) access and utilize treatments available in the culture; and (6) develop healing practices that promote resilience.

Campbell (1992) further outlines the four functions of mythology as follows: (a) spiritual-mystical; (b) cosmological; (c) sociological; and (d) psychological. Each of these functions is revealed within mythology and has direct parallels to the nature of psychological requirements in dealing with the impact of trauma to self and psychological functioning. For example, trauma and traumatic life-experiences form a reconciliation with unconsciousness and the meaning of life. This issue concerns directly the mythology of one's own life and the role trauma has played in it. For example, novels and autobiographies of war trauma of former combat soldiers typically characterize the horrific encounter with death, the existential questioning of the purpose of war and how such experiences subsequently shape life-course trajectory (Caputo, 1980). Traumatic experiences often force a self-effacing look at personal identity and consciousness. Trauma serves to put the individual in touch with their unconscious processes, including the disavowed, dark or 'shadowy' side of personality. By carefully analyzing the functions of mythology within a culture we can identify how it is that culture shapes posttraumatic adaptation, growth and the challenges of self-transformation.

Trauma, Culture and Posttraumatic Syndromes: The Core Questions

The concept of traumatic stress and the multidimensional nature of cultures requires a conceptual framework by which to address core issues that have direct relevance to understanding the nature of trauma as embedded within a culture and its assumptive systems of belief and patterns of behavioral regulation.

To be clear, in this discussion as well as throughout the book, the authors are not using the term posttraumatic syndrome as synonymous with PTSD, although it certainly includes the narrow, diagnostic definition of the disorder. Rather, posttraumatic syndromes involve a broad array of phenomena that include trauma complexes, trauma archetypes, posttraumatic self-disorders (Parsons, 1988), posttraumatic alterations in core personality processes (e.g., five-factor model); identity alterations (e.g., identity confusion) and alterations in systems of morality, beliefs, attitudes, ideology and values (Wilson, 2005). The experience of psychological trauma can have differential effects to personality, self and developmental processes, including the epigenesis of identity within culturally-shaped parameters (Wilson, 2005). Given the capacity of traumatic events to impact adaptive functioning, including the inner and outer worlds of psychic activity (Wilson, 2004), it is critically important to look beyond simple diagnostic criteria such as PTSD (Summerfield, 1999) to identify both pathogenic and salutogenic outcomes as individuals cope with the effects of trauma in their lives. As argued elsewhere (Wilson, 2005), the history of scientific research on PTSD is badly skewed (perhaps for reasons of historical necessity) towards the study of psychopathology rather than on human growth, self-transformation, resilience and optimal functioning.

When we address the question of how cultures deal with psychological trauma in its diverse forms, it is useful to examine commonalities and differences among approaches to counseling, healing, psychotherapies, treatments and traditional practices. If traumatic stress is universal in its psychobiological effects (Friedman, 2000; Wilson, Friedman, & Lindy, 2001) are therapeutic interventions, in turn, designed in culture-specific ways to ameliorate the maladaptive consequences of dysregulated systems of affect, cognition and coping efforts (Wilson, 2005; Wilson &, 2004; Marsella, Friedman, Gerrity, Keane, & Scurfield, 1996)? If so, what are the differences in therapeutic approaches across cultures to dealing with trauma? To answer this question requires further examination of the core questions pertaining to culture and the patterns of posttraumatic adaptation.

1. Is the experience of psychological trauma the same in all cultures?
This question addresses the issues of how cultural belief systems influence the perception and processing of trauma. For example, Kinzie (1988, 1993) noted that among Cambodian refugees who had suffered multiple life-threatening trauma during the Khmer Rouge regime, many who suffered from PTSD and depression understood their symptoms in light of their Buddhist beliefs in karma

as a station in life, an incarnate level of being and fate. Hence, Western psychiatric views of suffering and depression may not exist within a Buddhist ideology per se. Personal suffering may be seen from a religious-cosmological perspective of the meaning of life.

Among many Native American people a "good world" is one defined by harmony and balance in "all things" and "all relations" in the environment and amongst people (Mails, 1991). Illness is thought to result from imbalance, loss of harmony and being dispirited within oneself due to a loss of vital connectedness. Among some aboriginal native people, trauma is simply defined as that which causes one to lose balance in living with positive relations with nature and the human made world. Moreover, within this cosmology, it was well known that certain events, such as warfare, could cause profoundly altered states of well being (i.e., dispiritedness) and necessitated healing rituals for the restoration of wholeness (Wilson, 1989, 2005).

If a culture does not have linguistic connotations of a pathogenic nature (e.g., PTSD), how then does the person construe acute or prolonged effects of extreme stress experiences? In a discussion of depression and Buddhism in Sri Lanka, Obeyeskere (1985, p. 134) stated: "How is the Western diagnostic term depression expressed in society whose predominant ideology of Buddhism states that life is suffering and sorrow, that the cause of sorrow is attachment or desire or craving, that there is a way (generally through meditation) of understanding and overcoming suffering and achieving the final goal of cessation from suffering or nirvana?" Hence, sorrow, suffering, depressive symptoms, traumatic memories, disruptions in sleep patterns, and other trauma-related symptoms will likely be construed in a similar manner, especially since depression is a component of posttraumatic stress disorder (Breslau, 1999).

2. Are the emotional reactions to psychological trauma the same in all cultures?

Scientific evidence, especially neurobiological studies, have documented that affect dysregulation, right hemisphere alterations in brain functioning, and strong kindling phenomena are universal in PTSD (Schore, 2003; Friedman, 2000). If there is a common set of psychobiological changes associated with either PTSD or prolonged stress reactions, is the emotional experience universal in nature (e.g., hyperarousal, startle, anger, irritability, depressive reactions) or do cultural belief systems "override" or attenuate the magnitude or severity and intensity of dysregulated emotional states?

3. Does culture (i.e., cognitive-affective belief systems) act as a perceptual filter to the cognitive appraisal and interpretation of psychic trauma? If so, how do internalized belief system and culturally shaped patterns of coping and adaptation, govern the posttraumatic processing of traumatic experiences?

This question goes to the heart of the culture-trauma relationship. First, how does a culture define trauma? Is a trauma in one culture (e.g., natural disaster, incestual relations; traffic deaths; political oppression; motor-vehicle accidents; murder, etc.) necessarily viewed as a trauma in another culture? For example, in the 1988 Yunnan earthquake in a rural, peasant area of China, over 400,000 people were impacted by the event which had not been previously experienced by most inhabitants. However, among the common explanations for the earthquake was that a great dragon was moving beneath the earth because he was angry with the people (McFarlane & Hua, 1993). Does such a mythical attribution influence the subsequent psychobiological responses to the disaster once it terminates? What if the dragon returns to his 'rest' and 'sleep'?

Second, what sets of expectations for resiliency in coping does the culture possess? For example, after the July, 2005 terrorist bombings to transit systems in London, the general media and political leaders noted that the British people immediately returned to work the next day, rode the buses and subways, and manifest high levels of resilience. The prime minister, Tony Blair, made reference to how British resolve was evident during the bombing raids in WWII and that in 2005 such resilient resolve was once again transparent. Is this a cultural norm or expectation? How do cultural beliefs and values influence the post-event processing and cognitive interpretation of the traumatic stressor itself?

4. Are traumatic experiences archetypal for the species?

Research on PTSD has identified categories and typologies of traumatic life-events and the specific stressors they contain (Green, 1993; Wilson & Lindy, 1994). While there is agreement on the nature and types of traumatic events, a more fundamental question is whether or not they are archetypal in nature. Elsewhere, Wilson (2004, 2005) has discussed the unique nature of trauma archetypes and trauma complexes and suggested that the experience of trauma is both universal and archetypal for the human species. However, culture shapes the way that individuals form trauma complexes after a traumatic experience and, once formed, articulate with other psychic complexities. Dimensions (see Table 17.1) of the trauma archetype and how they influence posttraumatic personality dynamics and adaptive behavior have been delineated (Wilson, 2005).

5. Are there cultural-based syndromes (cf. not necessarily PTSD) of posttraumatic adaptation? If yes, what do they look like? What is their psychological structure?

This core issue is among the most fascinating to consider and interesting to conceptualize since there may be unique ways that posttraumatic adaptations occur within a culture or sub-culture (e.g., trance states, dissociative phenomena, somatic illnesses, mythical attributions, etc.). How does culture provide awareness for posttraumatic syndromes to exist and be expressed? Are these forms of adaptation pathogenic or salutogenic in nature (Marsella, 1982)?

6. How do cultures develop rituals, medical-psychological treatments, religious practices and other forms of institutionalized mechanisms to assist persons who experience psychological trauma?

This question attempts to identify the specific, institutionalized and non-institutionalized healing methods for victims of trauma that cultures develop. This question is of significant research interest as it defines the areas in which commonalities overlap and in which culture-specific differences exit.

TABLE 17.1. Trauma archetype (universal forms of traumatic experience)[©].

Dimensions:

1. The Trauma Archetype is a prototypical stress response pattern present in all human cultures, universal in its effects and is manifest in overt behavioral patterns and internal intrapsychic processes, especially the Trauma Complex.
2. The Trauma Archetype evokes altered psychological states, which include changes in consciousness, memory, orientation to time, space and person and appear in the Trauma Complex.
3. The Trauma Archetype evokes allostatic changes in the organism (posttraumatic impacts, e.g., personality change, PTSD, allostatic dysregulation) which are expressed in common neurobiological pathways).
4. The Trauma Archetype contains the experience of threat to psychological and physical well being, typically manifest in the Abyss and Inversion Experiences.
5. The Trauma Archetype involves confrontation with the fear of death.
6. The Trauma Archetype evokes the specter of self-de-integration, dissolution and soul (psychic) death (i.e., loss of identity), and is expressed in the Trauma Complex.
7. The Trauma Archetype is a manifestation of overwhelmingly stressful experience to the organization of self, identity and belief systems and appears as part of the structure of the Trauma Complex.
8. The Trauma Archetype stimulates cognitive attributions of meaning and causality for injury, suffering, loss, death (i.e., altered core beliefs) which appear in the Trauma Complex.
9. The Trauma Archetype energizes posttraumatic tasks of defense, recovery, healing and growth, which include the development of PTSD as a Trauma Complex.
10. The Trauma Archetype activates polarities of meaning attribution; the formulation of pro-social – humanitarian morality vs. abject despair and meaninglessness paradigm.
11. The Trauma Archetype may evoke spiritual transformation: individual ⟶ journey / "encounter with darkness: ⟶ return / transformation / re-emergence, healing (J. Campbell, 1949). The evocation of a "spiritual" transformation is manifest in the Trauma Complex as part of the Transcendent Experience and the drive toward unification.

Source: John P. Wilson, 2004©

For example, most Native American nations use the Sweat Lodge Purification Ceremony to "treat" states of dispiritedness, mental illness, alcohol abuse, depression as well as to instill spiritual strength (Wilson, 1989). The Sweat Lodge purification ritual has a unique structure and process and is embedded within the traditional cosmology of a tribe (e.g., Lakota Sioux). Under the guidance of a trained and experienced medicine person, the Sweat Lodge is used to restore "balance" through purification, sweating and emotional catharsis (Wilson, 1989; Mails, 1991). This is just one example of many that exist among and between cultures to facilitate "stress reduction" and to alleviate suffering, including prolonged stress reactions after traumatic life events.

As we will discuss later, it is our belief that each person's posttraumatic syndrome is a variation on a culturally sanctioned modality of adaptation which can be "treated" by either generic or culturally-specific practices.

7. Is it possible to standardize the assessment and treatment of trauma across cultural boundaries?

This is a core issue in terms of the "globalization" of knowledge about the relation of trauma to culture. At present, we have no standardized etic (universal) measurements of trauma and PTSD (Dana, 2005). Similarly, we do not have standardized cross-cultural treatment protocols for persons suffering from post-traumatic syndromes. There exist empirical and clinical voids in the knowledge base as to what "treatments" work best for what kinds of person and under what set of circumstances.

8. Do pharmacological treatments of posttraumatic syndromes work equally well in all cultures?

This question is intriguing because it posts the controversy as to whether or not the psychobiology of trauma is the same across cultures and therefore treatable by pharmacological agents designed to stabilize the dysregulation in neurobiolog-ical functioning caused by extreme stress experiences. However, to date, there are few comparative randomized clinical trials (RCT) of medications to treat PTSD in culturally diverse populations (Friedman, 2001). Yet, studies have shown that some anti-depressant medications are more efficacious in symptom reduction than others for non-Western populations with severe PTSD (Kinzie, 1988; Lin, Poland, Anderson, & Lesser, 1996).

9. Is the unconscious manifestation of posttraumatic states the same across cultural boundaries?

This core question is complex and fascinating because it demands a method to assess unconscious processes cross-culturally (Dana, 1999) and to discern if unconscious memory encodes trauma experiences in similar ways, perhaps in trauma complexes that are, in turn, shaped by cultural factors (Wilson, 2005).

10. What conceptual belief systems underlie cultural approaches to heal-ing and recovery from trauma?

In many respects, this issue deals with the most 'pure' consideration of the trauma-culture relationship. How does the culture view "trauma" and employ methods to facilitate healthy forms of posttraumatic adaptation? What set of assumptive beliefs does the culture "bring" to the understanding of trauma? Within a culture, is trauma idiosyncratic or synergistic in nature? Are there differences between individual and cultural trauma? What does damage to the structure of a culture mean in terms of posttraumatic interventions? For example, Erikson (1950) noted that among the Lakota Sioux Indians in the United States, the loss of their nomadic mystical culture oriented around the Buffalo meant a loss of historical continuity and collective identity which was profoundly trau-matic once the Lakota were interned on federal reservation lands that deprived them of their cherished patterns of living (Wilson, 2005).

Culture and Treatment for Posttraumatic Syndromes

The ubiquity of traumatic events throughout the world has raised global awareness of PTSD and other reactions to trauma as important psychological conditions that result from a broad range of traumatic experiences (e.g., war, ethnic cleansings, terrorism, tsunamis, catastrophic earthquakes, etc.). Economic globalization has "flattened the world" (Friedman, 2005) as technologies have changed the face of commerce and international marketplace. In a real sense, globalization has generated trends towards the homogenization of cultures and at the same time heightened awareness of distinct cultural differences. However, when it comes to the issue of cultural differences and posttraumatic syndromes (e.g., PTSD) it cannot automatically be assumed that advances in Western psychotherapeutic techniques can be exported and applied to non-Western cultures (Summerfield, 1999). Further, the literature on cultural competence has brought awareness of the need for knowledge, sensitivity and innovation when it comes to mental health treatment in non-Western cultures (White & Marsella, 1989). More recently, Moodley and West (2005) discussed the limitations of verbal therapies and presented a rationale for the integration of traditional healing practices into counseling and psychotherapy. It is worthwhile to point out that there are culture-specific healing practices as well as overlaps in conceptual viewpoints about the assumptions that underlie traditional healing practices across different cultural groups.

Let us consider five very different cultural views of healing: Native American; African – Zulu; Indian (Ayurveda), traditional Chinese medicine (TCM), and Western. What do each of these cultures assume about (traditional) healing and the cosmological (cf. one could also say mythological) assumptions they hold about physical and mental health?

Native American

In most North American aboriginal nations, healing is considered from the perspective of relations – balanced relations – between individuals and environment and the world at large (Mails, 1991). When sickness occurs it is generally assumed that there is an imbalance in the nature of "relations to all things;" that a loss of balance and harmony has occurred within the person and illness follows.

TABLE 17.2. Cultural convergence: similar principles?.

Principle/Assumption	Native American	African (Zulu)	India (Ayurveda)	Chinese (TCM)	Western Industrial Culture
1. Harmony in relations (earth, people, society)	Yes	Yes	Yes	Yes	No
2. Vulnerability within person	Yes	Yes	Yes	Yes	Yes
3. Balance of biological and mental forms	Yes	Yes	Yes	Yes	No
4. Illness is imbalance, loss of harmony	Yes	Yes	Yes	Yes	No
5. Health is restoration of balance, harmony	Yes	Yes	Yes	Yes	No
6. Healing empowers vital energy	Yes	Yes	Yes	Yes	Yes

Healing, then, is the empowerment of the individual spirit with the great circle of life; to restore balance and harmony with nature, others and the Great Spirit (God). The medicine wheel and traditional shamanic (i.e., medicine) practices are used as a guide to understanding. Through traditional healing practices, rituals and ceremonies, the designated "medicine" person facilitates the restoration of a persons' spirit and inner strength in order to restore their vital power to be in good balance i.e., to have good relations of balance and harmony. More specifically, trauma can cause a loss of centeredness in the person and lead to a loss of "spirit," resulting in various forms of "dispiritedness," which includes, according to the western medical terminology, depression, PTSD, dissociation, and altered maladaptive states of consciousness and being (Jilek, 1982; Mails, 1991; Wilson, 1989; Poonwassie & Charter, 2005).

South African (Zulu)

The Zulu culture in South Africa employs a view of mental and spiritual life that is intricately interconnected. Bojuwoye (2005, p. 63) states: "The interconnectedness of phenomenal world and spirituality are two major aspects of traditional African world views. The world view holds that the universe is not a void but filled with different elements that are held together in unity, harmony, and the totality of life forces, which maintain firm balance, or equilibrium, between them. A traditional Zulu cosmology is an individual universe in which plants, animals, humans, ancestors, the earth, sky and universe exist in unifying states of balance between order and disorder, harmony and chaos". In Zulu culture, then, traditional healing practices have respect for this view and attempt to facilitate the restoration of a harmonious state of being in relation to these dimensions of the persons' phenomenal world.

Indian (Ayurveda)

Indian healing, in the Ayurvedic tradition, views restorative practices as unifying mind, body and spirit within the context of social conditions. Kumar, Bhurga and Singh (2005, p. 115) state: "According to Ayurvedal principles, perfect health can be achieved only when body, mind and soul are in harmony with each other and with cosmic surroundings. The second dimension in this holistic view of Ayurveda is the social level, where the system describes the ways and means of establishing harmony within and in the society. Mental equilibrium is sought by bringing in harmony three qualities of the mind in sattva, vajas and tamas". Thus, traditional Indian healers use time-honored practices (e.g., touching, laying of hands) to facilitate helping a person restore unity in the psyche. After the 2004 tsunami, such practices were used with success by local healers to aid victims who suffer from the stress-related effects of the disaster in India (Siddarth, in press).

Traditional Chinese Medicine

In traditional Chinese medicine (TCM), "mental illnesses are said to result from an imbalance of yin and yang forces, a stagnation of the qi and blood in various organs, or both" (So, 2005, p. 101). He further elaborates that "the driving forces behind this relationship are the entities of qi (virtual energy) and li (order). The oft-cited concepts of yin and yang, oppositional yet complementary in nature, are characteristics along the meridian channels of that compound to the specific organ of the body" (p. 101). Thus, TCM views health and illness as related to a balance of vital forces and that disruptions which effect their critical balance can result in physical or mental illnesses.

Western Approach

The Western Judeo-Christian postmodern industrial culture overemphasizes individualism at cost of integrative tendencies. An individual feels balanced when there is a balance within him/herself. The harmony of the individual in relation to its surroundings, the society or the earth is less important than in other cultures. Consequently, illness is not viewed as a result of a loss of harmony, but as an individual problem, caused by disturbances and misbalance on the level of individual biology. Therefore, healing focuses on treatment of the individual mirroring the culture's preference of reductionism over holistic approach.

Cultural Convergence and Divergence in Healing

Table 17.2 compares the different cultural approaches to healing across five basic dimensions that represent assumptions about the nature of illness and health: (1) harmony in relations (e.g., with earth, others, nature, society; (2) personal vulnerability within the person due to imbalance caused by external forces or inner conflict; (3) the importance of balance in biological and mental processes; (4) illness results from imbalance and loss of harmony; and (5) health is the restoration of balance and harmony in mind, body and spirit. Thus, in all cultures healing empowers vital energies contained within the person. By comparing different cultural views and assumptions that underlie we can go further and ask how it is that culture deals with those who are severely traumatized by events of human design or acts of nature.

Western Scientific Colonialism: Does it Make Sense?

In an influential and important critique of mental health programs in war-affected areas (e.g., Bosnia, Rwanda, etc.), Derek Summerfield (1999, pp. 1452–1457) explicated seven fundamental assumptions that many of these programs embrace as justifications for interventions with programs derived from clinical efforts and research on psychotherapy in Western cultures, primarily the United States and Western Europe. These seven assumptions are as follows: "(1) experience of war and atrocity are so extreme and distinctive that they do not just cause suffering, they 'cause' traumatization; (2) there is basically a universal human response to highly stressful events, captured by Western psychological framework [cf. PTSD]; (3) large numbers of victims traumatized by war need professional help; (4) Western psychological approaches can be applied worldwide as victims do better if they emotionally ventilate and 'work through' their experiences; (5) there are vulnerable groups and individuals who react to a specific target for psychological help; (6) wars represent a mental health emergency: rapid intervention can prevent the development of serious mental problems, as well as subsequent violence and wars; and (7) local workers are overwhelmed and may themselves be traumatized".

This same set of assumptions could safely be generalized to non-warzone countries in which there are catastrophic natural disasters (e.g., tsunami; earthquake) or other conditions of human rights violations by political regimes: "the humanitarian field should go where the concerns of survivor groups direct them, towards their devastated communities and ways of life, and urgent questions about rights and justice" (p. 1461). Moreover he notes that "the medicalization of distress, a significant trend within Western culture and non-globalizing, entails a mined identification between the individual and the social world, and a tendency to transform the social into the biological. Consultants have portrayed war as a mental health emergency with large claims that there was an epidemic of 'post-traumatic stress' to be treated, and also that early intervention could prevent mental disorders, alcoholism, criminal and domestic violence and new wars in subsequent generations by nipping brutalization in the bud" (p. 1461).

More fundamentally, the question can be raised whether it is appropriate to refer to Western healing techniques as therapies and treatments, while we use terminology like traditional healing and rituals when describing non-western approaches. Are the western approaches just well structured rituals (in terms of focus and time management) embedded in the western culture, where efficiency, self assertiveness, highly individualized control over life and individual-centered worldview are the most important values and traits? At the same time, non-western approaches focus more on re-establishing harmony in relationship between the individual and the world around him/her, which fits better in a non-western worldview. Besides this, the question is whether western techniques like cognitive behavior therapy (CBT) or eye-movement desensitization and reprocessing (EMDR) must be praised for their efficiency, while there have been accidental reports of fast recovery after just one session of maraboutage or another non-western healing approach.

Western healers favor approaches that are evidence based, and often define non-western alternatives as mambo-jumbo practices. At the same time, there have been almost no studies of non-western healing approaches. Opportunity to do scientific research is a privilege of rich societies, as most of the western societies are. Therefore, the exclusion of non evidence based approaches from those that should be applied in intercultural trauma treatment does not seem appropriate. It reflects yet again the western scientific colonialism.

These views raise a number of critical questions when it comes to the proper and efficacious treatment of posttraumatic syndromes in different cultures in the world.

Posttraumatic Interventions: What Works Best for Whom Under What Conditions?

To focus the central issues rather sharply, what types of counseling, interventions, treatments, practices, rituals, medicines, ceremonies and therapies work best for whom and under what set of conditions? This seemingly simple and straightforward question turns out to be extraordinarily complex and multifaceted for several key reasons. First, we do not have sufficient scientific studies across cultures to begin to answer this question. Second, cultural competence has shown the need to explore assessment, diagnosis and treatment within a sensitive cultural framework that reflects knowledge and understanding of a culture. Indeed, the World Health Organization (WHO) published a global plan for culturally competent practices that included mandates to insure the availability of traditional and alternative medical practices in safe and therapeutically useful ways (WHO, 2005). Third, it cannot be assumed that well-documented Western psychotherapies for PTSD, for example, are necessarily useful in non-Western cultures, especially therapies that rely heavily on verbal self-reports (e.g., CBT, psychodynamic). Fourth, there are a broad range of individual responses to traumatic events. It cannot be assumed 'a priori' that PTSD is an inevitable outcome of exposure to extremely stressful life-events. It is entirely possible that the concept of PTSD (cf. Western in conceptualization) is foreign and not readily understood in many cultures that do not utilize psychobiological explanations of illness or human behavior. Fifth, to understand 'maladaptive' behavior consequences of trauma (and therefore traumatization) can only be meaningfully defined by cultural norms and expectations about "normal" and "abnormal" behavior. Human grief reactions are universal to death and loss but that does not make them pathological (Raphael, Woodling, & Martinale 2004). Acute adjustment reactions for a short period of time are entirely expectable after the 2004 tsunami that destroyed towns, cities, even cultures and more than 250,000 people. But that does not make adaptational requirements pathological or a posttraumatic stress symptoms an illness *per se* for the survivors. Sixth, it can be justifiably assumed that throughout centuries of human evolution, cultures have developed adaptive mechanisms and wisdom to deal with the human effects of extreme trauma. As noted earlier, the great mythologies of the world chronicle such events and the adaptational dilemmas they present for survivors. Such mythical themes point to the necessity of framing culture-sensitive perspectives on human resilience versus psychopathology (Wilson, 2005). These considerations allow us to now explore 10 hypotheses about the relation of trauma to culture to posttraumatic adaptations and how mental health "treatments" can be construed in culturally-competent ways.

Ten Hypotheses Concerning Trauma, Culture and Posttraumatic Mental Health Interventions

1. Each person's posttraumatic syndrome, state of psychological distress or adaptational pattern is a variation on *culturally sanctioned* modalities of behavioral-emotional expression. While the impact of trauma seems to be universal on a biological level, both attribution and conceptualization of traumatic experiences are culture-bound.
2. Healing and recovery from psychic trauma is *person-spe*cific. There are multiple pathways and forms of treatment within a culture. Help-seeking behavior is culture-bound.
3. Each culture develops specific forms and mechanisms for posttraumatic recovery, stabilization and healing (e.g., rituals, counseling practices, treatment protocols, medications, etc.). At any given time, cultures may not have available certain types of treatments that would be beneficial to people. These will either evolve in time or be adapted from other cultures.
4. Based on Trauma Archetypes, cultures contain the wisdom to develop mechanisms to facilitate the processing and integration of psychic trauma. Empathy, as a universal psychobiological capacity, underlies the development and evolution of culture-specific forms of healing (Wilson & Thomas, 2004; Wilson & Droždek, 2004).
5. The concept of "mindfulness" in states of consciousness (traditionally associated with Buddhism) is a key mental process to self-transcendence and the integration of extreme psychic trauma into higher states of consciousness and personal knowledge. Mindfulness, in this regard, is personal awareness of the impact of trauma to living in one's culture of origin and how trauma has impacted the quality of life.
6. There is no individual experience of psychological trauma without a cultural history, grounding or background. Similarly, there is no individual sense of personal identity without a cultural reference point. Anomie and alienation are commonly produced by severely traumatizing experiences and are associated with forms of anxiety, distress and depression (Wilson & Droek, 2004).
7. The rapid growth of globalization and mass migrations in the twenty first Century are creating new evolutions in a "world-universal" culture and the possibility of fusing cross-cultural modalities of treatment and recovery.
8. Healing rituals are an integral part of highly cohesive cultures. Healing rituals evolve in situations of crisis, emergency and threat to the social structure of society and culture. Healing rituals demand special roles and skills (e.g., shaman, crisis counselor, psychologist, medicine person, priest, etc.) to facilitate efforts for recovery and the psychic metabolism of trauma.

9. Western posttraumatic therapies and traditional healing practices, in *culturally-specific forms*, can facilitate resilience, personal growth and self-transcendence in the wake of trauma (Wilson, 2005).
10. The pathways to healing are idiosyncratic and universal in nature across cultures. The pathways of healing vary in form, purpose, duration, social complexity and utilization by a culture.

The 10 hypotheses concerning the relationship of culture and trauma provide a framework for understanding the diversity of posttraumatic psychological outcomes. As Summerfield (1999) noted, it is prejudicial and scientifically unwarranted to assume that traumatic events at the individual or cultural (collective) level will always produce PTSD and the clinical need to intervene with programs and procedures developed primarily in Western cultures. For example, cognitive behavioral therapy (CBT) is the most validated psychotherapy for PTSD in the USA (Foa, Keane, & Friedman, 2000). But is CBT be applicable to assisting victims of the 2004 tsunami who live in a non-English speaking culture in Ache, Indonesia? Or, the survivors of the 2003 catastrophic earthquake in Bam, Iran which killed over 30,000 people? Or, the mothers of genocidal warfare in the Sudan in 2005 whose children were murdered or starved to death? Or, Native American Vietnam war veterans living in traditional ways on the Navajo reservation in Arizona?

Clearly, posttraumatic adaptations fall along a continuum from pathological to resilient (Wilson, 2005). At the pathological end of the continuum we find PTSD, dissociative reactions, brief psychosis, depressive disorder and disabling anxiety states. In contrast, the resilient end of the continuum includes optimal forms of healthy adaptation, manifestations of behavioral resiliency in the face of adversity and the resumption of normal psychosocial functioning (Wilson, 2005). By examining the continuum of culturally sanctioned modalities of posttraumatic adaptation, the second and third hypotheses can be understood more precisely. Healing and recovery is *person-specific* and there are *multiple pathways* to posttraumatic recovery, if they are needed. Considered from an evolutionary and adaptational perspective, cultures develop rituals, helper roles, ceremonies and other modalities to facilitate recovery from distressing psychological conditions, including those produced by trauma (Moodley & West, 2005). Where such modalities of treatment do not exist or are inadequate, they will be developed and implemented as it is critical to culture to have functional and healthy members to carry out the critical day to day activities necessary to sustain commerce, family life and the functions that define the identity and essence of the culture itself. For example, a culture that is sick, self-destructive and dissolving due to warfare, political conflicts and revolution, massive natural disaster or illness, will not thrive or maintain itself in a viable way.

The viability of culture in the face of collective trauma illustrates the sixth assumptive principle that there can be no experience of psychological trauma without a cultural history, grounding or continuity of background. There is no individual sense of personal identity without a cultural reference point

(Wilson, 2005). Personal identity within a cultural context includes a sense of continuity and discontinuity in life-course development which shapes personality and the coherency of the self-structure. Thus, there is no sense of personal identity without a cultural reference marker to counterpoint and define those events which seem to shape the formation of identity for the person. As an extension of this viewpoint, it can readily be seen that anomie and alienation (e.g., feeling detached, separate, cut off, divorced, estranged, distanced, removed) from mainstream cultural processes is a potential consequence of severely traumatizing experiences and typically associated with anxiety, distress and depression since the traumatic experience can "push" the person "outside" the customary boundaries of daily living. The potential of trauma to dysregulate emotions and set-up complex patterns of prolonged stress cannot be dismissed as statistically infrequent (Kessler, Sonnega, & Bromet, 1995). As Wilson and Drožđek (2004) have noted, this is particularly true when: (1) the trauma is massive and damages the entire culture, (2) the nature of trauma causes the person to challenge the existing moral and political adequacy of prevailing cultural norms and values, (3) the trauma causes the individual to become marginalized within the culture and to be viewed as problematic, stigmatized, "damaged goods," or tainted by their experiences or posttraumatic consequences (e.g., physically disabled, disease infected, atomic radiation exposure; mentally ill, etc.).

The nature of how cultures deal with the social, political and psychological consequences of trauma raises the issue of the availability of therapeutic modalities of healing and recovery. Stated simply, what does the culture provide to assist persons recover from different types of trauma? Examining this question is instructive since one can analyze the nature of formal, organized and institutionalized mechanisms for recovery from trauma as well as informal, non-institutionalized or officially sanctioned modalities of care and service provisions. While a detailed analysis of these issues is beyond the scope of this article, it is nonetheless important when using a "crows nest" or "helicopter aerial" view of how cultures deal with those who suffer significant posttraumatic consequences of trauma. Clearly, there are levels of posttraumatic impact to the social structures of culture and to the inner-psychological world of the trauma survivor. There are primary, secondary, and tertiary sets of stressors associated with trauma. In the "big view" of traumatic consequences, they intersect to varying degrees in affecting the patterns of recovery, stabilization and resumption of normal living (Wilson, 1994).

Final Remarks

So what does globalization portend for trauma treatment in the twenty first Century as the world "flattens" due to technological advances and commercial homogenization? In brief, the ready availability of scientific data on international databases for posttraumatic stress disorders (e.g., P.I.L.O.T.S.@ncptsd.org) enable clinicians, researchers and patients to have instant access to information about PTSD, complex PTSD, treatment advances, pharmacotherapies, and much more. Second, the spread of knowledge has spurned unprecedented levels of international cooperation and the formation of international professional societies (e.g., ISTSS, International Society for Traumatic Stress Studies in 1985; Asian Society for Traumatic Stress in 2005) to share scientific data and clinical wisdom and to lobby for political and legislative changes on behalf of trauma victims. Third, globalization, to a certain extent, allows for homogenization, fusion and experimentation with different modalities of counseling, psychotherapy, traditional healing practices and modern medicine (e.g., traditional Chinese medicine). As this occurs, the answer to the question, "What works for whom and under what conditions?" will take on new meaning in terms of how we conceptualize the prolonged effects of extreme stress experience to the human psyche and as a holistically integrated organism.

Beyond doubt, nineteenth and twentieth Century conceptualizations of counseling and psychotherapy are cultural-bound in nature and origin. The twenty first Century will witness the development and emergence of global conceptualizations of what constitutes trauma and how it gets healed. There will be developed a matrix of databases which cross-list cultures and the diversity of techniques employed to cope with states of traumatization. Moreover, as this convergence begins to occur, the scientific 'gold standards' of what works for whom under what circumstances will take on meaning that transcends culture but not persons whose human suffering impels humanitarian care.

References

Bojuwoye, O. (2005). Traditional healing practices in South Africa: Ancestral spirits, ritual ceremonies and holistic healing. In R. Moodley & W. West (Eds.), *Integrating traditional healing practices into counseling and psychotherapy* (pp. 61–73). Thousand Oaks, CA: Sage Publications.

Breslau, N. (1999). Psychological trauma, epidemiology of trauma and PTSD. In R. Yehuda (Ed.), *Psychological trauma, epidemiology of trauma and posttraumatic stress disorder* (pp. 1–27). Washington, DC: American Psychiatric Press, Inc.

Campbell, J. (1949). *Hero with a thousand faces*. New York. Penguin Books.

Campbell, J. (1992). *Pathways to bliss*. New York: Harper.

Caputo, P. (1977). *A rumor of war*. New York: Holt, Rinehart & Winston.

Caputo, P. (1980). *A rumor of war*. New York: Holt, Rinehart & Winston.

Dana, R. H. (1999). *Handbook of cross-cultural and multicultural personality assessment*. Matwah: L. E. Erlbaum Associates.

Dana, R. H. (2005). *Handbook of cross-cultural and multicultural personality assessment*. Matwah: L. E. Erlbaum Associates.

Erikson, E. (1950a). *Childhood and society*. New York: Norton.

Foa, E. B., Keane, T. M., & Friedman, M. J. (Eds.). (2000). *Effective treatments for PTSD*. New York: Guilford Press.

Friedman, L. J. (2000). *Identities architect*. Cambridge. Harvard University Press.

Friedman, M. J. (2001). Allostatic versus empirical perspectives on pharmacotherapy. In J. P. Wilson, M. J. Friedman & J. D. Lindy (Eds.), *Treating psychological trauma and PTSD* (pp. 94–125). New York: Guilford Press.

Friedman, T. (2005). *The world is flat.* New York: Girraux, Strauss & Co.

Green, B. (1988). *The MMPI.* Boston: Allyn & Bacon Publications.

Jilek, W. G. (1982). Altered states of consciousness in North American Indian ceremonies. *Ethos, 6,* 326–343.

Kessler, N. C., Sonnega, A., & Bromet, E. (1995). Posttraumatic stress disorder in the national comorbidity survey. *Archives - General Psychiatry,* 52, 1048–1060.

Kinzie, J. D. (1988). The psychiatric effects of massive trauma on Cambodian refugees. In J. P. Wilson, Z. Harel, & B. Kahana (Eds.), *Human adaptation to extreme stress* (pp. 305–319). New York: Plenum Press.

Kinzie, J. D. (1993). Posttraumatic effects and their treatment among Southeast Asian refugees. In J. P. Wilson & B. Raphael (Eds.), *International handbook of traumatic stress syndromes* (pp. 311–321). New York: Plenum Press.

Kumar, M., Bhurga, D., & Singh, J. (2005). South Asian (Indian) traditional healing: Ayurvedic, shamanic, and sahaja therapy. In R. Moodley & W. West (Eds.), *Integrating traditional healing practices in counseling and psychotherapy* (pp. 112–123). Thousand Oaks, CA: Sage Publications.

Lin, K. L., Poland, R. E., Anderson, D., & Lesser, I. M. (1996). Ethnopharmacology and the treatment of PTSD. In A. J. Marsella, M. J. Friedman, E. T. Gerrity, & R. M. Scurfield (Eds.), *Ethncultural aspects of posttraumatic stress disorder* (pp. 505–529). Washington, DC: American Psychological Association.

Mails, T. E. (1991). *Fools crow.* San Francisco, CA: Council Oaks Books.

Marsella, A. J. (1982). Culture and mental health: An overview. In A. J. Marsella & G. White (Eds.), *Cultural conception of mental health and therapy,* (pp. 1–3). Boston, MA: D. reidel Publishing Co.

Marsella, A. J. (1989). Culture and mental health: An overview. In A. J. Marsella & G. White (Eds.), *Cultural conception of mental health and therapy* (pp. 1–3). Boston, MA: D. Reidel Publishing Co.

Marsella, A. J. (2005). Rethinking the 'talking cures' in a global era. *Contemporary Psychology,* November, 2–12.

Marsella, A. J., Friedman, M. J., Gerrity, E., & Scurfield, R. M. (Eds.). (1996). *Ethnocultural aspects of posttraumatic stress disorder: Issues, research and applications.* Washington, DC: American Psychological Association Press.

Marsella, A. J., & White, G. M. (1989). *Cultural conceptions of mental health and therapy.* Boston, MA: D. Reidel Publishing Co.

Marsella, A. J., & White, G. M. (1989). *Cultural conceptions of mental health and therapy.* Boston, MA: G. Reidel Publishing Co.

McFarlane, A. C., & Hua, C. (1993). Study of a major disaster in the Peoples Republic of China: The Yurnan earthquake. In J. P. Wilson & B. Raphael (Eds.), *International handbook of traumatic stress studies* (pp. 493–499). New York: Plenum Press.

Moodley, R., & West, W. (2005). *Integrating traditional healing practice into counseling and psychotherapy.* Thousand Oaks, CA: Sage Productions.

Obeyesekere, G. (1985). Depression, Buddhism and the work of culture in Sri Lanka. In A. Kleinman & B. Good (Eds.), *Culture and depression: Studies in anthropology and cross-cultural psychiatry of affect and disorder* (pp. 134–152). Berkeley, CA: University of California Press.

Parsons, E. (1988). Post-traumatic self-disorders. In J. P. Wilson, Z. Harel, & B. Kahana (Eds.), *Human adaptation to extreme stress:* From the Holocaust to Vietnam (pp. 245–279). New York: Plenum Press.

Poonwassie, A., & Charter, A. (2005). Aboriginal worldview of healing: Incusion, blending and binding. In R. Moodley & W. West (Eds.), *Integrating traditional healing practices into counseling and psychotherapy* (pp. 15–26). Thousand Oaks, CA: Sage Publications.

Raphael, B., Woodling, & Martinale (2004). Assessing traumatic bereavement. In J. P. Wilson & T. M. Keane (Eds.), *Assessing psychological trauma and PTSD* (pp. 492–513). New York: Guilford Press.

Schore, A. N. (2003). *Affect dysregulation and disorders of the self.* New York: Norton.

Schore, A. N. (2003). *Affect dysregulation and the repair of the self.* New York: Norton.

Siddarth, A. S. (in preparation). Ethnomedical best practices for international psychosocial efforts in disaster and trauma. In J. P. Wilson & C. Tang (Eds.), *The cross-cultural assessment of psychological trauma and posttraumatic stress disorder.* New York: Springer – Verlag.

Smith, M., Lin, M. K., & Mendoza, R. (1993). Non biological issues affecting psychopharmacology: Cultural considerations. In K. M., Lin, R. E. Poland, & G. Nalcasali (Eds.), *Psychopharmacology and psychobiology of ethnicity* (pp. 37–58). Washington, DC: American Psychiatric Press, Inc.

So, J. K. (2005). Traditional and cultural healing among the Chinese. In R. Moodley & W. West (Eds.), *Integrating traditional healing practices in counseling and psychotherapy* (pp. 100–112). Thousand Oaks, CA: Sage Publications.

Spiegel, D. E. (1994). *Dissociation.* Washington, D. C.: American Psychiatric Association Press.

Summerfield, D. (1999). A critique of seven assumptions behind psychological trauma programs in war-affected areas. *Social Science and Medicine, 48,* 1449–1462.

Wilson, J. P. (1989) *Trauma, transformation and healing: An integration approach to theory, research and posttraumatic theory.* New York: Brunner/Mazel.

Wilson, J. P. (1994). The need for an integrative theory of post-traumatic stress disorder. In M. B. Williams (Ed.), *Handbook of PTSD therapy* (pp. ????). New York: Greenwood Publishers.

Wilson, J. P. (2004). *The abyss experience and the trauma complex.* New York: Brunner-Routledge.

Wilson, J. P. (2005). *The posttraumatic self: Restoring meaning and wholeness to personality.* New York: Brunner-Routledge.

Wilson, J. P., & Droek, B. (2004). *Broken spirits: The treatment of traumatized asylum seekers, refugees and war and torture victims.* New York: Brunner-Routledge.

Wilson, J. P., Friedman, M. J., & Lindy, J. D. (2001). An overview of clinical consideration and principles in the treatment of PTSD. In J. P. Wilson, M. J. Friedman, & J. D. Lindy (Eds.), *Treating psychological trauma and PTSD* (Ch. 3, p. 59–94). New York: Guilford Press.

Wilson, J. P., & Lindy, J. (Eds.). (1994). *Counter-transference in the treatment of PTSD.* New York: Guilford Press.

Wilson, J. P. (2004). The abyss experience and the trauma complex: A Jungian perspective of PTSD and dissociation. *Journal of Trauma in Dissociation, 3,* 43–68.

Wilson, J. P., & Thomas, R. (2004). *Empathy in the treatment of trauma and PTSD.* New York: Brunner/Routledge.

World Health Organization (2002). *Traditional medicine strategy 2002–2005.* WHO Publication, WHO/EDM/2002.1. Geneva: Switzerland.

Index